Osteopathy In Britain

Osteopathy In Britain

The First Hundred Years

Dr Martin Collins

Principal
British School of Osteopathy

ISBN : 1-4196-0784-7

To order additional copies, please contact us.
BookSurge, LLC
www.booksurge.com
1-866-308-6235
orders@booksurge.com

Osteopathy In Britain

Contents

PREFACE

Writing this book has been a difficult conflict between providing a work that is of general interest, an exciting story, enjoyable to read, and one providing a comprehensive account of the material available as a resource at this important moment in the history of Osteopathy, before documents and recollections are lost forever. While much has been deleted through successive drafts, I have nevertheless veered towards the latter.

Rather like completing a complex jigsaw, producing it has been very exciting, as each new piece fell into place and a picture emerged. It has also been a great challenge. Unlike a jigsaw, the pieces were not readily available, scattered on the table. They have had to be sought and the picture will never be complete, as some pieces are lost forever. Some that once existed have long since been destroyed. I was saddened to read in the Board of Governing Directors' minutes of the British School of Osteopathy (BSO) for 1943, that records prior to 1936 were to be scrapped because of a shortage of space and the national demand for paper salvage. The hands of many osteopaths who knew what really happened in the past are now at rest. Between starting and completing this book, there were, however, a diminishing few with their recollections. Speaking to them and recording their stories was a great enjoyment and motivation to complete this work, for the profession owes them an inordinate debt.

My interest in the history of Osteopathy in Britain began with the enthralling lectures of John O'Brien in 1990, when I was a student at the BSO. History has an appeal to me as an inveterate gossip. John's lectures inspired me to begin to fill in some of the gaps. I began by interviewing senior members of the profession: Colin Dove (1991), John Wernham (1991), Jocelyn Proby (1992), Greg Currie (1992) and Alan Stoddard (1992). I only regret that I was unable to speak to 'Sammy' Ball, Douglas Mann and others who, though around in the early 90s, are no longer with us.

The library at the BSO has been of great value with its quite unique collection of osteopathic books and journals, some autographed by the authors. I am grateful to the librarians, Will Podmore and Les Fagan, for their assistance and particularly to Will for proof-reading of the manuscript. I am also grateful to Mark Anderson, ICT Technician, and Jill Skok, ICT Trainer, both of the BSO, for their assistance in the production of this book.

Colin Dove, one-time Principal of the BSO, mentioned old records of the School kept in the BSO library, but a thorough search revealed nothing. I suspected that they had been disposed of in the move from Buckingham Gate in 1980. As a last resort I spoke to the Services Manager, who knew every nook and cranny of the building. He referred to a box in the safe known as 'The Littlejohn Box'. John Martin Littlejohn was founder of the School and played an important part in the history of Osteopathy in Britain. I accompanied him into the small room in the Suffolk Street building in which the safe was kept and was shown the box. It was locked. It was suspected that the Finance Director had the key. She knew nothing about the box, but she did have some old keys. One fitted the lock. It was a moment of great excitement. The box was opened and inside were Littlejohn's ledgers in which he recorded the names of all his students, their background and educational experience from Elsie Wynter Wareing listed as student number one, together with a wealth of other archival material.

As a result of a water leak, I was obliged to clear a small storeroom adjacent to the library at Suffolk Street. On the top shelf, having miraculously escaped water damage, was a bound folder inscribed: 'Webber's Bequest'. ('Webber' was the nickname of the second Principal of the School, Shilton Webster-Jones). It contained personal letters from the 1940s and other valuable historical material.

Through making my interest known, people began to send me memorabilia. I am particularly grateful to Claude Dutton and Roderic MacDonald for allowing me to have access to the British Osteopathic Association (BOA) minutes from 1928, before they were lodged in the Wellcome Library for the History and Understanding of Medicine and to Michael Newman, a descendent of Littlejohn through a daughter, who provided me with some valuable Littlejohn memorabilia. Peter Leigh, clinic tutor at the BSO who knew a Mrs D. King, the niece of Joyce Canning, facilitated access to documents that belonged to the latter and to James Canning. David Gilhooley put me in touch with Dr Max Mitchell-Fox the son of Thomas Mitchell-Fox. I am grateful to Christian Fossum and the European School of Osteopathy for allowing me access to the material that once belonged to T. Edward Hall, found in the attic of the School.

I am particularly appreciative of the many osteopaths who have provided information that has added to the picture, or helped verify or correct that which I had gained from elsewhere, particularly Margery Bloomfield, Colin Dove, Claude Dutton, David Dyer, Malcolm Mayer, Hugh Hellon Harris, Ronald Harvey, Jane Langer, Dr Ian Drysdale, Lady Audrey Percival (nee Smith), Richenda Power and David Wainwright. Wendy Arnheim kindly sent me a copy of Margaret Chambers' '*The British Naturopathic Association The First Fifty Years*', which contained much useful information in piecing together the complex history of Naturopathy, which has a bearing on Osteopathy.

I am particularly grateful to Robin Kirk, who through experience at what is now the British College of Osteopathic Medicine, the Maidstone College and the European School of Osteopathy, is familiar with the history of these institutions. The numerous discussions I have had with him has been immensely helpful. I am also indebted to Chris Campbell who gave me access to his research on the early life of Littlejohn.

Sometimes in an unexpected place a missing piece of the puzzle is found, such as when laboriously reading the rigorous cross-examination of witnesses at the Select Committee of the House of Lords in 1935, the published minutes of which were kindly made available to me by Gareth Butler.

Back numbers of the *Journal of Osteopathy*, *Osteopathic Quarterly*, *The Osteopathic Newsletter* of the Osteopathic Association of Great Britain, *Osteopathic Review* and other publications have also been useful sources of information. Particularly revealing were the obituaries.

This book concentrates on the overall development of the profession. I have intentionally avoided discussing changes in theory and practice, from so-called '10-fingered Osteopathy' to the present day, interesting as they may be.

I am sure that some people on reading this book will be critical of what may be perceived as a 'BSO-centric' view. It must be recognised that the BSO and its graduates dominated much of the history of the profession during the greater part of the 20th century. The overemphasis on the history of the BSO is also in part due to my greater access to information on this School and its graduates. I have, however, made a serious attempt to obtain information from all quarters of the profession.

Much is included on the transactions that took place at the Select

Committee of the House of Lords in 1935. Summarising them was extremely difficult, but they revealed much about the profession at that time and the extent of bitter opposition to statutory regulation.

The emphasis is also on the early years, beyond the memory of the majority alive today. Events close to the turn of the millennium are still fresh in the minds of many. However, today's events will be the material for tomorrow's historians.I hope that this book will be one of many on the subject. Others will follow and make good my deficiencies, as is the manner by which knowledge progresses.

The cover photograph is by Mark Turnbull and Gary Weeks.

Martin Collins

London

To Those Osteopaths Past And Present Who Have Built The Piers Upon Which Osteopathy Has Bridged Three Centuries

Chapter 1

Before Osteopathy in Britain

I t is not the intention of this book to discuss in detail the origins of Osteopathy, but a little needs to be said to place the history of Osteopathy in Britain in context. Osteopathy was the brain child of Andrew Taylor Still, born in Virginia in 1828, but afterwards settling in Kirksville, Missouri. Still began to seek an alternative to the orthodox medicine of his time based on purging using potent minerals such as mercury compounds, arsenic and antimony mixed as an addictive cocktail with opium or alcohol. Even in Still's time there was a growing antipathy to this 'heroic' medicine. It was Still's disillusionment with medicine, particularly apparent to him during his time in the civil war and the death of three of his children from spinal meningitis in 1864, that drove him to seek an alternative path. His second wife, who came from New York State, and a Major Abbott he met in the army may have also influenced his views.[1]

Still believed that God had made humans as perfect machines and the role of Osteopathy was to restore the body to its perfect state. He had an interest in machines, not surprising in view of the impact of farm mechanisation in the US at that time and he himself invented a mowing machine and a butter churn. An early interest in anatomy from studying the bodies of animals he caught hunting was developed when he later in life dissected the bodies of dead Indians. The works of the evolutionist Herbert Spencer may have been important in his appreciation of the relationship between structure and function.[1]

Still claims he discovered Osteopathy at 10 o'clock in the morning on 22 June 1874. Evidence suggests at that time he was practising 'magnetic healing', a therapy based on the idea that illness was due to a blockage of flow of magnetic energy through the body. In the 1880s he was advertising himself as a 'lightning bonesetter'. By the end of that decade he had amalgamated these two therapies and developed them into one of his own.[1,2] In 1892 he founded the first school of Osteopathy, The American School of Osteopathy (ASO).

While Osteopathy and manipulation are not the same, they have been confused by some. Osteopaths may use manipulation as one of many techniques, but Osteopathy has a set of 'Principles' governing patient evaluation and management, which manipulation alone does not. However, manipulation and the treatment of the musculo-skeletal system has a long history that precedes Osteopathy.[3] In the Western world the craft of manipulation is known as 'bone-setting'. It is important in the development of Osteopathy, not only because Still practised as a 'lightning bone setter', but also because some bone-setters in Britain the first two decades of the century gained a considerable reputation and laid the foundation for the acceptance of Osteopathy in this country, for in the minds of many of the public and the medical profession, Osteopathy and bone-setting were synonymous. Dr Graham-Little MP, who was considered the chief spokesman of the medical profession in the 1920s on medical matters of public controversy, preferred the term bone-setter to the 'new fangled and shoddy American substitute of "Osteopath"'.[4]

Written descriptions of manipulation can be traced as far back as Hippocrates, who in 'Periarthron' described various manipulative techniques involving traction, walking up and down a patient's spine, the use of a wooden board to effect a 'thrust' and manual adjustment. The descriptions were reproduced down the centuries. They appear in the writings of the Roman physician Galen and in Arabic medical texts. Throughout the world there have been for centuries individuals with such skills, developed not through a formal training based on a study of anatomy but through apprenticeship, and who considered it a natural gift and not a scientific discipline. Bone-setters were generally rural and never organised into a medical cult (hence never in conflict with orthodoxy) and often practised secondary to other work, e.g. as blacksmiths in Cumberland and shepherds in Wales. The craft was conveyed from father to son (occasionally to a daughter). In the Scottish Highlands they were often a seventh son. A seventh son of a seventh son was considered to have special gifts.[3]

In 1656 Robert Turner wrote a treatise entitled, 'The compleat bone-setter wherein the method of curing broken bones, and strains and dislocated joints, together with ruptures, vulgarly called broken bellyes, is fully demonstrated'. It was based on a work by Friar Moulton that he revised, enlarged and translated from the Latin.[5] Even at that time there was criticism of bone-setters. Richard Wiseman (1622-1676) in 'Severall Chirurgicall Treatises' wrote, 'I have had occasion to take notice of the inconveniences many people have fallen into, through the wickedness of those who pretend to the reducing luxated joints by the peculiar name of Bone-setters...'.[3]

Sir Norman Moore, in his history of St Bartholomew's Hospital, mentioned that in the 17th century it employed a bone-setter and his assistant, though both were also members of the Barber-Surgeons Company.[6]

Profile: Sarah Mapp

The first bone-setter of whom any details are known was Mrs Sarah Mapp, who practised in the early 18th century. Known as 'Crazy Sally', or 'Cross-eyed Sally', she was the daughter of a bone-setter of Hindon, Wiltshire, named Wallin. The London Magazine of August 1736 refers to the, 'Fame of a young woman at Epsom, who, though not very regular it is said in her conduct, has wrought such cures that seem miraculous in the bone setting way....She gets near 20 guineas a day executing what she does in a very quick manner'.[3]

Her fame grew. She treated the Queen and the niece of Sir Hans Sloane, travelling from Epsom to London in a horse-drawn carriage with footmen, before moving to Pall Mall. A play was written in her honour, 'The Husbands Relief or the Female Bone-setter and the Worm Doctor' and a poem:

"You surgeons of London who puzzle your pates,
To ride in your coaches and purchase estates;
Give over for shame, for your pride has a fall,
The Doctress of Epsom had outdone you all.
Dame Nature has given her a doctors degree,
She gets all the patients and pockets the fee;
So if you don't instantly prove it a cheat,
She'll loll in a chariot whilst you walk the street."[3]

Sir Percival Pott, the English surgeon, however, had this to say of her: 'We all remember that even the absurdities and impracticability of her own promises and engagement were by no means equal to the expectations and credulity of those who ran after her; that is of all ranks and degrees of people from the lowest labourer or mechanic up to those of the most exalted rank and station; several of whom not only did not hesitate to believe implicitly the most extravagant assertions of an ignorant, illiberal, drunken, female savage, but even solicited her company; at least seemed to enjoy her society.' Her fame rapidly declined and she died in poverty in Seven Dials, London in 1737.[3]

In the 19th century, some 12 or so families had great reputations as bone-setters. Among them were: the Thomas's of Anglesey and then Liverpool (see below); the Taylors of Whitworth, Lancashire; the Matthews of the Midlands; the Huttons of Westmoreland; the Maltbys of Nottingham; the Masons of Lincolnshire; the Crowthers of Yorkshire and the Burbridges of Frimley, Surrey.[7,8]

Profiles: Evan Thomas and his Descendants

Bone-setting had a significant influence on the development of modern orthopaedic medicine. One of the great orthopaedic physicians of the 19th century was Hugh Owen Thomas (1843-1891), famous for developing 'Thomas's splints'. He was descended from a long line of bone-setters. His father Evan Thomas practised as a bone-setter in Liverpool where he was much respected by the dockers and went on to study medicine at Edinburgh, London and Paris.[9]

His nephew, Sir Robert Jones (1857-1933), began his career as apprentice, partner and successor to his uncle in the Liverpool docks.[10] He established orthopaedics and incorporated bone-setting skills into it, but was nevertheless considered a 'bone-setter' in Liverpool. Kelman MacDonald (an eminent Scottish osteopath, see chapter 5) regarded him as, 'The greatest orthopaedic surgeon that has ever existed.'[11] During the First World War, Jones, who had acquired the equipment of Wharton Hood (see below), instructed young orthopaedists based on Wharton Hood's treatise on bone-setting.[8]

The Medical Act (1858)

It was only 40 years before Osteopathy was introduced into Britain that the Medical Act of 1858 made a clear distinction between those who could and those who could not practise medicine. In effect, it exerted a monopoly on medicine.

Before that date, the distinction between orthodox and 'fringe' or 'heterodox' medicine was far from clear. The further one goes back in history, the more blurred the distinction becomes. 'Regulars' were only a small proportion of those engaged in healing in the 18th century, nor was there a single orthodoxy, nor single fringe medicine. A survey in 1842 of practitioners in one or more branches of medicine revealed that 11,000 were 'qualified' and 23,000 'unqualified'.[12] Those engaged in fringe medicine were popularly known as 'quacks'. Daniel Turner in 1718, described 'The Modern Quack; or the Physical Impostor Detected'.[13,14]

The lack of clear distinction between the 'regulars' and 'quacks' is evident from James Boswell's experience with 'Senior Gonorrhoea'. He resorted to Kennedy's Lisbon Diet Drink as a cure, advertised with a long list of testimonials to its effectiveness. Boswell, however, found it ineffective and described its vendor as a 'gaping babbler', yet Kennedy had been taught at distinguished medical schools and was a Fellow of the Royal Society! Other 'medical transvestites' adopted the manner of quacks.[15] Dr Theodor von Myersbach was a successful 'pisse prophet', and was attacked by Dr John Coackley Lettsom for being a 'quack'. In his defence, Myersbach criticised the regular medical practitioners for their use of, "Magical' words, claims of exclusive knowledge, affectation of mystery in their writing, shows of deep erudition, an air of absolute confidence, a solemn, self-important expression in a hope of captivating the ignorant'.[16]

The Apothecaries' Act of 1815 and the formation of the Pharmaceutical Society of Great Britain, which defined how health care professions should be regulated, laid the foundations for the Medical Act of 1858.[15,17,18] After 1858 an entrenchment occurred between those practising healing who were registered with the General Medical Council (GMC), formed as a consequence of the Act, and those who were not, such as bone-setters.

Paget and after

Over 100 years after Sarah Mapp died, the medical profession began to show an interest in what bone-setting might have to offer. In 1866, Sir James Paget gave a lecture at St Bartholomew's Hospital, *On the Cases that Bone-setters Cure*, which was published the following year.[19] He concluded:

> 'From all this you may see that the cases that bone-setters may cure, though more by luck than wit, are not a few. I think it very probable that those in which they do harm are still more numerous, but the lessons which you may learn from their practice are plain and useful. Be on the watch for them. Learn then to imitate what is good and avoid what is bad in the practice of bone-setters; and if you would still further observe the rule, *fas est ab hoste doceri**.'

* It is right to be taught, even by an enemy.

Paget's lecture followed the social stir and the 'professional indignation' resulting from the treatment of Sir Spencer Ponsonby by a bone-setter, Richard Hutton (1801-1871), but there was also a growing interest in manipulative therapy within orthodox medicine.[8] (See below). Hutton practised in Watford and was an upholsterer before becoming a bone-setter. He was descended from a famous family of bone-setters from Westmoreland, who had practised there for 200 years.[20] In about 1867, a Dr Peter Hood treated Hutton for a severe illness, but refused a fee, as Hutton had treated many poor people. By way of gratitude Hutton offered to explain his work as a bone-setter. Pressure of work prevented Hood accepting, but the offer was extended to his son, Wharton Hood, who considered it unjustified to publish what he learnt until Hutton's death. The account appeared in *The Lancet* in 1871.[21] There was considerable medical correspondence on bone-setting in the 1870s, especially in *The Lancet* and it was the principal subject of the Annual General Meeting of the BMA in 1882.[7]

R. Dacre Fox, Surgeon to the Manchester Southern Hospital and to the Manchester Police Force, related his experiences of bone-setting in a 15 page booklet published in 1883.[22]

In 1884 George Matthews Bennett, a bone-setter of Warwickshire, wrote, '*The Art of the Bone-setter. A Testimony & Vindication*', defending bone-setting against its critics and claiming it was not violent and not quackery just because it was based on accumulated experience.[7] He suggested that limited instruction from books actually intensifies the powers of observation. He was critical of Paget for his poor understanding of bone-setting and suggested that physicians, while dismissing bone-setters as quacks, were intent on learning their secrets to receive their fees. He claimed Paget's arguments were founded on conjecture and therefore many of his conclusions were wrong.

These publications may explain how the founder of Osteopathy, A. T. Still, obtained his knowledge of bone-setting. There is no evidence of his having gained it through apprenticeship. One of Still's competitors, Dr A. T. Noe, who practised 'Neuro Osteopathis' claimed that he had not stolen the idea from Still, as the latter had obtained his knowledge through reading Wharton Hood's works.[1]

Profile: Sir Herbert Barker

Herbert Atkinson Barker, born in 1869, learnt bone-setting at the age of 20 from his cousin John Atkinson, who worked at 12 Park Lane, London and who had treated, amongst others, the pianist Paderewski, the Duchess of Hamilton, the Duke of Cambridge and members of the Royal Family and who did make some attempt to learn anatomy. Atkinson was taught by Robert Hutton (1840-1887), a nephew of Richard Hutton (see above).[20]

When Barker was a young boy travelling to Canada by ship, a passenger slipped on the deck and dislocated his arm. Others attempted to reset it, but failed. Barker stepped forward and instinctively corrected it and despite his father's wish for him to become a lawyer like himself, he set out on a career as a bone-setter.[23] Having gained all he could from Atkinson, Barker practised in Manchester, Liverpool, Sheffield, Bradford and Leeds. He then returned to London, practising in Suffolk Place (just off the Haymarket, by a turn of fate virtually next door to where the BSO was to relocate in 1980). After working in the North, he settled in London in 1905, and took over Atkinson's practice at Marlborough Chambers, 71 Jermyn Street, London, when the latter died. Barker treated royalty, the nobility, famous writers such as H. G. Wells and John Galsworthy, as well as Members of Parliament and famous athletes and actors of the time, becoming the well-known 'society' bone-setter.

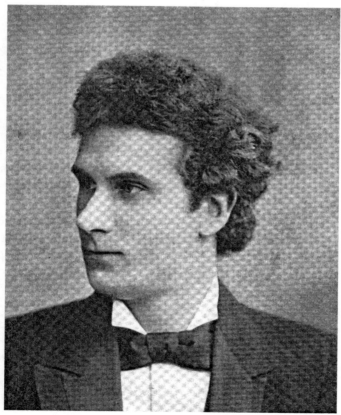

Sir Herbert Barker at the age of 20

From 1906 Barker was in bitter controversy with the medical authorities and there was a frequent exchange of correspondence in *The Times*, *The Medical Press and Circular* and with the BMA. He invited medical people to a demonstration of his Art, but few accepted. A Dr F. W. Axham was sufficiently impressed to return 45 times and to offer his services as an anaesthetist. Axham wrote, 'The paramount duty of my profession is the relief of suffering not the observance of any regulations that may interfere with that duty'. Brave words. On 25 May, 1911, *The Times* informed the public that Axham was struck off the Register for 'infamous conduct' in a professional respect. The 'infamous conduct' was assisting Barker. No appeal was possible. He had been in practice 49 years. Many newspapers came to his support, but the GMC claimed it was 'powerless in the matter'. He died aged 86, in 1926, his name not having been restored to the Medical Register, though the correspondence in the press indicated that public opinion was in his favour.[20]

A petition was signed by over 300 MPs recommending Barker for an honorary medical degree. This, not surprisingly, was refused, but George V created him a Knight in 1922. The BOA made him an honorary member and through the recommendation of Wilfrid Streeter of the Osteopathic Defence League, The Kirksville College of Osteopathic Medicine and Surgery, previously the ASO, gave him an honorary Doctorate of Osteopathy in 1925, which he referred to as his 'American Knighthood'.[24] In the Prospectus of the BSO of 1928-1929 he is listed as a 'Governing Director'. In 1936 Barker gave a demonstration to over 100 members of the British Orthopaedic Association on some 20 patients at St Thomas's Hospital.[3]

Barker succeeded in bringing manipulation to the attention of the public. Thus when Osteopathy was introduced into Britain, manipulative therapy was well-known. At the turn of the 20th century, the sharp divide between 'medicine' and other therapies was still comparatively recent, but the former's desire for monopoly resulted in a backlash against the unorthodox, as experienced by both Hugh Owen Thomas and Sir Herbert Barker and was later to be experienced by Osteopathy.

References

1. Trowbridge C. (1991). <u>Andrew Taylor Still 1828-1917</u>. (Kirksville, Missouri: The Thomas Jefferson University Press).
2. Gevitz, N. (1982). <u>The DOs. Osteopathic Medicine in America</u>. (Baltimore: The Johns Hopkins University Press).
3. Schiotz, E.H. & Cyriax, J (1975). <u>Manipulation Past and Present</u>. (London: Heinemann).
4. Barker, H. (1926). *The Times,* 23 January. In Streeter, W. (1929). <u>The New Healing</u>, pp. 143-145. (London:Methuen & Co).
5. Turner, R. (1981). <u>The Compleat Bonesetter</u>. (1656). Republished. (Isleworth: Tamor Pierston Publishers).
6. Report from the Select Committee of the House of Lords appointed to consider the Registration and Regulation of Osteopaths Bill [H.L.] together with the proceedings of the Committee and minutes of evidence. (1935). 5993, p. 426. (London: HMSO).
7. Bennett, G. M. (1884). <u>The Art of the Bonesetter—a Testament and Vindication</u>. (London: Thomas Murby).
8. Cooter, R. (1987). Bones of contention? Orthodox medicine and the mystery of the Bone-setter's craft, in Bynum, W.F. & Porter, R. (1987). <u>Medical Fringe & Medical Orthodoxy 1750-1850</u>, pp.158-173. (London: Croom Helm).
9. Vay D. le. (1956). <u>The Life of Hugh Owen Thomas.</u> (Edinburgh and London: E. & S. Livingstone Ltd).
10. Watson, F. (1934). <u>The Life of Sir Robert Jones</u>. (London: Hodder & Stoughton).
11. Report from the Select Committee of the House of Lords appointed to consider the Registration and Regulation of Osteopaths Bill [H.L.] together with the proceedings of the Committee and minutes of evidence. (1935). 2136-2137, pp. 152-153. (London: HMSO).
12. Report from the Select Committee of the House of Lords appointed to consider the Registration and Regulation of Osteopaths Bill [H.L.] together with the proceedings of the Committee and minutes of evidence. (1935). 5611, pp. 380-389. (London: HMSO).

13.   Porter, R. (1989). Health for Sale. Quackery in England 1660-1850. (Manchester: Manchester University Press).

14.   Bynum, W. F. (1987). Treating the wages of sin: Venereal disease and specialism in Eighteenth Century Britain. In Bynum, W. F. & Porter, R. (1987). Medical Fringe & Medical Orthodoxy 1750-1850, pp.11-12. (London: Croom Helm).

15.   Loudon, I. (1987). "The vile race of quacks with which this country is infested'. In Bynum, W.F. & Porter, R. (1987). Medical Fringe & Medical Orthodoxy 1750-1850, pp. 106-128. (London: Croom Helm).

16.   Porter, R. (1987). 'I think ye Quacks'. The controversy between Dr Theodor Meyersbach and Dr John Coakley Lettsom In Bynum, W.F. & Porter, R. (1987). Medical Fringe & Medical Orthodoxy 1750-1850, pp. 57-58. (London: Croom Helm).

17.   Porter, R. (1987). Disease, Medicine & Society 1550-1860. (Basingstoke: Macmillan).

18.   Holloway, S. W. (1987). The orthodox fringe. The origins of the Pharmaceutical Society of Great Britain. In Bynum, W.F. & Porter, R. (1987). Medical Fringe & Medical Orthodoxy 1750-1850, pp.129-157. (London: Croom Helm).

19.   Paget, J. (1867). Cases that Bonesetters Cure. *The British Medical Journal*, January, 5 (1):1-4.

20.   Barker, Sir H. (1927). Leaves from my Life. (London: Hutchinson & Son).

21.   Hood, W. (1871). So-called "Bone-setting," its nature and results. *The Lancet.*11 March: 336-38; 18 March: 372-4;1 April: 441-443; 15 April: 499-501.

22.   Fox, R. Dacre. (1883). Bone-setting so called and the treatment of sprains. (London: John Heywood).

23.   Barrow, Curzon G. R. (1950). Obituary of Sir Herbert Barker. *The Osteopathic Quarterly*, 3(4): 96-100.

24.   Adler, P. & Northup, G. W (Eds.) (1977). 100 Years of Osteopathic Medicine. Part 3, 1925-1949, p.14 (USA: E. R. Squibb & Sons).

Chapter 2

The First 30 Years

The Early Years

What must it have been like to be the first osteopath to practise in Britain? Even today, after the Osteopaths' Act of 1993, one still meets many people who do not know what 'Osteopathy' is. At the turn of the century Osteopathy was virtually unknown in Britain. Would it have been difficult starting a practice? The bone-setters may have paved the way. It is perhaps not insignificant that the first osteopaths chose to practise in the provinces, where bone-setting was familiar, or in the heart of the West End of London, where Sir Herbert Barker practised.

Osteopathy was introduced to the UK in July 1898. As a result of correspondence with literary and scientific friends in Great Britain, John Martin Littlejohn delivered a lecture on, 'Osteopathy in line of apostolic succession with Medicine', at the Addison Hall, London, to the Society of Science, Letters and Art, of which he was a Fellow and for which he was awarded the Society's Gold Medal (inscribed to the Rev J. Littlejohn Sept.1898).[1,2] So successful was this lecture that the following July another was given to the same Society on 'Osteopathy as a Science'. In the Bulletin of the Society of 19 April 1899 it was recorded, 'Osteopathy was applied by Dr Still to the new Science on account of the fact that the displacement of bones occupied the first place in the order of discovery by himself of causes of lesions producing diseased conditions'.[2] Regrettably, no other evidence of the existence of this Society has as yet been found.

On 24 August 1899, Littlejohn wrote a letter in defence of Osteopathy in *The Scotsman*, Edinburgh, entitled, 'Osteopathy in America', in reply to the claim of an American correspondent on 27 June that Osteopathy was medical charlatanry. Littlejohn wrote:

'If your correspondent knew anything of the system, he would not make such a statement....This is an age of progress and if you could see our school at Kirksville, Mo., a large institution with over 600 students, fully equipped and splendidly taught, you would realise that we meant to give the largest amount of knowledge...We have no kindred with any form of faith cure or charm cure, but rely wholly on nature and the resources of nature which are inexhaustible. (Dean of the American School of Osteopathy, Kirksville, Mo.).'[1]

He treated patients in London in 1899 and in 1900.[3,4] On 17 July of the following year, a further lecture was delivered to the Society of Science, Letters and Art, entitled, 'Osteopathy, A new view of the Science of Therapeutics' and the Society distributed several thousand copies of the lecture all over Britain.[1]

A slightly different account appeared in a Foreword to *The Reflex*, the Yearbook of the Chicago College of Osteopathic Medicine and Surgery in 1923, where he claimed to have 'hoisted the flag of Osteopathy in Great Britain' in the Holland Hall, Kensington in 1898 and to have lectured in the same hall in 1899 and 1900 on 'the prophylactic and curative value of Osteopathy' and 'Osteopathy, a new view of the science of therapeutics'. Copies of the lectures were apparently presented to members of the BMA at its Annual General Meeting in 1900.[3]

Among the earliest American-trained osteopaths to practise in the UK were William Smith, Franz Josef (later changed to Francis Joseph, no doubt as a result of the war with Germany) Horn, L. Willard Walker, Jay Dunham, and Ray Harvey Foote. William Smith, the first teacher of anatomy at Kirksville, returned to Scotland in 1901 and practised there until his death in 1912.[5] His sister married David Littlejohn, the brother of John Martin Littlejohn. (See Chapter 3). F. J. Horn and L. Willard Walker came to the UK in the Spring of 1902 encouraged by a wealthy American. Horn, a life-long friend of Littlejohn, established his practice at 1 Hay Hill, London. L. Willard Walker practised in Glasgow.[6] Dunham, from Lyons, Kansas went to Ireland in October 1903 at the request of a wealthy Irish-American patient living in Kansas, who wished him to treat his sister, who was bedridden. This he achieved and stayed on in Ireland. He practised in rooms in a hotel at Portadown, County Armagh. His success and fame spread throughout the country and two years later he set up a clinic in Belfast, after a brief return to Kansas.[7,3] Dunham cabled Harvey Foote, 'Cut your cards for Ireland'.

Foote sailed from New York on 4 May 1904 and practised at 71 Harcourt Street, Dublin.[8]

The first woman to practise Osteopathy in England was Dr Georgina Watson in 1907, but she returned to the US.[9] The same year Wilfrid Streeter and Elmer Pheils came to the UK to practise in Glasgow and Birmingham respectively. A Dr Barker came over to practise in Liverpool in 1909.

Friends of Osteopathy in those days included the Duke of Argyll, Dr Krause, the friend and physician of Cecil Rhodes, and the Principal of Glasgow University.[3]

Early support from the medical profession

In 1910 Alexander Bryce published in the *British Medical Journal* an article entitled, 'Remarks on mechano-therapy in disease: with special reference to Osteopathy'. He was interested after the, 'Remarkable improvement of several of my own reputedly incurable patients' and decided to inform himself of the, 'Good and bad points of such a potent method of treatment'. Having read widely on the subject and obtaining such practical knowledge as was possible in this country he visited Schools of Osteopathy in the US. He provided a definition of Osteopathy and explained lesions and subluxations and claimed, 'The chief function of an osteopath is to reduce the subluxations and to correct the lesions, though he was relieved that one osteopath indicated that he rarely found them and another never thought of looking for them!' He considered that the benefits of osteopathy may be consequential to relief of 'contractured muscle' or muscular fibrosis, though osteopaths denied indignantly that massage had anything to do with manipulative efforts. He was critical of those devotees who claimed too much and also of dogmatism. He considered that acute conditions may be aggravated by manipulation. Allegedly medical journals and daily papers had reported cases of injury following osteopathic treatment. He considered that, 'There must be some virtue in a method which had such vitality as to spread all over a continent in a few years' and that, 'It was of striking benefit in select cases'. He stated, 'I do not hesitate to plead for the admission of this new form of scientific bone-setting among the recognised methods of treatment practised by the medical profession'.

In the same issue an anonymous article claimed that, 'In the sphere of medicine there is a vast area of ' "undeveloped land" which Lloyd George somehow failed to include in his budget.' Reference was made to how Harvey, Pasteur and others were ridiculed and that damage was done to the profession by neglect of things which if properly applied, held within them large possibilities of usefulness for the relief of suffering. While Osteopathy was considered in this context, attention was drawn to the Flexner Report of the same year in which the US osteopathic Schools were severely criticised. Rather like Paget, the author concluded that, 'If there is anything in Osteopathy that may help to ease a sufferer of some pain the cause of which is not a patient, the practitioner should not hesitate to use such aid...These things, therefore, should not be dismissed with a foolish contempt; they should be studied, and the secrets of whatever good there may be in them should be discovered'.

The Formation of the British Osteopathic Association

By 1910, there were sufficient osteopaths in Britain to form a British Osteopathic Society.[9] 12 members attended the first meeting.[6] On 1 July 1911 at a meeting in Manchester, it became the British Osteopathic Association (BOA), the formal wing of the American Osteopathic Association (AOA), for American trained osteopaths, 'To uphold the professional ethical standards and to provide the public with a list of trained and qualified osteopaths, to advance Osteopathy and to maintain a professional spirit'. BOA members were also eligible for membership of the AOA. As in the case of other associations, membership was purely optional and there were, 'Doubtless osteopaths with equal qualifications outside its ranks'.[10] From the minutes of the BOA in the late 1920s and 1930s it is evident that members had to pay an additional fee to the AOA and there was representation at the AOA conferences. However, while AOA members could practise in this country, unless BOA members had undertaken the State Examinations, they could not do so in the USA. An example of such a person was Kelman MacDonald, who graduated in Medicine from Edinburgh and in Osteopathy from Kirksville, but could practise neither in the USA.[11] By 1925 the BOA had over 50 members and six were also registered medical practitioners.

In 1914, the BOA appointed a committee to try and secure the registration of the Association under the Companies Act, as a Scientific Society without the use of the word Limited. The case for Osteopathy was presented to the Board of Trade. The President of the Board said, 'You have told us the standing of your profession in USA. What is your standing here? What have you done?' Because of the GMC's opposition, the Board of Trade refused the application. A letter was then prepared and sent to the GMC and the British Medical Association (BMA), but neither body paid any attention to it.[6]

The first School of Osteopathy

In 1903 Littlejohn visited cancer hospitals in France, Germany and Austria and treated patients in the UK.[6] On passing through Britain he discussed with Horn and Willard Walker the establishment of a British School of Osteopathy. Dunham and Harvey Foote agreed to help. Among its aims was, 'To set up a standard of Osteopathic Science, to show the public what the Science is and clinically to demonstrate its efficiency'.[12]

Littlejohn returned permanently to the UK in 1913 and lived at Thundersley (North Benfleet), Essex and resumed discussion regarding a School with Horn and Walker. There was certainly a need for the formal education of osteopaths at this time. L. N. Fowler & Co published in 1914, 'A Home Study Course in Osteopathy, Massage and Manual Therapeutics', though each page is headed 'Osteopathy'. Such 'Teach Yourself' guides enabled the unqualified to set up in practice. How was the public to know the difference?

In 1914, Littlejohn and J. Stewart Moore (on behalf of the BOA) wrote privately to the President of the GMC regarding a School of Osteopathy and the teaching of the subject to medical students, medical graduates and others. In his reply, Sir Donald McAllister recognised that the right to practise the art of healing is based on qualification and that no restrictions can be imposed upon any theory of Medicine.[1,2]

'Any one who pursues the course of study and examinations prescribed by any of the licensing bodies in this country may obtain a qualification admitting him to the Medical Register and so bringing him under the jurisdiction of the General Medical Council....It would therefore appear that the legislature has already provided for the registration of the practitioners that you have in mind on the conditions that they offer the statutory guarantees that they possess the knowledge and skill required for the efficient practice of Medicine and Surgery and Midwifery.'

In March 1915, an attempt was made to incorporate a British School of Osteopathy. A Memorandum and Articles were drawn up, but the Treasury refused to sanction the organisation of any body involving capital in a field not actually associated with war service. This date has been quoted as the actual date of the foundation of the School.[1]

The BSO first germinated in the early years of the war as a clinic at Thundersley.[13] The first building was a hut, built entirely by the first students of the School. It then relocated to Central Hall, Kiln Road, Thundersley, a building dedicated to public welfare, where the osteopathic table was screened off from the audience room. While this clinic was in progress, a new centre was opened at 15, The Ridgeway, Enfield. From 1915-1917 30-50 patients were treated a week. The Enfield centre was affiliated with the Osteopathic Institute at Torquay.

During the war, from 1915-1917, the School provided treatment for distinguished naval, military and aviation officers, including Lord Jellicoe, Lord French and Earl Beatty, as well as ordinary soldiers, seamen and airmen. One major had a dislocated shoulder which was said to be incurable. It was successfully treated. A naval surgeon arrived at Victoria Station unable to walk. He was successfully treated in the Grosvenor Hotel for a week. A young lady ambulance driver injured in France and in the Far East was put in a mental home as a certified patient until she was rescued by osteopathic treatment.[14]

Through the assistance of solicitors, the BSO was incorporated on 7 March 1917. A 6 page (probably incomplete), hand-written letter by Littlejohn exists explaining how the School was founded, 'At the first meeting of the Governing Directors on 17 March, 1917. The second meeting was held on 13 April at which Bye-Laws were presented and passed'. The incorporation of the School was on condition that not more than two shares, each of £1 be issued during the continuance of the war. Horn and Littlejohn held these as Governing Directors. Thus, although Littlejohn is considered the founder of the BSO, he was actually a co-founder.

J. J. Darlison[15] has provided an account of the early years of the incorporated School. It was then housed in Littlejohn's consultancy rooms at 48, Dover Street, London W1, but the clinics were still at Thundersley and Enfield for patients unable to pay full fees. There were clinical demonstrations upon volunteers enlisted in war service, as well as other patients. In 1918 more than 50 patients a week were being treated. The students were composed almost entirely of those who, having received substantial benefits from Osteopathic treatment, had decided to make it their career, just as in the early years of the ASO. 'Progress was slow at first for the work was encompassed by much hindrance and obstruction and its promoters had to overcome the repressive bias which, as the history of mankind shows, has ever been the lot of pioneers.'[15]

After the war the restriction on shares ceased and one share was sold to the BOA. An attempt was made to follow this up by co-operation with them, but the BOA insisted on ownership of the School. This was refused because it was considered, 'Not the province of the BOA, any more than it would of the BMA or AOA to own schools. Schools and Colleges are controlled by governing bodies...conformable to legal standards of Education'.[1]

In 1921, Littlejohn had completed the organisation of a four year course of theoretical and practical work, as outlined by the Associated Colleges of Osteopathy in the US, that excluded materia medica and surgery. The first and second years were devoted to fundamental subjects. A premedical course in chemistry, physics and biology was followed by anatomy, physiology, histology, embryology, dissection, microscopic and analytical demonstration of foods, drugs, poisons, hygiene and bacteriology, at Chelsea Polytechnic. Some students studied instead at the University of Sheffield or King's College, London.[12] The 3rd and 4th years were devoted to Osteopathy.

Graduates and students in medicine and surgery were credited with work previously undertaken and were required only to complete the final two years.[16]

Another provision of the original Charter of the School was that it must be a 'non profit' organisation. At the Select Committee of the House of Lords in 1935 there was an implication that Littlejohn benefited financially from the School. He claimed nothing could be further from the truth.[1] Although he was a teacher and administrator at the School, he apparently never received any profit or salary.

On February 13, 1922, at a Special and Extraordinary Meeting of the Directors, a 'Committee of Clinique and Sanitorium' was initiated, with J. Stewart Moore as Superintendent. In that year a part-time Faculty was established of BOA members.

Dr Kelman MacDonald, in a lecture given in a Committee Room in the House of Commons on 31 March 1925, on, 'Osteopathy and its position in the British Isles', specified that one of the BOA's aims was to obtain a Royal Charter or a similar official recognition for the BSO. It emerged that that the BOA actually sought this for themselves.

The BSO attempted to comply with the requirements of the law regulating osteopathic schools in the provinces of Canada and the United States, where Osteopathy was fully recognised. The Board of Regents of Ontario, Canada recognised the School as one of the reputable Schools of Osteopathy.

By 1925, more space was required and the School moved to Vincent Square, a house given rent-free for two years by Horn, from where the first practitioners graduated. Friends of Osteopathy raised the money to provide running expenses.[6] The first Diploma was issued to Elsie

Wynter Wareing on 1 August 1925. Her sister had received treatment from Littlejohn, but died. As he could not issue a death certificate an inquest was held, but after hearing his evidence the case was dropped. The reporting of it brought him many more patients.[3]

The New Era Illustrated in October 1926 carried an article on the BSO, with a photograph of Littlejohn in a small room treating a patient with two female assistants. The patient is on the plinth fully dressed, with shoes. Littlejohn was in shirtsleeves and waistcoat and with a winged collar and tie.

In 1926 the BOA still desired to gain control of the School and to model it on the American School of Osteopathy, which by that time had an allopathic curriculum. The Charter of the School was therefore expanded to make the School, 'A perpetual Trust under the control of Governing Directors as Trustees'. Stewart Moore and Dr William Cooper were Directors. By 1928 the Directors included Sir Herbert Barker, Harvey Foote, W. A. Martisus, W. C. Minifie and Arthur D. Wareing (an ex-head-master and teacher of science and mathematics, with a First Division Certificate of the Board of Education).

In 1927, due to the demand for osteopathic treatment and the need for larger clinic rooms, the School moved to Abbey House, two Victoria Street, Westminster, London SW1. Dr Wareing was superintendent of the enlarged clinic.[12] In 1929, 200 patients were treated weekly.

In the Prospectus for 1931-32, it is indicated that following the Companies Act of 1929 the Articles of Incorporation were modified in view of the, 'Possibility in the future, as funds increase and the School enlarges, to arrange for the full Collegiate Curriculum in Science... similar to the Medical Schools. In order to provide for the Hospital Osteopathic School contemplated in the new arrangement...and the higher field of research...we decided to incorporate the College of Osteopathic Physicians and Surgeons. All graduates of the British School of Osteopathy will become members'.

In 1930 the School moved to 16, Buckingham Gate, London SW1, its home until it moved to Suffolk Street in 1980. This was made possible by a loan from John Martin Littlejohn that was not repaid until 1946. In 1890, the building had been the residence of the Grand Duchess of Meckleburg-Stelitz, cousin of Queen Victoria. The lease was for 21 years. The yearly rent was £650. A further lease was issued in 1949 for 21 years, with a yearly rent of £1,750.

At Buckingham Gate a growing number of students had to be accommodated.[16] Structural alterations were carried out in order to provide greater and more comfortable cubicle space for patient treatments. In addition to large lecture rooms, the school acquired several demonstration rooms, a small chemical laboratory, a minor surgery room and other facilities. There were four rooms that could be fitted with beds as a nucleus for an 'indoor department and receiving ward' for a planned hospital.[17]

Arthur Millwood (see below) claimed that in the Winter of 1930/31 he discussed with Dr Littlejohn the value of an X-ray for the School and launched an appeal in April 1931. The response was not very good. A few years later another effort was made and in due course he was able to hand over £283 16s 6d. Admiral Taylor opened the X-ray Department.

Profile: J. Stewart Moore

J. Stewart Moore was the first Superintendent of the 'clinique and sanitorium' (1922) and on the Council of Education and a Director of the School (1924-1925), before which he had been President of the BOA. Born in Londonderry, Northern Ireland, he was educated there and in Belfast and trained as a chemist. After emigration to the US 'in early life', he became interested in Osteopathy and studied at the Boston School of Osteopathy. Even before he graduated he was assistant to the Dean. He then practised at Falmouth, Cape Cod, often not charging his patients who became his friends. Apparently 'Money meant little to him'. He then decided to practise in London at 69 Piccadilly, where he was joined by Littlejohn when the latter returned to the UK in 1913. Together they moved to 48 Dover Street. 'He was a genial, kindly, considerate man, whose one fault was his over-generosity'. He had some quite original inhibitory techniques. He died of pneumonia on 17 September 1939, at the age of 66.[18]

Profile: Dr William Charles Minifie

W. C. Minifie PhD, DO was a Director of the BSO and among the 'special demonstrators' in 1928. The following is based on information supplied by Mrs Violet Fussell, Dr Minifie's daughter, and from the records of the School.

He was educated at Sherborne School. On coming to London he became involved in the Young Men's Christian Association. He developed an ambition to become a medical missionary and began studying anatomy, physiology and First Aid at London teaching hospitals and the Royal College of Surgeons and studied in the British Museum Library.

The Missionary Society, however, decided that his health was not sufficiently robust to withstand conditions in the tropics. He then entered Spurgeon's College to train for the Baptist Ministry and later became one of Dr. Spurgeon's private secretaries. Together with Littlejohn, he formed the Bible Institute and undertook lecture tours in England, the USA and Canada.

He accepted the pastorate of one of the leading churches in Boston, Massachusetts, and while there studied at Harvard University. He became infused with the desire to combine healing with preaching. While in America he studied for the degrees of PhD and LittD and also Osteopathy. In 1918, he entered the BSO and in 1926 he was awarded the 9th Diploma, having returned to the USA during 1920-24. Later he was a lecturer at the School and a member of its Council. With the co-operation of Littlejohn, he established the first osteopathic clinic in the UK. He practised Osteopathy successfully both in London and on the French Riviera, even at the grand age of 91.

The Looker School of Bloodless Surgery

The history of this School is pertinent to the history of Osteopathy in Britain, as some of its graduates later qualified from the BSO, after being credited for work undertaken at the Looker School. This provided the ammunition needed by opponents of the Osteopaths Bill in 1935 to question the soundness of the qualification issued by the BSO, the only school of Osteopathy in existence at that time and upon which statutory recognition depended.

William Looker had spent many years in America, practising in Pennsylvania, before returning to England. He established an osteopathic practice in Manchester in 1920[5] and founded 'The Looker School of Bloodless Surgery', registered in 1921. In 1923 the name changed to the Looker College of Osteopathy and Chiropractic,[19] but the majority of its graduates elected to practise only Osteopathy. It then transferred to London as the Looker College. It 'taught the science in an admirable manner and...did most excellent work and turned out many able and efficient practitioners.' The Prospectus apparently outlined a three year course. Hill and Clegg[19] claim it was of only three to six months' duration, but their book contains many inaccuracies. Littlejohn claimed it was a three year course.[1]

Looker was a regular contributor to *"Health and Efficiency"*. When he died in 27 July 1926, his obituary in the Journal noted:

'We record with unfeigning sorrow the untimely passing of the well-known osteopath, Dr William Looker, whose articles for practitioners have been a feature of this journal for many months past. A forceful personality, gifted with that buoyant and positive temperament which is so great and valuable an asset to a healer, Dr Looker was just beginning to unfold his full powers, and there can be no doubt that he was only on the threshold of a remarkable and beneficial career. Unusually many-sided, he was an accomplished musician, as well as a mender of broken men—indeed, if medicine claimed his energies to the point of exhaustion, he found a restorative in his passionate devotion to music. Many were the plans and projects he had formed for realisation in the near future, many his honourable ambitions, now with tragic swiftness the strong and willing worker has had to lay his burden down, and those who knew him most intimately will feel most keenly this abrupt conclusion to a half-told tale.'[9]

In 1925, a few of the graduates of the Looker College formed the 'Incorporated Association of Osteopaths Ltd' (IAO), as they were unable to join the BOA. As Littlejohn explained in 1935, 'The object of that Association was first of all, to support, advance, maintain and carry out investigation into the principles, theory and practice of Osteopathy; to train, teach and graduate students therein. They set themselves to work in 1925, to teach themselves and to be taught by others, who went and lectured to them from time to time'.[20]

'It met with much adverse criticism in a certain section of the press (details unknown),[14] but made progress, conducting study circles, periodic meetings, lectures and clinics to assist in the development of the profession.[15] Members were granted the privilege of the title of 'osteopathic physician', 'osteopathic surgeon' or both.'

After Looker's death, the Looker College closed and in 1926 some of its graduates, all members of the Incorporated Association and in practice for several years, applied to the BSO to qualify for the BSO Diploma. Negotiations between the IAO and BSO commenced in 1927.[10] The son of John Leary recollected his father speaking of 12 such students and consequently Littlejohn referred to them as 'the Disciples'. From details of the background of students recorded in Littlejohn's ledger of graduates, it would seem that 19 joined the BSO accredited with work at the Looker School. 15 were mentioned at the Select Committee of the House of Lords (1935).

Accreditation of IAO members with work at the Looker School was consistent with the regulations regarding credited work of the Associated Colleges of Osteopathy in the US, of which Littlejohn had been President for three years. There was a record of some 20 'irregular' schools in the US in which the same plan and principles were carried out.[20]

IAO members were obliged to attend monthly study circles in Manchester, conducted by BSO graduates. From time to time even Littlejohn taught there. On 14 July 1928 he conducted a formal practical examination in the Milton Hall, Manchester.[18] After 12-18 months, during which eight test papers were set which students worked through at home, they sat a final examination in accordance with the requirements governing all the other students of the School.[19] Those who passed were granted a Diploma. The same requirements applied to graduates of the British College of Chiropractic (see below).[14] All became successful practitioners and some, such as Willis Haycock and Arthur Millwood, made significant contributions to the profession.

Not all members of the IAO agreed to this arrangement with the BSO and some who considered that they already held 'reputable' qualifications were not willing to spend further time and money and either resigned from the IAO or allowed their membership to lapse.[13] In due course, they ceased to be any longer eligible for membership, as it was later only open to graduates from the BSO.

At the Select Committee of the House of Lords held in 1935 to discuss the possible statutory recognition of Osteopathy, (See Chapters 5 and 6), Littlejohn was one of the witnesses called to defend Osteopathy, but the lawyers representing those opposing legislation were intent on demonstrating that the Dean of the only school in existence was dishonest. Sir William Jowitt accused Littlejohn of issuing diplomas to Looker graduates who had not completed 'a full and rigorous' four years at the School.[20, 21]

Jowitt read out the certificate of George Spencer, a Looker graduate, who was taught at the BSO for one year:

> 'To whom this may come, Greeting. Be it known that George Spencer having completed the required study and attended the full course of Lectures, Clinics and Demonstrations during the regular 4 years' course, and having passed satisfactory examinations in all branches of training taught in this school including Clinics and other practical demonstrations, is hereby admitted to the Diplomate in Osteopathy D.O., given at London 22 December 1928.'

Littlejohn explained that in accordance with the conditions of the Associated Colleges of Osteopathy, students were credited with three years' work, but were required to undertake one further year's work, pass an examination and undertake clinic work in Manchester. They also had undertaken three years' work as graduate members of the IAO.[1]

It is ironic that it is now quite commonplace for students to join institutions with credit for work undertaken elsewhere. In the year 2000 some students transferred to the BSO from the John Wernham College of Classical Osteopathy (later the Surrey Institute of Osteopathic Medicine), which had not at that time received Recognised Qualification status from the General Osteopathic Council, and the students were credited with work previously undertaken.

The British College of Chiropractic and The Western Osteopathic School

The British College of Chiropractic was founded in 1925 with temporary headquarters in London. Dr T. Mitchell-Fox, a graduate of the Looker College, transferred it to Plymouth. Incorporated with it, but kept quite separate, was the Western Osteopathic School. Apparently it, 'compared favourably with American Colleges regarding its entry requirements and curriculum'.[10] It was a three year (27 month) course, costing 100 guineas and leading to a Diploma in Chiropractic. There was also a postgraduate course, for those of other therapies, of nine months' duration. The first graduation ceremony took place in 1928 in the presence of the Mayor of Plymouth. The course had difficulty in obtaining suitable resident staff and sufficient students. Several graduates expressed an interest in Osteopathy and after negotiation these were admitted to the BSO and credited with previous work undertaken.[14] The British College of Chiropractic then suspended its teaching. Graduates also became members of the British Chiropractic Society and affiliated to the British Naturopathic Association (BNA).[10]

The Incorporated Association of Osteopaths Ltd (IAO)

The origin of the IAO as an association for graduates of the Looker School is described above. Graduates of the BSO later became eligible for membership, the first ones joining in 1927. However, before 1929, in accordance with Article XXIV, subsection 5 of the Articles of Association of the BSO, the corporate body for BSO graduates was 'The Association of British Osteopaths'. After 1929, this was replaced by the IAO.

A special resolution was passed on 16 March 1929 and confirmed on 13 April, that the Memorandum of Association of the IAO be altered and amended to read: 'To incorporate into a united organisation the graduates of the British School of Osteopathy'.

In a letter to graduates on 15 May 1929, Littlejohn wrote:

'The Incorporated Association of Osteopaths Ltd has been transferred to the British School of Osteopathy and it has been so amended that it represents the organisation of the Graduates of the British School of Osteopathy for the purpose of preserving and publishing a professional Register of Graduates to maintain a code of Ethics and to perform such other duties including the election of one member of the Board of Directors of the British School of Osteopathy. In order to organise and function this body, a meeting is hereby called of all Graduates of the BSO to take place in Abbey House, two Victoria Street on 1 June 1929 at 3pm.'

In 1936 the IAO changed its name to the Osteopathic Association of Great Britain (OAGB), a title suggested by Shilton Webster-Jones (later the second Principal of the BSO). In 1964, Clem Middleton and Audrey Smith, the latter then President of the OAGB, urged Arthur Millwood to record the early history of the Association. At that time only he and Patrick Saul of the founder members were still alive. In his article, 'The early beginnings of the Association', Millwood wrote:

'The graduates of the last two decades can have little idea of the conditions and prejudices of the 1920s...It was in the Autumn of 1924 that I talked to one or two about forming some sort of body. It must be remembered that there were very few of us. Ernest Davis of Liverpool suggested that I call a meeting. I did this, asking them to meet in Manchester. Some of them wrote back to say they hardly knew the city. So I suggested meeting in the first class waiting room at the Central Station, Manchester. From there, we adjoined to the Deansgate Hotel...I often say that our association first started in the waiting room of a railway station!
The Articles and Memorandum were drawn up by a Manchester solicitor, Mr Davies, 'a real Dickensian character'...and signed by 7 osteopaths and dated the 12th of May, 1925....
It wasn't until 1929 that the first dinner was arranged. Dr Littlejohn was President that year and I helped to organise the event which was held at the Hotel Cecil in the Strand. The Shell-Mex building stands there now. The dinner was on Friday, October 18th...From the Hotel Cecil we went to

the Trocadero. The Mayfair Hotel held sway for a long time. Others were held at the Savoy and at Claridges.

...In 1930 the Annual Meeting and the Dinner (were held in the Midland Hotel), Manchester on 17 October. Dr Harvey Foote was the President. On the Saturday after the dinner Galli Curci was singing at the Free Trade Hall. Harvey Foote would have me go up to her suite in the Midland Hotel....In spite of Dr Foote's persuasiveness, she would not come to the dinner. A few weeks after this...she gave a concert in New York and the whole of the proceeds were given to osteopathic clinics.'

The IAO had 67 members in 1934.

Profile: Harvey Ray Foote (1880-1937)

Dr Harvey Ray Foote had been President of both the BOA and IAO and was one of the Committee that promoted the Osteopaths Bill in the 1930s. He was born in Kansas on 25 June 1880 and studied medicine in Chicago. On a country holiday he was practising the high jump and felt an acute pain in his right side, initially diagnosed as pleurisy and then tuberculosis, from which he suffered considerable pain for eight months, eventually being unable to raise his arm. He was treated by Dr Dunham, who located a downward displacement of the 3rd rib on the right side. Improvement was rapid. He went on to study Osteopathy at Des Moines and graduated in 1904.

After nearly two years of practice in Belfast with Dunham, Foote set up practice in Dublin where he remained until 1913. In 1912 Dr William Cooper, who became a prominent BOA member, became his assistant. The week when war was declared, Foote moved to London and practised for nine months at Harewood House, Hanover Square, returning to Dublin three days a week, but moved to 40a Park Lane in 1920 and then later 33 Hertford Street. In 1921 he set up the first osteopathic hospital at 12 Wigmore Street and later at 35 Manchester Street. Foote contributed to the BSO as Chair of the Governing Directors, assisting in administration and in teaching technique, 'Which although that of the older and more direct than delicate school, never failed to achieve its purpose'. His funeral was on 6 August 1937.[22,23]

The BOA in the late 1920s

In 1927 the BOA opened a clinic in Vincent Square to bring Osteopathy to all sections of the community. It was purchased and given to the BOA by Dudley Docker. Patients paid according to their means and gave voluntary contributions. In 1931, it moved to 24-25 Dorset Square, London NW1 (Andrew Still House).

Minutes of the BOA Council from 1928 exist and are now lodged in the Wellcome Library for the History and Understanding of Medicine. The BOA Council had Legislative, Clinics, General Information, Membership, Education, Ethics and Programme Sub-Committees.

The minutes record that in 1928 Dr George MacDonald was President of the BOA. The Council discussed bringing Osteopathy before Parliament (See Chapter 4). A publicity and propaganda group was to be set up with the object of controlling all propaganda from the profession and starting an official journal. A decision was made to collect all available evidence regarding the BSO, over which the BOA had failed to gain control, to ascertain details of management, educational standards and the granting of diplomas.

The minutes of the BOA Council for 1929 record that Pheils and Semple proposed that Council recommend to the General Meeting that the question of Dr Littlejohn's school be discussed, with a view to demanding from him a report of his instructional course and mode of issuing diplomas. The same year, Lord Clifford of Chundleigh was anxious to amalgamate herbalists with the BOA and to start a joint college. The Ethics Committee of the BOA were concerned about a newspaper advertisement in which Littlejohn's name appeared. The AOA was anxious for still closer working between them and the BOA. Pheils and Gilmour were to rewrite the affiliation agreement and the AOA was to be invited to hold a convention in London.

George Bernard Shaw and Osteopathy

George Bernard Shaw opened the BOA clinic in Vincent Square. The relationship between Shaw and Osteopathy is explained in an article entitled, 'Thank you, Mr Shaw', by Murray T. Pheils, the son of Dr Elmer T. Pheils[24] who was a prominent osteopath and a friend of Shaw.

Elmer Pheils was born in Toledo, Ohio in 1879 and trained at Kirksville. He visited London in 1907 for a working vacation with Horn, but stayed on and then moved to Birmingham. In the BSO Prospectus for 1924-1925, Pheils is listed as a member of the BSO Faculty. He suffered from poor vision following retinitis pigmentosa, which he claimed, 'Enhanced his sense of touch and contributed to his skills in joint manipulation'.[24]

In a letter to *The Times* (October 23 1925: The case of Dr Axham) Shaw, defending Axham, the anaesthetist to Herbert Barker, who had been struck off, makes the casual comment that in 1924 he injured his back while walking in Ireland:

> 'It took me 10 days to get to Birmingham, where an American D.O. [Doctor of Osteopathy] also classed as black-leg by the GMC, set me right after 75 minutes' skilled manipulation.'

Pheils and his family went to live in Malvern, where Shaw holidayed. Pheils and Shaw would walk and talk together about politics, science, religion, history, theatre, music, boxing and baseball and occasionally Shaw and his wife Charlotte would lunch at the Pheils. Unlike Shaw, who was a teetotaller, vegetarian and non-smoker, Pheils apparently was rumbustious and fond of food, whisky and cigars.

By 1926 Pheils was keen to get another School of Osteopathy started in London. He became President of the BOA and Chairman of the Appeal Committee.

Shaw commented on the Appeal pamphlet and on 18 December 1926 wrote a response to Pheil's invitation to attend a banquet at the Dorchester Hotel in aid of establishing a school of Osteopathy:

> 'I'd rather die. I refuse all banquets. The fact is notorious; and if I made an exception for the Yosteops nobody would ever believe that I am unbiased on the question afterwards.'

Pheils even attempted to enlist the help of Lady Astor in persuading Shaw. (The Astors were later to feature in the life of another osteopath, Stephen Ward). He also requested that Shaw's wife, Charlotte, be Patron of the appeal, to which Shaw replied on 4 March 1928:

> 'My wife is in bed with one of her bronchial attacks, and asks me to write to you very nicely to explain how, hampered as she is with a celebrated name, she must not sign appeals for money, as there would be no end to it if she did. Also, her husband tells her never to sign anything except a cheque, and then as far as possible by way of endorsement. In short, to put it nicely as I can, she- - - -won't.'

In 1940, Pheils treated Queen Elizabeth (later the Queen Mother). On two August 1950, when Pheils had congestive heart failure, Shaw wrote to him for the last time:

'I am all right except my legs, which are so groggy that I can only walk round the garden with a stick, and an attack of lumbago which you could perhaps have cured, but failing you I had to try radiant heat. Finally, I left it to nature, which did the trick slowly.
For heart trouble walk up to the Beacon three times a day. No immobilisation: no whisky. Cut out protein and live on raw vegetables as I do. Too much nitrogen is killing the human race.'

Shaw died in 1950; Elmer Pheils in 1952.[24]

Osteopathic Publications in the 1920s

Some of the first British books on Osteopathy were published in the 1920s. In 1927, L.C.Floyd McKeon wrote, 'Osteopathy and Chiropractic Explained' and in the same year Harvey Foote wrote, 'The Science of Osteopathy'. Captain Gerald Lowry wrote 'A Place Among Men' with a foreword by Viscount Allenby in 1928 and Wilfrid A Streeter wrote 'The New Healing' in 1929.

In 1929, Littlejohn published the *Journal of Osteopathy*, which continued until the war years. It was the official journal of the BSO, to satisfy the persistent demand from the public and especially prospective students for a statement of Osteopathy's fundamental principles. Over 200 copies were sent out bi-monthly to enquirers, including to China, India, Africa, Australia, Canada and the United States.

Profile: Capt. Gerald Lowry

Lowry was blinded in 1914 during the First World War, a bullet having passed through one temple and out of the other severing his optic nerves. After qualifying from the Institute Examination of Chartered Societies as a masseur, he eventually enrolled at the BSO and was the second student to graduate in 1925. Apparently despite his blindness he was a keen sportsman and rode, swam, skied, played golf, boxed, played bridge and was a yachtsman. He opened a free clinic in Stepney, East London with the support of the Chairman of the British Legion and worked there two nights a week.[25]

Natural Therapeutics in the UK (1900-1930)

A brief history of nature cure and naturopathy is relevant in that one of the opponents to the Osteopaths Bill at the Select Committee of the House of Lords in 1935 was the Nature Cure Association. They claimed that Osteopathy was a part of nature cure and the Bill would restrict the practice of Osteopathy solely to those describing themselves as 'osteopaths'. This close association between the two therapies is evident in the curriculum of the BSO in the 1920s, when hydrotherapy, climatology and dietetics were taught, and was later to find expression when in 1961 the titles of the British Naturopathic Association and British College of Naturopathy were changed to include Osteopathy.

The following has depended heavily on the account of the first 50 years of the British Naturopathic Association by Chambers,[26] aided by the research of Richenda Power[27] and an historical chart of William Spenceley.[28]

Nature Cure established itself in the UK at about the same time as 'pure' Osteopathy, initially by individuals who were self-taught, had attended courses abroad, or who had served an 'apprenticeship'.

Bernarr Macfadden is credited with being among the first to have brought Nature Cure to the UK. Initially working in the US, he opened a London office to publish an *Encyclopaedia of Health Culture* and a British version of his magazine, *Physical Culture*, first published in the US in 1899. He then edited *Health and Efficiency*. About 1909 he personally came to the UK and set up a health clinic in Brighton for about 50 patients, but on the outbreak of the First World War it closed and he returned to the US.[29,26] Macfadden also opened a health home at Orchard Leigh, Chesham, Buckinghamshire, which was taken over by Stanley Lief (See below). In 1913 the Pitcairn-Knowles' founded the Riposa Nature Cure Hydro near Hastings, Sussex.

James C. Thomson, who was wrongly diagnosed as having a fatal disease of the lungs, stayed at Macfadden and Kellogg's sanitoria in the US and then trained with Lindlahr of Chicago and became his chief assistant and superintendent of his sanitorium. A Scotsman by birth, Thomson returned to Edinburgh in 1913 and founded the Edinburgh School of Natural Therapeutics in 1919.[27] This survived until 1964 as a full time, four year course. In the 1920s, together with his wife, Jessie, he set up a free clinic for children and their parents for, 'The prevention and correction of deformities.' In 1939, he opened the Kingston Health Home, which at one time accommodated 45 residents.[26] Thomson died in 1960.

Milton Powell, the principal founder of the Nature Cure Association (NCA), was inspired by the writings of Macfadden. He worked at Macfadden's Brighton sanitorium (1909-1910) and then in London for Eustice Miles who taught and practised Nature Cure. Powell worked as a 'physiotherapist' during the First World War. In 1919 he set up a Nature Cure Health Home in Northampton. In Edgar

Saxon's *Healthy Life* Powell urged the formation of a Nature Cure Association[27], which was founded in 1920, 'To improve standards of education, promote changes in the law, compensate members who had been victimised and promote health education through publication'. James Thomson was President and Joseph Allen Patreionex, Andrew Pitcairn-Knowles and Edgar Saxon were also important contributors. The first NCA conference was held in 1921 at Northampton organised by Milton Powell and Edgar Saxon.[26]

On 18 June 1925, The Nature Cure Association of Great Britain and Ireland was incorporated as a non-profit making company limited by guarantee.

The witness to his signature makes it clear that Saxon's real name was actually Ernest John Savage, a London journalist. His family business was tea trading, but for economic reasons it turned to mail order of vegetarian products. He wrote on health for *The Christian Commonwealth* in 1906 and was a regular contributor to *The Healthy Life* in 1911, which he later bought. He also ran the Vitamin Cafe, a school of food reform and a guesthouse in the Cotswolds.[30]

James and Jessie Thomson considered the part-time courses inferior to that of their School in Edinburgh. They wanted the NCA to establish its own full time course, but the NCA did not have the resources. In 1928 they and their associates resigned from the NCA and founded the Incorporated Society of Registered Naturopaths.[26] A British Society of Naturopaths, or Society of British Naturopaths was evidently also founded by them in 1927.[27]

In 1920, Harry Clark and Ward Allen set up the part-time British Naturopathic College (British College of Naturopathy) in Ranelagh Gardens, London. In 1929 the graduates founded their own Association, the British Association of Naturopaths, led by Harry Clark, William Bone, Daley-Yates, Johnson-Drowfield and Percival Scarr.

The Therapeutic Institute was formed in Manchester in the early 1920s by Joseph and Lillian Patreionex.[27]

In 1928, Milton Powell and Harry Clements (a graduate of the New Jersey School of Chiropractic) founded the London School of Natural Therapeutics, in Kensington. The former was Principal. It was a part-time course, but with the same curriculum as the Edinburgh School. It closed in 1936 or 1938[27] to make way for the larger school of the NCA that was in existence by then.[26] Several graduates became members of the Register of the NCA.

In 1928, Victor Stanley Davidson, who trained with Lindlahr, founded Victor Davidson's College of Natural Therapeutics, providing an intensive course at Jesmond, Newcastle, but it closed in 1937 when Davidson went to South Africa.

Profile: Stanley Lief (1890-1963)

Stanley Lief was instrumental in setting up the British Naturopathic College, now the British College of Osteopathic Medicine (BCOM) and was its first Dean and Director of Studies. He was born in Lutzen, Latvia, one of the five children of Isaac and Riva Lief, who emigrated to South Africa at the turn of the century, where they opened a trading store at Roodeport, East Transvaal. Lief was a sickly child. After a basic education he started work in the store. One of the publications sold there was that of Macfadden. Lief followed the advice in the journal and his health improved. He worked his passage over to the USA and succeeded in persuading Macfadden to sponsor his education in Naturopathy and Chiropractic and he trained at Macfadden's School.

About 1914 he moved to the UK, becoming Assistant Director of Macfadden's Health Home in Brighton, before enlisting. After the war he continued to practise at Orchard Leigh and became director and proprietor in 1921. He helped to establish the Nature Cure Association of which he was President four times.

Lief married Stella Naylor Hollingsworth in March 1921 and their son, Charles Graham Lief, became a student at the BSO, but was killed in action in March 1945.

Orchard Leigh closed in 1926 as it was too small for the demands made upon it. Lief obtained financial support from a patient at Orchard Leigh to purchase 'Champneys' in 1925, the Rothschild mansion near Tring, which he converted to a Nature Cure resort for the rich and famous, the income from whom subsidised those of lesser means. He retained this until the late 1950s. He also had a clinic in Park Lane. In 1927 he founded the monthly magazine *Health for All* with John Wood, a student of William Looker, who apprenticed with Lief, acting as his 'ghost writer' and editor.[27,31,32] It continued until the 1960s when it was absorbed by *Here's Health*.

References

1.   *The Journal of Osteopathy.* (1935). June-August, VI(3 & 4).
2.   Littlejohn, J. M. (1932). Editorial. *The Journal of Osteopathy*, October, IV(1):2.
3.   Littlejohn, J. M. (1923). Osteopathy in Britain. *The Reflex*: 96-97. (Chicago College of Osteopathy).
4.   Littlejohn, J. M. (1935). *The Journal of Osteopathy*, January-April, 6 (1 & 2): 3.
5.   *The Journal of Osteopathy.* (1929). December, 1(2):3.
6.   Puttick, R.W. (1956). Osteopathy, p. 44. (London: Faber and Faber).
7.   Foote, Harvey R. (1906). Osteopathy in Ireland. *Journal of the American Osteopathic Association,* 6(IX):117-18.
8.   Littlejohn, J. M. (1937). Obituary: Harvey Ray Foote. *The Journal of Osteopathy*, July-September, VIII(3): 7.
9.   McKeon, L. C. Floyd (1938). Osteopathic Polemics. (London: C. W. Daniel Co).
10. McKeon, L. C. Floyd (1933). A Healing Crisis, pp. 109-110. (Weston super Mare: Michell Health products).
11. Report from the Select Committee of the House of Lords appointed to consider the Registration and Regulation of Osteopaths Bill [H.L.] together with the proceedings of the Committee and minutes of evidence. (1935). 3040, p. 209. (London: HMSO).
12. British School of Osteopathy. Prospectus 1928-1929.
13. British School of Osteopathy. Prospectus1931-1932.
14. Editorial. (1939). *The Journal of Osteopathy*, July-September, X(3): 3-4.
15. Darlison, J. J. (1935). British Osteopathy. The school and its founder. *The British Osteopathic Journal.* July, pp. 3-11.
16. British School of Osteopathy. Prospectus 1924-1925.
17. *The Journal of Osteopathy.* (1930). December, II(2):2.
18. Littlejohn, J. M. (1939). Obituary: J. Stewart Moore. *The Journal of Osteopathy*, October-December, X(4): 6.

19. Hill, C. & Clegg, H. A. (1937).<u>What is Osteopathy?</u> (London: J M Dent & Sons).

20. Report from the Select Committee of the House of Lords appointed to consider the Registration and Regulation of Osteopaths Bill [H.L.] together with the proceedings of the Committee and minutes of evidence. (1935). 3623-3647, pp. 237-239. (London: HMSO).

21. Report from the Select Committee of the House of Lords appointed to consider the Registration and Regulation of Osteopaths Bill [H.L.] together with the proceedings of the Committee and minutes of evidence. (1935). 3325-3381, pp. 222-225. (London: HMSO).

22. Littlejohn, J. M. (1937). Harvey Ray Foote. *The Journal of Osteopathy,* VIII(3): 7.

23. *The Osteopath.* (1937). Obituary Dr Harvey Foote. December, 1(2): 5.

24. Pheils, M. T. (1994). Thank you, Mr Shaw. *The British Medical Journal*, 309 (6970): 1724-1726.

25. Lowry, G. (1928). <u>A Place among Men</u>. (London:Mondiale).

26. Chambers, M. M. (1996). <u>The British Naturopathic Association. The first fifty years</u>. (The British Naturopathic Association.)

27. Power, R. (1984). A Natural profession? Issues in the professionalisation of British Nature Cure, 1930-1950. Dissertation submitted as course requirement of the CNAA MSc in Sociology, Polytechnic of the South Bank.

28. Spenceley, W. Historical flow chart. In Power, R. (1984). A Natural profession? Issues in the professionalisation of British Nature Cure, 1930-1950. Dissertation submitted as course requirement of the CNAA MSc in Sociology, Polytechnic of the South Bank.

29. Rumfitt, A. (1967). Looking back 1927-1967. *Health for All*, Summer:19.

30. Jenner, A. (1956). A teacher of the art of living. Serialised in *Here's Health*.

31. Wood, J. (1977). Tribute to Stanley Lief. *Health Messenger*, 13, Spring/ Summer.

32. Powell, M. (1963). Obituary: Stanley Lief. *British Naturopathic Journal and Osteopathic Review*. Spring, 5(8):252.

Chapter 3

Profile: John Martin Littlejohn (1865-1947)

This chapter is devoted to John Martin Littlejohn as Osteopathy owes much to him. He had a major influence on osteopathic education not only in this country, but also in the US through his positions at the ASO and the Chicago College. He participated in developing the first curriculum for a course in Osteopathy; he provided a physiological explanation for Osteopathy; he introduced Osteopathy into Britain and he founded the BSO. Littlejohn's unique philosophy, which viewed Osteopathy as, 'the science of adjustment' in its broadest sense and a complete system of medicine, produced many of the great osteopaths who were to follow and enhance the reputation of Osteopathy in this country.

It is ironic that a person so academic as John Martin Littlejohn, educated in divinity, law, oriental languages and political history and a prolific writer, should leave behind for his biographers so much that is enigmatic. The first detailed biography was by T. Edward Hall, delivered as the first John Martin Littlejohn Memorial Lecture on, 'The contribution of John Martin Littlejohn to Osteopathy', at the Mayfair Hotel on 3 October 1952. Hall had corresponded with a number of people in the USA who knew Littlejohn.[1]

Littlejohn's cross-examination at the Select Committee of the House of Lords in 1935 revealed information on his background and qualifications that is useful in piecing together his life.[2] More extensive research into Littlejohn's early life has been undertaken by Chris Campbell.[3] I am indebted to him for permitting me to refer to his unpublished work, before its reproduction in S. John Wernham's book on Littlejohn.[4] Campbell's research revealed that Hall's account of Littlejohn's life was not entirely accurate.

Background and Early Years (1865-1881)
Littlejohn was born at 27 Taylor Street, Glasgow on 15 February

1865, the son of Elizabeth and James Littlejohn. The family had poor beginnings. Two children died from scarlet fever before John Martin and his brothers William, David and James were born. His father was then a probationary preacher in the Reformed Presbyterian Church of Scotland, before becoming a city missionary and supply preacher in the provinces,[2] travelling long distances, rather like the father of A. T. Still.

In 1870, they moved to Gaelic-speaking Seil in the Western Islands of Scotland, where his father became a minister.[1] The congregation dwindled following a conflict of allegiance in the sect. The family then moved to Garvagh, Co. Derry, Ireland in 1876, where Littlejohn's father became minister the following year. In 1879 Littlejohn attended the Upper School at Coleraine Academical Institution and undertook the examinations of the Intermediate Education Board, gaining honours and prizes.

He was a frail boy, but strove to employ his academic talents to the full to fulfil his destiny, 'divine predestination' being a central tenet of the Reformed Presbyterian Church.[3] This may have been his driving force throughout his life.

Glasgow University (1881-1885)

In 1881 (at the early age of16) he entered Glasgow University, with his brother William, to undertake an MA, studying arts, theology, Hebrew and oriental languages,[1] as a necessary prerequisite to studying theology, with a view to a career in the Reformed Presbyterian Church. The following year they registered as students at the Theological Hall in Belfast. According to Edward Hall, he did not choose to graduate in 1885, but left the University.[1] In a letter to Chris Campbell in 1993, the acting deputy archivist of Glasgow University explained that while he was eligible for graduation, he may not have done so either because of the cost, or because testimonials at that time were considered just as useful as a degree certificate.[3] He certainly depended on testimonials for gaining positions at Columbia College, Amity College and the ASO,[1,5] (see below). A more likely explanation is that he, like other non-conformists, refused to take an oath of allegiance to the University. Members of the Reformed Presbyterian Church, as covenanters, would not take any oaths outside of the faith, e.g. to the Crown, educational institutions, or in Court.[3] It is, however, claimed elsewhere that he obtained Honours and First Class in Mental Philosophy in 1884 and Honours and First Class in Divinity with special prizes in Oriental Languages in 1885.[6] It would seem that subjects relevant to a career in the church were not all that he studied at this time. He became University

Foundation Scholar in Mathematics and Philosophy in 1884 and was also a tutor at Glasgow University from 1883 to 1885.[6] Little is known regarding William Littlejohn, who was apparently the 'black sheep' of the family.

Ireland (1885-1888)

Campbell[3] has managed to piece together some of Littlejohn's life between 1885 and 1892 when he left for the United States. He returned to Ireland and on 7 September 1886 was ordained a Minister at Creevagh, Ballybay, Co. Monaghan.[3] It is also claimed he was a lecturer in theology at Ballybay Union Hall in the winter of 1886-7.[6] He also wrote articles for the *Covenanter Magazine* on the church and missions at this time. Within the first six months of 1888, he resigned his post, evidently because of the 'unwanted attention' of three women of the parish, and possibly because of a conflict between himself and the congregation, many members of which stayed away from his services.[3]

Back to Glasgow (1888-1892)

It must have been shortly after his return to Glasgow in 1888 that he had a serious fall down a flight of concrete steps at the Faraday Laboratory and lay unconscious for four hours with concussion and a fractured cranium.[7,2] Shortly after that he started having 'haemorrhages from his throat',[7] requiring periods of convalescence. On account of his ill-health he visited the US in 1889,[2] as recommended by Dr Matthew Charteris of Glasgow and Sir Morell Mackenzie of London and stayed at a sanatorium on Long Island. He attended Columbia College only periodically, as his research there did not require him to be present daily.[2]

At Glasgow University he specialised in Divinity. He took his Licentiate in Arts[3] (a lesser degree than an MA), the reason for which is unclear, but he received an MA that year in classical languages, (there was no BA at that time), possibly completing his previous studies at the University.[2] In 1889, he was made a Life Member of Glasgow University Council.[6] He also studied for a BD which he obtained the following year. He then studied law, gaining an LLB in 1892, the first place in Legal Science and the William Hunter Gold Medal in Forensic Medicine from the legal department.[1,6] He received the University Medal in Jurisprudence, the Special Prize in Federal Law and the Henderson Prize in Theology of 20 guineas for his thesis on, 'The sabbathism of Hebrews iv 9'.[6]

He must have been a very busy man at this period, as in addition to these diverse studies, in 1891-2, he was a lay member of the Students'

Representative Council and joint editor of the Glasgow University
Magazine. It is claimed from 1890 to 1892, he was also Principal at
Rosemount College, a School for young ladies.[1,6] He also studied in
three European seminaries.[4]

It must have been at this time that he gained his knowledge of
physiology. Hall writes, 'It has been stated, however, on good authority
that these years were devoted to the study of anatomy and physiology at
Kelvin Hall under the eminent Scottish physiologist, Dr McKendrick.'[1]
At the Select Committee of the House of Lords (1935), Littlejohn
claimed (of that period), 'I had no degrees in medicine, but that did not
prevent me from studying'. He claimed that he trained in chemistry and
elementary philosophy under Professor McKendrick and in anatomy
and physiology at the Anderson's Medical College. The *Journal of
Osteopathy* for 1934 refers to a visit Littlejohn made to Scotland with his
son, James and his return to the McKendrick School of Physiology in
Glasgow, his 'alma mater'.[8]

Columbia College (1892-1894)

In October 1892 (aged 27) he enrolled for a PhD at Columbia College
(later Columbia University), New York. According to Hall,[1] following the
'haemorrhages in the neck', he was advised by the eminent physician Sir
Morrell MacKenzie to seek a warmer, drier climate otherwise he would
not last more than seven months. Mackenzie allegedly said, 'May God
make it possible for your student life to be prolonged in the summer
climes of the New World.'[1,5] It is likely that this account referred to an
earlier visit (see above). Anyone who is familiar with New York will know
of its winter climes. It is not the sort of climate in which one would
choose to live for the sake of one's health! It was also a poor prognosis
for someone who lived to the age of 82. It is difficult to imagine the
attraction of the United States to a man like Littlejohn, other than as an
opportunity for 'missionary' work on behalf of his church.

At Columbia College he was a University Fellow in Philosophy. He
studied political philosophy, political economy and finance[1] and took
examinations in the various required subjects as part fulfilment of a PhD
Course.[5] At the Select Committee (See Chapter 5) he was questioned as
to how he became a Fellow. Sir William Jowitt, representing the BMA,
presumed that this was equivalent to being a 'Fellow' at Oxford and
challenged Littlejohn's honesty. 'Do you know what it means to be a
Fellow?' Littlejohn replied, 'I know because I was one.'[2] His research
topic was 'The Political Theory of the Schoolmen and Grotius'. It
was inspired by Professor Lorimer of Edinburgh University and he

may have began this work before leaving Scotland.[3] It required him to travel around the universities of Europe studying medieval literature. In the summer and autumn of 1893, he was, 'A student in Cathedral and University Librarian of England, France, Germany, Switzerland and Italy'.[6]

In 1893, due to continued ill-health, he temporarily gave up work and never sat the written examinations. After his illness, he spent some months under hospital treatment in Philadelphia, then at a sanatorium in Waukesha, Wisconsin, then at Denver, Colorado and at Waco, Texas, where he met Dr Lowber.[7] When at Waukesha, he started as a Research Fellow in Psychology at the National University, Chicago and continued research at Chicago University on, 'The fee system of payment of officials in contrast with salaried service'.[5]

Amity College (1894-1897)

References from Columbia College secured him in November 1894 an appointment as President of Amity College, College Springs, Iowa, a co-educational institution empowered to grant degrees in Arts, Science, Philosophy, Letters and other subjects.[1] At 29 he was one of the youngest college Presidents in the US. He served as the college's Chief Executive Officer and extended the course. 'The scope widened in conformity with the spirit of liberal education.' He also taught mental philosophy and Hebrew.[2] He must have either liked the US, or saw a greater opportunity there than in his native Scotland.

It is likely that while at Amity College he completed his PhD. The thesis was presented early in 1894 and considered a work of scholarship and 'rare merit'.[1]

When challenged by Jowitt as to whether it was from Columbia University, he denied it, but then the College did not become an independent University until 1894.[2] This is the date given for his PhD in the BSO Prospectus of 1924-5. Elsewhere it is stated that it was from Chicago National University in 1895.[6] The thesis is still in existence, and was published at College Springs, Iowa in May 1895. Campbell suggested that the PhD may have been an Honorary Degree from Amity College on the basis of his achievements as President of the college and work undertaken at Columbia.[3] That he should have received such a qualification from his own college is not so far-fetched. A PhD was awarded to his brother, David Littlejohn, by Amity College.[9]

In early 1897, he left Amity College and took up a teaching post at the ASO, Kirksville, Missouri, with the founder of Osteopathy, A. T. Still. The problems with his neck and throat ('haemorrhages for 9 years')[5] led him to visit Kirksville regularly to receive personal treatment from Still. He also apparently had thyroid problems, which is consistent with a photograph of 1890 showing him very slim with bulging eyes. The trustees of Amity College were reluctant to accept his resignation and paid a tribute to him at a meeting, stating:

> 'We recognise in Dr J. M. Littlejohn one of the ablest ministers and ripest scholars. And as an educator he has no superior. A refined gentlemen, a true Christian, his influence has always been on the side of right and the best interest of education, his aim in life being to lift up and stimulate the educational interests of the whole community'.[5]

At the ASO (1898-1900)

In February 1898 he was appointed Professor of Physiology, Psychology and Dietetics at the ASO[3] and Dean of the Faculty, with an outstanding commendation from Amity College. Such a prestigious appointment was possible as Amity College was larger than the ASO at that time.[2] His appointment, however, is surprising as he had no qualifications in physiology, though what he taught as 'physiology' was probably very different from what we understand by the term today.

He later wrote, 'Being an enthusiast in the study of anatomy and physiology and myself a sufferer, and exiled from my native land by the medical profession on the ground of ill health, I was fascinated by Still's ideas...'.[10]

He was joined by his brothers David and James. James had graduated in medicine from Glasgow University in 1892[11] and worked as a surgeon in the UK before joining John Martin Littlejohn, first as Vice-Principal at Amity College and then as Professor of Major Surgery at Kirksville. As well as teaching, the three brothers were students of Osteopathy. On 27 October 1898 John Martin Littlejohn addressed the graduating class, claiming, 'Osteopathy is certainly an independent system of medicine'. He undertook research in a barn, subjecting animals to lesions under anaesthesia and attempting to correct them. He also explored the toxicity of chemicals foreign to the body: morphine, quinine, iron and arsenic, and the lymphatic system and its capability of flushing lungs in pneumonia.

Within one year of taking up his appointment he had written three books on physiology and a book on 'Psycho-physiology' and had inaugurated '*The Journal of the Science of Osteopathy*' (later '*The Osteopathic World*').[1,5]

It was during this period that he re-visited the UK, where he lectured in London and treated patients in Scotland. (See Chapter 2).

From Kirksville to Chicago (1900-1913)

The ASO curriculum broadened, under the guidance of William Smith, who taught anatomy and the Littlejohn brothers, an inevitability following the legislation passed in Missouri in 1897 enabling ASO graduates to receive state licences as physicians, but requiring the School to conform to the allopathic medical curriculum. As a consequence the course began to shift from the 'Evangelical Osteopathy' of A. T. Still to so-called '10-fingered Osteopathy'. Littlejohn, 'Took Still's Osteopathy and we gather, against much opposition, dipped it well and truly in a bath of physiology and, what is more, kept it there.'[1] Still was opposed to the teaching of 'medical' subjects such as physiology. A conflict was inevitable. On one occasion Still stormed into a class and furiously wrote on the blackboard: 'No physiology'.[9]

Littlejohn was awarded a DO (Doctor of Osteopathy) from the ASO, but he wanted the title 'Doctor of Medicine (MD), Osteopathic'. This was refused. Smith and Littlejohn were further angered as Arthur Hildreth, Still's chief promoter of pure Osteopathy, returned from St Louis[9] to support Still, despite assurances from the trustees he would not. Furthermore he was appointed Dean in 1900, a position until then held by J. M. Littlejohn. Hildreth considered that four men on the Faculty who were of the 'allopathic School of medicine' (William Smith and presumably the Littlejohn brothers) were opposed to him because he was 'ultra-osteopathic' and Hildreth would tolerate nothing other than the strictest adherence to the teaching of Still and he was not medically qualified and had not graduated from a University.[4] Smith was dismissed. Money was also owed to Littlejohn by the School. Angry letters were sent from the Littlejohn brothers to the ASO trustees and Littlejohn then engaged in a law suit against the School that lasted two years.[3,9]

On 23 November 1899, the Littlejohn brothers and William Smith wrote to the Trustees of the ASO that, 'Arthur Hildreth has made himself objectionable to us in many ways. He is in the School in violation of a contract made with us last term....He has been installed without our consent being even asked, as our superior to the office of Dean'.

On 9 December the Littlejohn brothers wrote to A. T. Still's son, Charles Still, 'We beg to notify you that we request a settlement of the matters presented to you in our previous communications before 6pm today'. On 10 February 1900, Littlejohn resigned as Professor. On 15 June he wrote to Warren Hamilton, the Secretary and Treasurer of the School, regarding the refusal on 1 June to pay his salary.

Allegedly, there was also a difficulty over Still's daughter, Blanche. Littlejohn had courted her and had sent her a set of encyclopaedias, but Blanche was the kind of girl who preferred flowers.[9]

In May 1900 the Littlejohn brothers moved to Chicago and founded the American College of Osteopathic Medicine and Surgery and the Chicago Osteopathic Hospital, at 405 West Washington Boulevard, Chicago, which was opened in September 1900. The Faculty was composed of several MDs and local osteopaths. By 1905 they had graduated 114 students from the college and had published a number of books, pamphlets and charts.

On 7 August 1900 Littlejohn married Mabel Alice Thompson, the daughter of a grocer and eleven years his junior, at Ipswich, England and they settled at Lake Bluff, Illinois,[1] where his mother also lived until her death in 1911. They had six children, three boys and three girls. James born in 1905 and John Martin Littlejohn Jr born 1908 were both closely involved with the BSO, though James became an ENT surgeon. Edgar Martin, born in 1907, was killed in the Second World War.

In 1902, the Chicago College joined the Associated Colleges of Osteopathy and for three successive years (1908-1910) Littlejohn was its President. The American Association for the Advancement of Osteopathy (founded in 1897) became the American Osteopathic Association (AOA). Littlejohn wrote the first scientific article for the Journal. In 1908 the AOA set up the A.T. Still Research Institute. Littlejohn worked on neoplasms. The No.1 Bulletin of the Research Institute contained his paper on the relationship between neoplasms and Osteopathy.

Littlejohn also attended Dunham Medical College at West Adam Street, Chicago, from March 1897 until the following year, where he dabbled with homeopathy. He completed his training in 1900 and obtained an MD in May 1902.[2,6] Chicago University was still in its formation.[2] It was a four year course and he spent two years of that at Cook County Hospital, Chicago, apparently one of the largest and best equipped hospitals in the US. He received several state licences to practise medicine, surgery and obstetrics and was admitted in full standing as a physician in the Cook County Hospital.

Dunham was taken over by Hering Medical College in 1904,[2] The training at Cook County Hospital was considered too general, whereas

Hering had its own hospital. 40 graduates from Dunham received a certificate from Hering, so that they could be members of an existing medical institution. This explains why Littlejohn also had a MD from Hering in 1904.

His name appeared for over ten years in the Medical Directories as a fully qualified and registered MD. In 1913, the GMC challenged his right to use the MD degree. He presented his Diplomas to Sir Donald McAlister, President of the GMC, who confirmed his entitlement to use his MD degree in the UK.[5]

The American Medical Directories also record his position as a teacher of applied physiology.[5] He was Professor of Physiology at Dunham in 1901 for two years, even before he received his medical degree, and later Professor of Applied Physiology at Hering Medical College, Chicago National Medical University Chicago (1904-6) and the Hahneman Medical College.[6]

He also received an (Honorary) Doctor of Law from the Ad-Ranx Christian University of Texas (in existence ten years before the University of Texas) at Waco. Littlejohn had consulted Dr Lowber, (See above), the Chancellor, a literary man and writer on political science, in connection with his thesis at Columbia. This must have been just before his period at Amity College. Ad-Ranx was founded by 'The Disciples', who retained a 'chapel exercise' for ten minutes at the start of each day, as at Amity College, but that had been dropped by other Universities. Littlejohn became a member of the Executive Committee in connection with, 'Chateauqua lecture work' and lectured at practically all the centres in the Middle West from Cleveland, Ohio to Denver, Colorado; from the University of Minneapolis to Selma, Alabama. It was in connection with this work that he received his honorary degree.[2]

Littlejohn in the UK (1913-1947)

The American College was obliged to change its name in 1909 to receive recognition by the State Board of Health and became the Littlejohn College and Hospital.[12] In October 1912 a group of osteopathic physicians in Chicago met the leading osteopath Carl McConnell to consider the future of the College. At a meeting with trustees of the Littlejohn College it was agreed to form a new college 'independent of individuals'. In 1913 the work of the college was suspended. Following a further meeting of osteopaths, the Chicago College of Osteopathy was formed.[12,13] This may explain why in 1912 Littlejohn ceased to be President of the College and why he returned to the UK the following year, despite the fact that his children were born in the USA, he had become a citizen there and war was looming in Europe. According to a Dr Comstock of the Chicago College of Osteopathy, in communication with Edward Hall,[1] Littlejohn was, 'Most severely criticised by the majority of our profession'. His wife also wished to return.[4]

David Littlejohn (1876-1955) withdrew from the College in 1906 to follow a career in public health and sanitation. James Buchan Littlejohn (1869-1947) and his wife Dr Edith Williams Littlejohn remained at the College. A rift may have occurred between James Littlejohn and John Martin Littlejohn, as it is probable they never communicated after the latter returned to the UK.

Littlejohn, his wife and six children returned to the UK by sea on the SS *Corinthian* that set sail on 29 June 1913, probably a worrying experience given the *Titanic* disaster a few months earlier. They settled at Badger Hall, Thundersley (North Benfleet), Essex. It was an early 19th century farm house onto which in 1895 a Victorian manor house was built, but with limited facilities. Water was pumped from a well and oil lamps and candles were used for lighting.[4] He initially practised at 69, Piccadilly, London W1, then at 48, Dover Street, with further clinics at Enfield, Thundersley and Thorpe Bay, Essex.

As described in Chapter 2, Littlejohn made a major contribution to Osteopathy in the UK. After founding the BSO in 1917, his time was devoted to developing the curriculum and running the School. The first students graduated in 1925. That same year, he was President of the BOA, but his relationship with this organisation became strained (See Chapter 2) and he resigned from it. The School grew in strength, but in 1935, at the age of 70, he was severely criticised by the opponents of the Osteopaths Bill at the Select Committee of the House of Lords. (See Chapters 2, 5 & 6). A spirited defence appeared in *The Journal of Osteopathy* for June-August of 1935[5], which detailed Littlejohn's personal contribution to Osteopathy in this country, to reassure the profession that the criticisms of him and the School were unjustified.

Littlejohn delivered sermons at Thundersley and lectured to the Sunday afternoon Men's Brotherhood.[3] He was also a local councillor for Benfleet Urban District Council from 1929. The minutes of the Council from April 1931 record him being responsible for sewerage, town planning, recreation grounds, housing, allotments, general purposes and bathing pools. He sent a letter to the Council on 25 March 1939 confirming his retirement. The Council responded by expressing a hope, that, 'He will enjoy many years of health and happiness in retirement'. Reference was also made to his many years of public service.

From 1940, although Dean in name, his involvement with the School was very limited. He was suffering ill-health and ceased teaching. He wrote a letter to Shilton Webster-Jones, a principal teacher at the BSO, indicating that he was seeking medical advice. Webster-Jones and Clem Middleton, another teacher, took over his teaching at short notice. (See Chapter 9). One suspects that his pride was severely damaged by the proceedings of the Select Committee. He had also lost his son Edgar in the war.

Littlejohn died at Badger Hall on 8 December 1947. The funeral took place at St Peter's Congregational Church, Thundersley, on 11 December. The registration of his death states that the cause was carcinoma of the prostate. His wife Mabel Alice died in January 1968 aged 88, of bronchopneumonia and old age. She was then living in Hornchurch. Badger Hall was demolished in the 1960s for housing development, but the name remains in Badger Hall Avenue.[4]

Littlejohn's obituary in a local newspaper stated he was:

'A keen supporter of many local activities, he was a member of the Benfleet Parish Council before its amalgamation and later a member of Benfleet Urban District Council for many years. At one time he was also on the Rochford Rural Council. An active member of Thundersley Congregational Church he several times conducted services there in the absence of the Minister. He was a keen Liberal and helped the late Mr G. T. Veness (prospective Liberal candidate for S.E. Essex) in his election campaigns. Dr Littlejohn was also interested in the local League of Nations movement and was speaker many times at their meetings.'

References

1. Hall, T. E. (1952). The contribution of John Martin Littlejohn to Osteopathy. The John Martin Littlejohn Memorial Lecture. (London: British School of Osteopathy).

2. Report from the Select Committee of the House of Lords appointed to consider the Registration and Regulation of Osteopaths Bill [H.L.] together with the proceedings of the Committee and minutes of evidence. (1935). 3058-3107, pp. 210-212; 3174-4111; pp. 216-259. (London: HMSO).

3. Campbell, C. Notes on the Life of Littlejohn. (Unpublished).

4. Wernham, S. J. (1999). The life and times of John Martin Littlejohn. A biography. (Maidstone: John Wernham).

5. *The Journal of Osteopathy.* (1935). June-August, VI(3 & 4):4-7.

6. Statement of verification by J. Canning and T. E. Hall of Littlejohn's List of Degrees and diplomas in chronological order.

7. John Kemp. Personal communication.

8. *The Journal of Osteopathy.* (1934). V(1):1.

9. Trowbridge, C. (1991). Andrew Taylor Still (Kirksville: The Thomas Jefferson University Press).

10. *The Journal of Osteopathy.* (1932). October. IV(1):1.

11. Addison's Graduates of the University of Glasgow 1727-1987, p. 335. (Glasgow, 1898).

12. Unknown. (1923). Historical Sketch of Chicago Osteopathic College. *The Reflex:* pp. 16-17. (Chicago College of Osteopathy).

13. Gifford, R. O. (1939). History of the Chicago College of Osteopathy. *The Reflex* pp. 13-14 (Chicago College of Osteopathy).

Chapter 4

The Road to Legislation

The Osteopathic Defence League

Dr F. W. Axham, anaesthetist to Sir Herbert Barker, was struck off the Register of the GMC in 1911 (See Chapter 1). In 1924 the GMC issued a 'Warning Notice' banning anaesthetists from assisting unregistered practitioners:

> **'Association with Unqualified Persons**
> Any registered medical practitioner, who, either by administering anaesthetics or otherwise, assists an unqualified or unregistered person to attend, treat, or perform an operation upon any other person, in respect of matters requiring professional discretion or skill, will be liable on proof of the facts to have his name erased from the Medical Register.'

It was not prohibited for anyone to administer an anaesthetic, but for a medically qualified person to assist an unqualified person to practise as if they were a registered medical practitioner. This was largely instigated because of the medical assistance given to unqualified dentists.[1]

One osteopath very much affected by this was Dr Wilfrid A. Streeter, who was educated at Kirksville, under A. T. Still. He had practised since 1902, in Glasgow from 1907-1925 before moving to 71 Park Street, London. A distinguished 'osteopathic aurist', he established the first free osteopathic clinic for the deaf in Europe at Bush House, Aldwych, London.[2] He operated on ears with the assistance of an anaesthetist.

On the date the notice was issued, Streeter had several operations planned for the next day. He was phoned by his anaesthetist, who felt obliged to withdraw his assistance. Streeter then had to cancel a fortnight of operations before he found a medically qualified person brave enough to help him. Among Streeter's patients was Sir Walter Runciman, who wrote to the press in protest.[3] The *Daily Sketch* carried an article on 29 November,1924, which read: 'BATTLE FOR RIGHT TO HEAL DEAF. Famous Aural Surgeon's Work held up by Medical Council's Threat to Doctors.'

Streeter began a protest for the amendment of the Medical Act and against the monopoly of the medical profession. He, 'Waged incessant, but always ethical and polite, warfare against the powers arrayed against his beloved profession, who would either see it ruled out of existence, or would permit it to be tacked on as a kind of subsidiary to medicine and surgery'.[4] The Osteopathic Defence League was formed with him as Honorary Secretary. Its aims were to alter the law to place Osteopathy on a footing of legal equality with orthodox medicine, and also to make more widely known the principles of Osteopathy, 'As a system of bloodless surgery and drugless medicine' and, 'To educate the public in other methods than those of drug therapeutics for maintaining bodily health and curing disease'.

A new Act of Parliament was sought for the recognition and independent regulation of Osteopathy, to maintain the highest qualifications for osteopathic practitioners and to confer on osteopaths the right to develop along their own lines instead of being made subservient to the medical profession which was considered antagonistic to Osteopathy.

'The public of Great Britain is entitled to the benefits of Osteopathy, and no one has the moral right to deny them these advantages. Yet this is being done under the present law.

We also wish to educate the public to understand the principles of Osteopathy so that they may be ready to avail themselves of its incontestable benefits...

A new profession which challenges the dominance of the older and monopolistic school of therapeutics must not only be ready to fight for its own rights, but also refute the attacks of those who oppose it—whether that hostility arises from ignorance, stupidity, or self-interest. The League will do its part in this domain. It will also endeavour to remove misunderstandings now prevalent in the public mind—some of which are common to most new ideas, whilst others are deliberately fostered by those who are hostile. Osteopathy has a stern struggle in front of it if it is to obtain due recognition from the public. Until there is a wide public recognition of the true facts we cannot achieve our ideals.

It is to be understood that the Osteopathic Defence League does not seek in any way to interfere with the regular medical profession. It does not desire to see established standards of medical training lowered. Nor does it aim at securing admission of osteopaths into the ranks of the regular medical profession.

On the contrary, it is the definite intention of the organisers of the League to establish the highest possible standard of education and professional training for all who hold themselves out to the public as practitioners of Osteopathy; and to secure for our system of healing the same opportunities of development as eclectic medicine has enjoyed.'[4]

Thousands of signatures were obtained supporting the aims and objects of the League for a petition to Parliament. The 'Warning Notice' was never enforced, no doubt due to this public opinion.

Support for Osteopathy also came from Arthur Greenwood, MP, who had been Parliamentary Secretary to the Minister of Health in the Labour Government of 1924. In the House of Commons on 5 March 1925, on behalf of the BOA, he asked the Prime Minister whether he was aware of the warning notice and of the feeling of dissatisfaction amongst the general public and also amongst many medical practitioners, and whether he was prepared to set up a Commission or Committee of Inquiry into the operation and administration of the varied Medical Acts, and the function of the GMC with a view to the introduction of legislation to ensure the recognition and legal regulation in this country of Osteopathy, to safeguard both qualified practitioners and the general public.[5]

The Secretary of State for Foreign Affairs, Austen Chamberlain, replied that while the application of the principles laid in the notice to particular cases may have given rise to criticism, there was no evidence of any general dissatisfaction among the public or the medical profession, and he saw no necessity for the appointment of any Commission or Committee.

Greenwood then asked him to ask the Prime Minister whether he would receive a deputation of some members of the House of Commons. Chamberlain suggested that the most convenient and practical course would be for Greenwood to make representations to the Minister of Health.[5]

On 31 March 1925 Kelman MacDonald delivered a lecture in the House of Commons on, 'Osteopathy and its position in the British Isles'. He was asked by the BOA to lay before the House of Commons the objects of the Association, one of which interestingly, was to obtain a charter for the BSO, or some such official recognition. After doing so and outlining the history of osteopathy in the US and UK and explaining osteopathy, he claimed he had a list of over 100 registered practitioners with some personal knowledge and experience of the benefits of osteopathic treatment. 20 were willing to testify before a parliamentary committee of inquiry, but others feared reprisals from the GMC.

By 1925 British-born graduates were emerging from the BSO. On 9 June 1925 Littlejohn, as spokesman of the BOA, of which he was then President, presented to Neville Chamberlain, Minister of Health, a statement:

> 'In the interests of Science as well as of public protection only those qualified should hold themselves out as qualified to practise. As there are no medical schools teaching Osteopathy, we wish to establish our own schools on the highest basis of educational equipment and requirement.'

He referred the development of osteopathic teaching and the existence of the BSO.[6]

On 7 August, Chamberlain wrote:

> 'It is not clear on what principles Osteopathic practitioners could be selected for admission to any register without compelling the registration authority to accept as evidence of qualification diplomas or certificates issued by the American Institutions, the efficacy of whose teaching the authority would be unable to test and whose examinations it would have no power to inspect. The practical difficulties of compiling a register on this basis of qualifications which have not been obtained in the United Kingdom is too obvious to need elaboration.'[7]

A party of more than 100 US osteopaths visited the UK, France and Germany in 1925 to share experiences and encourage European osteopathic societies and education. Streeter wrote an essay in the *Empire*

Review (London) drawing attention to the dangers that would result if the GMC succeeded in obtaining control over British Osteopathy.[8]

In a letter to *The Times* on 23 January 1926, Sir Herbert Barker emphasised:

> 'We want as earnestly as any medical man, to protect the public from irregular practitioners; we want to prevent the intrusion into the medical profession of incompetent and unqualified persons. To do this, as Mr Streeter had persistently urged, we need to establish a school of mechano-therapeutics, and to set up a board of registration to regulate its practice, prescribe its standards of training and professional competence, and give its practitioners the privileges, responsibilities and immunities enjoyed by practitioners of the dominant school of therapy in this country.'

Chamberlain in the House of Commons on 9 February 1926 reiterated his concern regarding the registration of American-trained osteopaths and to accept diplomas, 'The value of which we could not pretend to examine, and over the qualifications for which we have no control'. Basil Peto, a supporter of Osteopathy, interrupted that they were not asking for American degrees in Osteopathy to be recognised in the UK. He pointed out that what was proposed was the creation of a separate Board, the establishment of their own institutions and the conferment of degrees.[3] The Minister replied that he saw no reason why the British osteopaths should not follow this course, and it seemed to him the only way in which they could achieve what they had in view:

> 'If they want to have a register of osteopaths set up in this country, the first thing for them to do is to start colleges of their own....They will be forced, eventually, I prophesy to do what has been done in America, and what the honourable member who moved the motion said they were going to do: that is to say, their curriculum would gradually have to conform to something very nearly approaching the normal curriculum in this country.'[3]

Further support for Osteopathy came from Cyril Atkinson MP, a distinguished KC and parliamentarian and John Bromley MP. Atkinson asked for, 'Regulation and registration of manipulative practitioners, having approved qualifications'.[3]

On the same date, Dr Graham-Little, MP for London University, proposed an inquiry into, 'The whole position of irregular practice in medicine and surgery'. He applauded the laws of Brazil, where the unorthodox are given one month's solitary confinement. This was seconded by Hilton Young (shortly afterwards to be appointed as a lay member of the GMC).[2] Colonel T. Sinclair, a member of the GMC, talked the motion out and hence prevented the House from voting on the question.[3]

On two June 1927 F. A. Macquisten MP asked the Minister of Health whether he would appoint a Royal Commission to inquire into the Medical Acts with a view to the alterations of the laws, especially with reference to the powers and privileges of the GMC. Chamberlain replied that he did not think such a revision was necessary and the President of the GMC shared his view.[3]

The Osteopath in June 1927 reported that on 7 April 1927 Monteith Erskine MP gave a large dinner party in honour of Viscount Curzon and Wilfrid Streeter in the Strangers' Room at the House of Commons. Erskine and members of his family were patients of Streeter. Many of the most influential people in Britain were present.[9] Streeter explained why osteopaths were badly in need of a law protecting their rights.

In 1928 the BOA accepted Streeter's suggestion for a conference to discuss their differences and to recommend a parliamentary policy. The BOA Council minutes indicate that Elmer Pheils, Cyril Atkinson of the BOA and Erskine were to attend.[10]

On 19 January 1928 the BOA decided to continue its policy of bringing Osteopathy before Parliament with a view to recognition and to do everything possible to establish an independent osteopathic school of an educational status equivalent to existing medical institutions. It was agreed to determine which MPs would be willing to introduce a resolution in favour of osteopathic legislation. Pheils, Cooper and George MacDonald were authorised to handle the matter.[11]

By March, Pheils had sounded out several MPs. It was agreed that Pringle would draft a resolution to be submitted for the consideration of members. A Unity Committee framed an agreed policy on parliamentary questions,[12] renamed the Osteopathic Legislation Committee in September.[13]

In 1930, the Committee prepared a legislative programme and planned to organise public opinion and then approach government.[14] There was also a need for a parliamentary agent to glean information and other necessary work. A parliamentary draftsman had drafted an 'idealistic' Bill. Pheils was watching affairs in the House of Commons and was in, 'Close touch with parliamentary friends'.

As a result of the differences had arisen between the BOA and Streeter, the BOA wrote to him: 'In reply to your letter of March 3rd, the BOA ...unanimously agree to place their confidence in Dr Pheils and Mr Atkinson in acting for them as the Osteopathic Legislative Committee. If you cannot see your way to co-operate any further on this joint committee, the Council will have no option but to accept your implied suggestion of dissolution.'[15]

A Royal Charter for the BOA

The BOA in March 1930 sought via Arthur Greenwood to obtain a Royal Charter to incorporate it as a legal entity and to give registration and protection to the title 'osteopath'.[15] The title RO (Registered Osteopath) would be conferred. Presumably in so doing only BOA members would be eligible and other 'osteopaths', including BSO graduates, would be excluded. It was considered essential to have a new clinic before a Royal Charter was granted.[16]

In June 1931, Pheils reported to the BOA Council that Greenwood had discussed the matter with Lord Palmer, President of the Privy Council, and there would be a great deal of opposition. Greenwood recommended that representatives should meet with the 'Medical Committee' to affirm that the Charter was only to enable the BOA to prevent impostors from posing as osteopaths and that they did not seek medical rights.[17]

By October 1931[18] the application for a Royal Charter had been refused, but it had raised a good deal of interest and discussion. There were six counter petitions lodged. It was claimed by the medical profession that osteopaths were encroaching on its ground. The BOA denied this. They stated they only wanted a Board with the authority to say who were good osteopaths and who were not.

Responses to the counter petitions were drawn up and were to be sent to the Privy Council.[19, 20] Examiners of London University were to be used to ensure standards. Some BOA members had signed the counter-petition. Pheils proposed that Christmas Humphreys, advisor to the BOA, should write to them and that they must decide whether they were petitioning for a Charter or counter-petitioning. If the latter, they must resign from the BOA.[19] Martisus withdrew his signature.[21] The medical profession were concerned that many members of the BOA would not come up to the qualification which they themselves had laid down and the BOA were asked what right they had to condemn other osteopathic bodies. On 4 May 1932, the BOA Council minutes record that the Privy Council had refused the BOA a Royal Charter.[22]

Towards The Osteopaths Bill

In January, 1930 an MP had put a question to members of the House of Commons regarding legislation for osteopaths. Following discussion with Cyril Atkinson and Arthur Greenwood, it was considered not an appropriate time, 'In the light of the recent newspaper publicity' and the question was withdrawn.[14] However, on 28 May 1930 Atkinson was given permission to present a draft Bill when he saw fit.

The *Daily Sketch* on 4 August 1930 referred to a 'Bill to give status to bone-setters'. The *Daily Express* was rather more supportive and claimed, 'More and more the belief is strengthening among orthodox Medical men that the osteopaths have discovered in their manipulative methods the clue to certain disorders that refuse to yield to older forms of treatment'.[23]

1931

The Bill 93, officially designated the 'Registration and Regulation of Osteopathy Bill', obtained a First Reading in the House of Commons on 11 February 1931, introduced by W.M. Adamson, MP. Its main objects were to, 'Regulate the Practice of Osteopathy and to prescribe the qualifications of osteopathic practitioners'.[7]

Clause 6 specified that within 12 months of the Act a Board should admit to the Register persons that are: (a) graduates of a British School of Osteopathy who, conform to the educational standards and regulations laid down by the Board, and satisfy the Board by examination or otherwise of competence to practise as an osteopath; or (b) hold some recognised certificate granted in some British Dominion or Foreign Country, or (c) prior to the passing of the Act had been engaged in the practice of Osteopathy for three years and, in the opinion of the Board, were fit and proper persons to be registered.

For Registration, it was stated that the course of training should be of not less than four years' duration with terms of not less than nine months in each year, such courses to include the subjects and the minimum hours of study in each year as set out in the Second Schedule of the Act or as prescribed by the Board.[4,7]

The Bill was instigated by Streeter. The BOA Council considered its position. The Board's control of examinations was an issue. It also had objections to the Bill in that it, 'Admitted to the Board representatives from various nebulous and at present non-existent organisations'. The BOA also intended to withdraw its support for the Bill if the right to grant birth and death certificates was not included.[24] As a consequence of the BOA's concerns the Bill was withdrawn. Agreement by the profession was essential as a strong medical opposition was forecast.

The Times and the Daily Telegraph carried articles on the Bill on 12 February and the Daily Express on 18 February. The Daily Telegraph commented that, 'The struggle between the medical profession and the unorthodox practitioner is old standing'. All three articles were discussed in The Journal of Osteopathy that month.[25]

Streeter wrote to the press:

'The public has shown no little interest in the efforts made by this League to secure recognition for that branch of the healing art known as Osteopathy. They will, however, regret to learn that Mr Adamson, MP, has felt obliged to withdraw the Registration and Regulation of Osteopathy Bill which obtained a First Reading in the House of Commons on February 11th. The Bill for some mysterious reason has not been received with favour by a section of the profession, represented by the British Osteopathic Association, and until there is agreement in the ranks of the profession it is but natural that Mr Adamson should feel that the proposed legislation...is hardly likely to be achieved in the face of the strong medical opposition which was forecast during the debate on the First Reading.

If the osteopaths can come together and agree upon a Bill, I am assured by Mr. Adamson that he will do his utmost to help it to reach the Statute Book. It will be necessary to make such an effort because of the large number of British-born students now studying Osteopathy—the entry of American osteopaths having been restricted by the Home Office—and these workers for health are anxious to see such a Bill passed in order to give them security in the exercise of their calling.'[4]

The BOA considered that this was not factually correct and they were not responsible for the withdrawal of the Bill, that the Bill never had a chance and they had merely stated that they would not support it if they were not given control of the Board.[17]

On 24 March, the Evening News referred to, 'A Bill to Register the Bonesetters—The doctors oppose it and so do the bonesetters'. On 5 June, the Daily Express mentioned that the British Medical Journal had refused to accept an advertisement from Streeter for an anaesthetist.

1933

The Bill was re-introduced (with only slight amendment) by Robert Boothby MP. The BOA's concerns were addressed. The proposed Board was to consist of, 'A chairman appointed by Privy Council, two representatives of Science, (one appointed by the Ministry of Health, and one by the Scottish Board of Health); 8 who were, or had been, engaged in the practice of Osteopathy, of whom 5 should be appointed by the BOA, one by the Osteopathic Defence League, and one by the British School of Osteopathy'.[7]

In introducing the Bill, Boothby said that persons admitted to the Register should have followed a prescribed course of study and should have acquired a prescribed standard of professional competence. Under the Bill an unqualified and incompetent charlatan and quack would be debarred from practising Osteopathy. Further, osteopaths qualified under the provisions of the Bill would be in a position to employ an anaesthetist without the latter falling under the ban of the GMC.[7]

At a BOA Council meeting in May, Dr Deiter spoke of the necessity of co-operation with the Incorporated Association, which had five objections to the Bill.[26] It was felt that the two Associations should present a united front. It was noted that the Bill also did not specify how an 'osteopath' was to be defined.[10] Due to its controversial nature, or pressure of government business, this Bill was unsuccessful.

At a BOA Council meeting in November 1933, Dr Mellor pointed out that the BOA could never benefit by contact with the BSO, but that equally Osteopathy could not obtain recognition as long as everyone was obliged to go to the USA to obtain a Diploma that was up to standard. It was possible that a Bill would be passed by the medical profession to limit the osteopaths in their work, or bring manipulation into medicine.[27]

1934

A debate was organised between osteopaths and medical profession by the 'New Health Society'. The BOA considered it essential that there was a united front and for them to support the reintroduction of the Bill to Parliament. Streeter had broken with the BOA, but the BOA acknowledged that he was 'anxious to do something for Osteopathy'.

Following a dinner at the House of Commons, Streeter wrote to Pheils stating that Sir Nicholas Grafton Doyle had asked him (Streeter) to chair an Osteopathic Parliamentary Committee, which would also include Foote and Littlejohn. He asked Pheils if he would serve on the Committee. Pheils replied that it would be necessary for him to have a ruling from the BOA and that the BOA would insist on an equal representation with the other three groups and an independent Chairman. The BOA considered that they should have three representatives: Pheils, Cooper and Sikkenga, who were already on their Legislative Committee.

In February 1934, *The Evening News*, *The Times*, the *Daily Mail*, the *Daily Express* and The *Practitioner* carried articles supporting Osteopathy.[28] The *Evening News* on 20 April referred to the antagonism of the BMA to Osteopathy.[29]

On 17 October 1934, Dr A. G. Timbrell Fisher wrote an article in the *Medical Press and Circular* entitled, 'Manipulative surgery: Its uses and abuses in medical and surgical practice, with some criticisms of osteopathic theory and practice'. He claimed that osteopaths believe that the osteopathic lesion was the sole cause of all disease. 'If the [osteopathic] theories were harmless one could safely ignore the cult and allow it to die a natural death, but unfortunately there are in many cases most dangerous.' He then cited cases in which people received useful and harmful treatment. 'Osteopaths pay little or no attention to diagnosis, and patients with malignant disease or other serious conditions often waste precious time and incidentally much money in this futile 'treatment'.[30]

Owing to pressure of public business the House of Commons had no time to discuss the Bill. Arrangements were therefore made to bring it before the House of Lords.[7] It came up for a Second Reading there on 11 December 1934. Viscount Elibank, who was sponsoring the Bill, requested Streeter to obtain the support of all osteopathic parties.

The Bill passed the Second Reading by 35 votes to 20, on the understanding it would be referred to a Select Committee that should hear counsel for and against it and examine witnesses on oath. This met on 4 March 1935. (See Chapters 5 and 6).

Lords Gainford and Ernle were supporters of the Bill. Lord Moynihan, a well-known surgeon, said that before the Bill could become effective the Medical Act of 1858 would have to be repealed. 'Medicine and Osteopathy', he declared, 'Were in hostile opposition: If the teachings of Osteopathy were true, then the foundations of the science of medicine had not been well and truly laid'. Lord Dawson said that the Bill aimed to give a short-cut to a body of people who wanted to get the status of a doctor. 'They would bring down the whole fabric of the healing art.'[31]

On 14 January 1935, the *Daily Telegraph* carried a letter against the

Bill from Sir Ernest Graham-Little MP, accompanied by one from Harvey Foote on behalf of the IAO, in support of the Bill.

Pheils said at a BOA Council meeting in December that it would be contrary to the policy of the College Committee for the BOA to support the Bill, as it would prejudice the negotiations regarding teaching osteopathy to medical students as a stepping stone towards a college run on the lines of osteopathic Schools in the US.[32] He claimed the BOA had nothing to do with the introduction of the Bill in the House of Lords and if the BOA supported it, he would resign from the Legislative Committee and College Committee. He then left the meeting. No action was taken regarding the threat of resignation, but clearly the profession was again divided in its support for the Bill.

The Medicines and Surgical Appliances (Advertisement) Bill

This Bill was presented by a Private Member on 27 March 1936 to the House of

Commons.[33,34] It had the support of the BMA, the pharmaceutical industry and numerous other organisations, which depended for their existence on the patronage of registered medical practitioners. Its original purpose was to stop certain types of advertising, but it prohibited unregistered practitioners from stating, or implying by any means whatsoever (publishing articles, addressing meetings, answering questions in public etc.) that they were dealing with, preventing, relieving or treating any disease.

A four page printed notice headed, 'Private and Confidential' and, 'Not for Publication' was produced by the Osteopathic Legislation Committee and signed by Littlejohn, Streeter and Harvey Foote (then President of the IAO). In pencil at the end is an indication it was to be sent to MPs, and for patients to sign an accompanying post card. It read:

'Dear Colleague,

We have been placed in possession of a copy of the Draft Bill bearing this title, which the medical authorities and allied interests are promoting as a counter-blast to the Bill, in charge of Mr Robert Boothby, MP for the Regulation of Osteopathy.

As you are aware, the leaders of the medical profession have opposed the recognition and legal regulation of Osteopathy as an independent system of therapy. On the other hand, they have hitherto remained indifferent to the question of altering the law with a view to dealing with the scandal of unqualified practice.

The Bill they have now in preparation must, we think, be taken as their answer to our claim that we are entitled, as a profession, to protect ourselves against unqualified and incompetent persons who call themselves osteopaths and bring our calling into disrepute.

The Bill deals with the question in such a way that if it became law it would, in our opinion, make it impossible for any osteopath who is not also a registered medical practitioner to continue in practice. Ostensibly, the Bill is aimed at those who advertise quack remedies for a certain group of diseases. We do not deny that legislation is required to stop such advertising. But we are satisfied that this Bill goes far beyond the import of its title, and we have fortified ourselves with legal opinion as to the proper construction to be placed upon its provisions....

The Bill in its present form, whether intentionally or otherwise, creates the conditions of a complete medical monopoly....It provides that no person shall advertise any medicine, surgical appliance, or treatment. (Those who could advertise were enumerated in the Bill).

It would certainly prohibit propaganda by osteopaths to the effect that the manipulative technique is effective for cure or prevention of any of the diseases mentioned (in section 1), or that it will have a salutary influence upon the course of any of them....This would mean that no irregular or non-registered practitioner could set up a name-plate or give hours of consultation on his letter-paper, or use a visiting card, or enter his name in any directory (even the telephone book!) with any addition whatsoever which suggests that he is available for consultation on matters of health.'

It ended: 'Our strength lies in the justice of our case, in the growing appreciation of the public, and in the distrust of monopoly where matters of health and disease are concerned and finality has not been reached in science and technique.'

The supporters of the Bill were aware that the osteopaths, herbalists, naturopaths and other unregistered practitioners were opposing it. As far as the osteopaths were concerned, it was considered that their two or three objections might easily have been overcome in Committee.[33]

They claimed it was not aimed at worthy, unregistered practitioners, but this claim was not evident in the draft, nor could they impress MPs that was so.[33] According to Christmas Humphreys, adviser to the BOA, 'The only way the Bill was killed was to get members to leave to make it inquorate'.[35]

The Bill evidently had predecessors in 1914, 1920 and 1931. O. B. Deiter, Editor of *The British Osteopathic Review*, indicated that according to the Editorial in one of the principal medical journals, the World War caused the death of the 1914 edition and another matter of national importance (the Grand National) caused the defeat of the 1936 attempt at a Second Reading, as the majority of MPs were at Aintree instead of the Commons![33]

Deiter considered that the real opposition to the 1936 version came from the MPs themselves, in that the Bill asked for too much and that its original purpose to stop certain types of advertising, seemed to be entirely lost in some of the clauses.[33]

References

1. Report from the Select Committee of the House of Lords appointed to consider the Registration and Regulation of Osteopaths Bill [H.L.] together with the proceedings of the committee and minutes of evidence (1935). 5752-5758, pp. 398-400. (London: HMSO).

2. Report from the Select Committee of the House of Lords appointed to consider the Registration and Regulation of Osteopaths Bill [H.L.] together with the proceedings of the committee and minutes of evidence. (1935). 1-14, p. 15. (London: HMSO).

3. Streeter, W. A. (1929). The New Healing. (London: Methuen & Co).

4. McKeon, L. C. Floyd (1933). A Healing Crisis. (Weston-Super-Mare: Michell Health Products).

5. Hansard 5 March 1925. In Streeter, W. A. (1929). The New Healing. pp. 203-204. (London: Methuen & Co).

6. *The Journal of Osteopathy.* (1935). June-August, VI(3 & 4).

7. McKeon, L. C. Floyd (1938). Osteopathic Polemics. (London: The C. W. Daniel Co Ltd).

8. Walter, G. A. (1981). Osteopathic Medicine—Past and Present. (1925-1949) p. 11.

9. Anon. (1927). Osteopathy Honored Again. *The Osteopath,* June: 30.

10. Minutes of the Council of the British Osteopathic Association. 19 January, 1928.

11. Ibid. 22 March 1928.

12. Ibid. 19 June 1928.

13. Ibid. 19 September 1928.

14. Ibid. 4 February 1930.

15. Ibid. 19 March 1930.

16. Ibid. 9 December 1930.

17. Ibid. 3 June 1931.

18. Ibid. 20 October 1931.

19. Ibid. 17 November 1931.

20. Ibid. 8 December 1931.

21. Ibid. 8 December 1931.

22. Ibid. 4 May 1932.
23. *The Journal of Osteopathy*. (1930). August, I(6):1.
24. Minutes of the Council of the British Osteopathic Association 25 February 1931.
25. *The Journal of Osteopathy*. (1931). February, II(3):1..
26. Minutes of the Council of the British Osteopathic Association. two May 1933
27. Ibid. 10 November 1933.
28. *The Journal of Osteopathy*. (1934). February, V(1)
29. *The Journal of Osteopathy*. (1934). April, V(2):1.
30. *The Journal of Osteopathy*. (1934). October, V(5):1.
31. Minutes of the Council of the British Osteopathic Association. 5 December 1934.
32. *News Chronicle*. (1934). 12 December.
33. Deiter, O. B. *(1936)*. Notes by the Editor. *The British Osteopathic Review*. May 3(2):112-113.
34. House of Commons Official Report (1936). 27 March, 310 (59). In *The British Osteopathic Review*. (1936). May, 3(2):125-135.
35. Christmas Humphreys. Minutes of the Council of the British Osteopathic Association. 10 November 1944.

Chapter 5

The Select Committee (1935)

On 4 March 1935, the Select Committee of the House of Lords met to consider the Registration and Regulation of Osteopaths Bill. Evidence was heard over 12 days. The Report, together with the proceedings and Minutes of Evidence, run to 490 pages and 6,347 statements.[1] Summaries of the proceedings were published in the *Lancet* and by the British Medical Association[2] and extracts appeared in the *British Osteopathic Review*.[3]

The Select Committee was chaired by Lord Amulree. Other members were: Viscount Esher, Viscount Elibank, Lord Redesdale, Lord Marley, Lord Carnock and Lord Dawson of Penn who was the King's physician. As the poem went: 'Lord Dawson of Penn has killed thousands of men, that's why we sing God save the king!'[4]

The four main parties supporting the Bill were: The Osteopathic Defence League, represented by Wilfrid Streeter, The British Osteopathic Association (BOA) represented by Dr William Kelman MacDonald; The British School of Osteopathy (BSO), represented by John Martin Littlejohn and The Incorporated Association of Osteopaths (IAO), represented by Harvey Foote, though he was never called as a witness.

The Bill was prepared by Streeter on behalf of the Osteopathic Defence League. When it was first introduced into the House of Commons, a copy was sent to the BSO and its opinion asked, but the comments provided apparently were ignored. Arrangements were then made for the Bill to be introduced into the House of Lords. The BSO was asked to support it, but the only notice it received was a telephone message. Just before the Bill was introduced Littlejohn met Streeter and Foote and gave unqualified support. The BOA refused any collaboration, up to the point at which the Select Committee was appointed and arrangements had been made for the hearing.[5]

Several meetings of the four parties took place in a Committee Room of the House of Commons, chaired by Robert Boothby. Discussions were amicable and there was agreement on a united front. The BSO recognised that Streeter had worked unselfishly for Osteopathy for many years and was willing to follow his leadership in legislation. It was expected that bygones were bygones, and that all were marching under the banner of A. T. Still. Littlejohn later wrote, 'United we stand, divided we fall was engraved on our banner'.[5]

Counsel appearing on behalf of the supporting parties were J. H. Thorpe and H. L. Murphy. Counsel for the parties opposing the bill were: Sir William Jowitt KC and H. C. Dickens, representing the British Medical Association, the GMC and a number of universities and medical schools; C. J. Radcliffe and D. L. Jenkins, representing The Royal College of Surgeons of England and the Royal College of Physicians of London; M. Fitzgerald, representing the Chartered Society of Massage and Medical Gymnastics; St John Raikes, representing The British Chiropractors Association and R. O. Jones, representing the Nature Cure Association.

Both supporters and opponents called additional witnesses. (See next chapter). A list was prepared of over 100 registered medical practitioners with some personal knowledge and experience of the benefits of osteopathic treatment, but only 20 were willing to testify before a parliamentary committee of inquiry. The others feared retribution from the GMC.

The witnesses were cross-examined under oath and with a vigour as great as in any murder trial at the Old Bailey. The proceedings of the Select Committee therefore provide a considerable insight into Osteopathy in the 1930s.

Of the principal witnesses defending a statutory Register, Foote was never called to the witness box. Littlejohn's cross-examination was discussed in Chapter 3. The cross-examinations of Streeter and MacDonald are provided in some detail below (though with considerable editing), as they reveal a great deal about Osteopathy in Britain and the medical profession's vicious opposition to it.

REPORT

FROM THE

Select Committee of the House of Lords

APPOINTED TO CONSIDER THE

Registration and Regulation of Osteopaths Bill [H.L.]

TOGETHER WITH THE

PROCEEDINGS OF THE COMMITTEE AND MINUTES OF EVIDENCE

Ordered to be Printed 13th February and
17th July 1935

LONDON
PRINTED AND PUBLISHED BY HIS MAJESTY'S STATIONERY OFFICE
To be purchased directly from H.M. STATIONERY OFFICE at the following addresses:
Adastral House, Kingsway, London, W.C.2; 120 George Street, Edinburgh 2;
York Street, Manchester 1; 1 St. Andrew's Crescent, Cardiff;
80 Chichester Street, Belfast;
or through any Bookseller

1935
Price 15s. od. Net

(29) (130)

Objections by the Nature Cure Association

A 17 section Memorandum on the Bill was produced by the Legislative Committee of the NCA of Great Britain and Ireland. It claimed that the legislation would, 'Interfere with those who have the right to use manipulative methods, and who, by virtue of training and conviction in their efficacy, have the right to practise them. The Nature Cure movement in this country is much older than the osteopathic movement. Manipulation has...always formed a part of the equipment of the Nature Cure Practitioner....The Osteopaths Bill seeks to destroy this traditional freedom of practice and choice.'

The NCA considered the Bill included no clear definition of Osteopathy and accordingly had no real basis for special legislation. The object of the Bill was stated to be, 'To place the practice of Osteopathy as a developing system of treatment of disease by manipulative methods....This phrase covers the practice of Nature Cure....The restrictive legislation...would be employed to limit unfairly competitive methods.'

As osteopaths purport to treat syphilis it was concluded that it would be by recognised medical methods, i.e. drug medication. 'The public have no clear definition in mind of what is meant by Osteopathy as distinct from other methods of manipulative treatment....If Osteopathy is manipulation...how can it be established as a complete therapeutic system?'

The cross examination of Wilfrid Streeter

The first witness to be called was Wilfrid Alberto Streeter. He was first examined by Harold Murphy to establish the background to the Bill and to explain how he became involved in seeking legislation. Streeter confirmed that the registration of osteopaths would not involve lowering educational standards but would improve them.

He considered that the principal difficulty in improving the educational standards and qualifications of those practising Osteopathy was the absence of standards to which to make them conform. He claimed they had no control over anyone who wished to call himself an osteopath and that there were no means of enforcing discipline amongst those practising Osteopathy. Membership of the professional associations was voluntary. That anyone could practise Osteopathy without a qualification was undesirable. There was no means by which a patient could know if a practitioner was qualified or not. At that time, of the some 3,000 osteopaths, 175 were qualified and he could see no means of protecting the public other then by registration. The registration of osteopaths would not impair the GMC's authority.

The questioning then centred on the importance of securing a status enabling consultation with medical men. Streeter confirmed that he did not have as much difficulty in this regard as he used to.

He explained that he was assisted by an anaesthetist, who was running a risk by being associated with him. If the anaesthetist ceased to do so there was no assurance he could be replaced. He related the case of the wife of an army captain with 'lung trouble' who needed to be re-examined. She saw Streeter who asked a Wimpole Street surgeon for a list of consultants and Streeter then arranged an appointment for her with one, indicating it was by way of referral and requested a report back. The consultant told the patient's husband that he could not communicate with Streeter as he was liable to be struck off the Register if he did so. The patient and her husband were very upset and sought a further two consultants, who disagreed with the diagnosis recommended by Streeter. This created friction between the family and Streeter.

Streeter was asked why those practising Osteopathy should not go through the ordinary medical course. He replied, 'I have never been able to understand why if I study Gray's Anatomy...I become a sound, safe, scientific practitioner, whereas if I study the same textbooks and something else in an osteopathic institution, I am a quack and an outlaw and just a craftsman'.

He confirmed that an osteopath studies nearly everything contained in the medical curriculum, 'But does not pay so much attention to the Materia Medica'. A proposed length of course of four years was recommended (as compared to five for medicine) given that Major Surgery and Materia Medica were excluded.

Further questioning centred on a definition of Osteopathy that had been read earlier. Streeter was asked to describe in his own words its distinctive features. He emphasised the importance of the structural integrity of the body as being the most important single factor in the cause and cure of disease and the importance of the bony framework and spinal column ('imperial storehouse of imperial structures'). Osteopathy involves removing the cause of disease wherever found. 'We recognise antiseptics, antidotes, radical surgery, dietetics and psychology.'

He confirmed that Osteopathy is in harmony with modern scientific pathology, but explained that the body has within itself, 'All the substances necessary for the cure of disease'. It was necessary, 'For that machine (man) to be in a fairly good state of adjustment in order that the body structure should work properly'.

When asked about his attitude to 'bacteriological phenomena' he explained that while the presence of bacteria was recognised, 'We do not think they are the primary cause of disease in all cases'. He was then asked what range of diseases and bodily infirmities he regarded as outside the sphere of Osteopathy and what he regarded as inside. Streeter would not agree to this divide. He stated, 'I think the Principle of the osteopathic concept is applicable to all illness', but he acknowledged that Osteopathy might not get all patients better without any other help. When asked about the osteopathic attitude to dysentery, he claimed an osteopath would employ orthodox treatment, in addition to his own particular treatment.

Lord Dawson of Penn sought confirmation that Streeter believed that the body contained all substances necessary to cure disease, that he recognised bacteria as a cause of disease, but not the primary cause and that he would adopt the ordinary medical treatment of dysentery, i.e. emertine. 'So far as I know the human body does not contain emertine. You say you would use emertine having previously stated that the human body contains all substances necessary to cure disease?'

Streeter: I hold that it does under ordinary conditions.
Penn: Does the human body contain emertine?
Streeter: I did not wish to imply it did contain emertine.
Penn: As regards dysentery, I put it to you that the human body does not contain the cure for dysentery?
Streeter: I could not say that it does not. I have treated many cases of dysentery myself without the use of emertine.
Penn: At any rate you do agree.... You would use the ordinary medical treatment in the treatment of dysentery and the ordinary medical treatment we know by unanimity is the use of emertine...In that particular case the human body does not contain the necessary substance to cure the particular disease.... You agree that the human body does not contain emertine.

Streeter was then asked what diseases he included as coming within the purview of Osteopathy. He replied he would not exclude any case.

Penn then referred to the reason for the osteopathic curriculum's being four years' long was that surgery and therapeutics were excluded. Streeter emphasised that they were not asking for the right to do major surgery under the Bill. He was in favour of including major surgery, but conceded that the course would then have to be six to eight years' long.

Penn again demanded to know what diseases would be included in the four year curriculum. Streeter stuck to his guns. 'As I said before... the osteopathic concept applies to all patients.'

Penn then moved to another specific example, asking whether he would treat pernicious anaemia. Streeter argued, 'We believe that osteopathic lesions predispose to anaemia...that in treatment liver and dietetic advice would be given'. Penn asked if that was consistent with the body making everything that was required for the cure of a disease. Streeter replied, 'I think so'.

Streeter emphasised that not all cases were treated by manipulation alone. Penn then sought confirmation that Osteopathy involved treatment by manipulation of the spinal column. Penn stated, 'I put it to you that in the case of pernicious anaemia the treatment (liver therapy) does not include manipulation, nor can the body provide the cure'. Streeter responded, 'I do not know how to answer the question in any other way than I have answered it'.

Lord Marley further asked him whether Osteopathy could prevent pernicious anaemia. Streeter emphasised that there was evidence that osteopathic lesions predisposed to anaemia. He affirmed that if a patient developed pernicious anaemia he would refer the patient to a general medical practitioner. Penn queried how he would know a patient was likely to develop pernicious anaemia before the symptoms developed. Streeter indicated that he did not undertake laboratory tests, but would arrange for them to be done. Penn asked, 'What is the disharmony in the body which warns that pernicious anaemia is on the way?' Streeter replied, 'Any spinal maladjustment'. Penn probed deeper. 'Would it not be a particular spinal lesion that would give you a particular warning of a particular disease?' Streeter: 'No,...osteopaths have never claimed that maladjustment of one particular vertebra meant pernicious anaemia and a maladjustment of another vertebra meant diphtheria.' Penn: 'Therefore in fact we have no means of knowing what the particular dysfunction is that warns us that pernicious anaemia is on the way?' Lord Marley came to the rescue, suggesting Streeter's point was that disharmony could lead to a large number of different diseases, but if treated early might prevent pernicious anaemia as well as other diseases. Streeter agreed that was a fair statement.

Viscount Esher asked if the thousands of unqualified practitioners were a danger to the community. Streeter replied that it was quite possible that many of them were. There was agreement between Esher and Streeter that everyone who undertakes diagnosis and treatment should be qualified.

Penn then referred to the exclusion of the Materia Medica from the four year course. He mentioned that the founder of Osteopathy had excluded drugs and he asked Streeter whether he would use them. Streeter again confirmed that some drugs were useful and Penn again took this as confirmation that there were cases when the body does not manufacture its own remedies.

He then asked if Streeter would employ anaesthetics as something outside the body yet necessary in the treatment of disease. Streeter argued that that the idea that the body had its own drugs applied to ordinary conditions, not to emergencies and not to all conditions.

Penn then explored Streeter's treatment of the deaf. Streeter explained it involved the reconstruction of the Eustachian tube, blocked by adenoid intumescences, removed by finger surgery. 'Am I right in supposing you jam your finger into the Eustachian tube?' Streeter corrected him. 'I manipulate it.' Penn sceptically enquired of the size of the Eustachian tube. Streeter offered to demonstrate if he would care to go along to his operating room. Penn: 'I understand the Eustachian tube is smaller than a finger; that is so is it not?' Streeter: 'Not mine. You could not put a finger that size into it.' (Holding up a thumb). Lord Esher confirmed that Streeter did not pretend to cure all cases of deafness, nor could the medical profession. In both cases there was no infallible cure. Streeter emphasised that he had never used the word 'cure'. Esher asked if he found his method effective. Streeter claimed that, 'I think we have the best treatment in the world for catarrh and deafness'.

Elibank's questions provided clarification. 'You do not profess to cure everything do you?' Streeter replied, 'I have never professed to cure anything...We believe our treatment is applicable to all disease in theory.' Elibank encouraged Streeter to admit that he treated only certain diseases, but relied upon the natural resisting resources of the human frame and that he had no hesitation in referring to medical practitioners and that the lack of willingness of the medical profession to refer to him was one of the objects of the Bill. Elibank re-established the difficulties of collaboration with medical practitioners and in obtaining an anaesthetist. While Streeter stated he could do major surgery if necessary, it was not intended that the Bill should sanction this.

Lord Redesdale proposed that the short answer to all the questions about drugs was that Streeter was not narrow minded and appreciated that in certain cases they were necessary.

When asked the difference between Osteopathy and manipulative therapy, Streeter indicated that the latter was only a small branch of the former. The Chairman asked whether the Bill would prevent manipulative surgery by anyone who was not an osteopath. Streeter explained that the Bill was never intended to interfere with other practitioners, but to protect the good name of Osteopathy.

Streeter denied that the bulk of the practice of Osteopathy was connected with 'sprains and ailments of that kind', but went on to claim that osteopaths treat tonsillitis, pneumonia and influenza by manipulation. Lord Dawson enquired about typhoid and appendicitis and Streeter affirmed this.

Viscount Elibank questioned the four year training in the Second Schedule of the Bill. Streeter said he had no objection to a five year course. Thorpe indicated that while there would be no objection, it was considered inappropriate.

Jowitt then questioned Streeter on behalf of the BMA. He argued that anyone in England can practise the healing arts, the only exception being midwifery, treatment of venereal disease and the prescription of dangerous drugs without a qualification, i.e. registration was unnecessary. There was no law preventing the administration of anaesthetics and he was surprised that Streeter did not know this. It was argued that there was wisdom in allowing freedom, subject to one check, that a man must not represent himself as being qualified when he was not qualified.

Jowitt: 'Osteopaths are asking for complete liberty of practice as physicians (other than surgery, anaesthetics and midwifery) and for the treatment of every sort of disease. That Osteopathy concerns itself merely with manipulation is a misapprehension.' Jowitt asked, 'Would you be content to be registered as manipulators?' Streeter replied, 'No'. Jowitt re-emphasised that he (Streeter) claimed to have the right to treat every disease—but did not claim the right to sign a death certificate. 'If a physician is trained to diagnose what a patient is suffering from, why should he not be able to diagnose what the patient died from?' Jowitt thus forced Streeter into agreeing with him.

Questions then centred on the definition of Osteopathy and 'structural integrity'. It was confirmed this was not confined to bones, but included all tissues, the entire body and keeping the person in a fit condition. Streeter was asked, 'Can you conceive of anybody who does not (place the chief emphasis on structural integrity)?' He replied, 'Every physician who says there is no good in Osteopathy'.

The discussion then moved on to major surgery. 'Is appendicitis or removal of a gland major surgery?' Streeter admitted it was difficult to define. Jowitt argued that under certain circumstances a physician may need to undertake emergency surgery and what is minor surgery becomes major surgery. Streeter considered that a year course should equip an osteopath to refer and admitted the difficulty in including minor surgery, but not major surgery. He was asked, 'What would happen if minor surgery was conducted, but the practitioner was obliged to undertake major surgery?'

Jowitt then moved on to the writings of A.T. Still claiming that Osteopathy was given to him by divine revelation and quoted examples of Still regarding himself as clairvoyant.

Streeter indicated that he knew Still but did not see evidence of, 'Remarkable powers of clairvoyance and clairaudience'. 'I think Dr Still was a highly religious man, but I do not think that had anything to do with the foundation of Osteopathy.' Jowitt implied that Osteopathy had no scientific basis. He quoted, "All the remedies necessary to health exist in the human body" as being one of Still's tenets. Streeter argued, 'I think modern Science confirms Dr Still's Principles all along the line'. Jowitt: 'Is there any passage in this book here suggesting it is legitimate or proper to use any drug?' Streeter replied, 'Yes'. Jowitt demanded: 'Now give me the passage.' Streeter claimed he could not remember the passage off-hand. Thorpe explained that Streeter had not read the book for 10-15 years.

Jowitt quoted Still (1915) that, 'The enemy has broken though the picket', implying that Still's pupils realised there were cases when drugs should be used, but Still did not.

Streeter affirmed that Still considered there were cases when drugs should be used. Jowitt again demanded evidence. Jowitt stated, 'Are you asking their Lordships to pass a Bill authorising you gentlemen to practise as physicians to cure all diseases without any knowledge of drugs?' Streeter replied, 'The curriculum specifies toxicology, poisons, antidotes and so on'. Lord Dawson interjected, 'Did you say toxicology or Materia Medica?' Jowitt claimed that toxicology was not the study of drugs.

Lesions were then considered and Still's theory that the cause of all diseases was what he called a 'lesion'. Streeter protested he did not say 'all diseases' and that he had been misquoted.

Jowitt asked what was Still's new theory of the causation of disease. Streeter said that under ordinary conditions the human body contains within itself the elements and substances necessary to cure disease. Jowitt then quoted Streeter from 'The New Healing'. "In no case could disease originate without a broken or suspended current of arterial blood." Streeter objected, 'I have never known him say that he could cure every case regardless of the condition'. Jowitt replied, 'Do I understand you to say that the statement in your book is incorrect?' Streeter claimed it was never intended to be a textbook. 'I think what you have read should be taken in conjunction with other passages. I have never maintained, and Dr Still never maintained that you could take any and every case, cancer or tuberculosis, regardless of the condition of the accident or injury and twiddle the backbone and cure it.'

Jowitt: I am delighted to hear you utter such words of robust common-sense.

Streeter: I have never done anything else.

Jowitt: You do not predicate that all disease is caused by some osteopathic lesion?

Streeter: I never said that.

Jowitt then stated, 'I am talking to you as a scientist and I want nothing popular here. I want a scientific exposition. Do you agree that diseases are not necessarily caused by spinal lesions or any other sort of lesions?' Streeter replied,' I certainly do not claim that all diseases are due to spinal lesions'. Jowitt asked if, ' It is that which differentiates you from the orthodox school?' Streeter replied, 'The osteopathic spinal lesion differentiates us from the orthodox school. We believe that these lesions predispose to most of the trouble in the body—the most important single factor.'

Jowitt argued that Science has progressed since 1874 (the year Still claimed to have 'discovered' Osteopathy). 'Have you now a complete explanation of immunity?' Streeter said he thought he had a fairly general one.

Diabetes, diphtheria and measles were then discussed. Streeter agreed that insulin was the proper treatment for diabetes and he would refer a patient to receive this. He clarified that in the case of diphtheria he would give anti-toxin in conjunction with his own treatment.

In the case of malaria, he would give the orthodox treatment, but that Jowitt had nearly exhausted the list of specifics. Jowitt asked, 'What do you think malaria is caused by? An osteopathic lesion? Was the bite of the mosquito an osteopathic lesion?' Streeter replied that osteopaths have never maintained that a mosquito could not bite you on the wrist unless your vertebrae was misplaced! Jowitt: 'You mean to say that the bite of the mosquito is the lesion?' Streeter: 'I say the structural integrity of the body is interfered with at the site of that inoculation.... Any abnormality anywhere in the body I would call a lesion.'

He was asked: 'Supposing you have a small boys' school and at the beginning of the term someone comes back who is suffering from measles. The probability is that (it) will run through the school and 50 of the100 boys will get it....Have they all got osteopathic lesions?' Streeter was then asked whether osteopathic lesions were catching.

Jowitt claimed it is ridiculous to say that the cause of all disease is an osteopathic lesion. Streeter considered that in measles there is a lower vitality which enables a person to contract it.

Lord Dawson asked: 'Are you prepared to produce evidence of that? It is notoriously against the weight of knowledge.' Jowitt continued: 'What has led you to demonstrate (I want you to answer with the weight and responsibility which you must have speaking to their Lordships) that the small boys at the private school who get measles have some kind of predisposition by reason of some structural maladjustment or something of that sort ? What is your ground for saying that? It is important to get this clear...this is a vital part of the enquiry from a scientific point of view.'

Streeter explained that, 'Interference with the nerve and blood supply predisposes to a lower vitality', but pleaded that for 27 years he had not accepted cases of acute ailments.

Jowitt stated, 'So it comes to this, that you are asking that your colleagues...shall have the right not merely to manipulate but to treat disease....There are cases of disease which you agree are introduced by the bite of some animal....You accept bacteriology? Surgery?...and agree that there are a number of diseases which require the use of drugs ?'

Streeter: There are a few specific drugs that have proved empirically to be valuable and we certainly want to give the patients the benefit of that doubt in every emergency and borderline case.
Jowitt: In pneumonia does your treatment differ from orthodox treatment?
Streeter: Apart from drugs, we have something extra which we think is better. I will tell you briefly if you would like me to do so....

Lord Carnock ascertained from Streeter that osteopaths do not object to inoculation or vaccination.

They then returned to malaria. Jowitt quoted the osteopathic textbook by McConnell and Teal that, 'The most common lesion found is a marked lateral deviation between the 9th and 10th dorsal vertebrae and a consequent downward displacement of the 10th rib'. 'Do you really believe that?' He quoted, 'Disturbance will always be found in the region of the 8th to 11th dorsal vertebrae inclusive or the corresponding ribs on the other side.' Streeter claimed he was taking it out of context and he had great confidence in Doctors McConnell and Teal. Streeter argued that a correlation between spinal lesions and tuberculosis was claimed to have been found by Louisa Burns. 'Do you really think that malaria is caused by that? I shall go with a much lighter heart on my summer holidays knowing that I have an assurance that so long as I do not have something the matter with my spine it does not matter what mosquitoes bite me.' Streeter claimed that was not so.

Streeter was again asked if he accepted the works of bacteriology. He affirmed this. Jowitt then quoted a reference from Streeter's book: 'The great medical superstition of bacteriology.' Streeter claimed the superstition is that it is the primary cause of disease in all conditions. Bacteria only enter if continuity of tissue is broken and when they get to their work there are predisposing causes. Osteopathic spinal lesions interfere with vitality and blood supply and give them a chance to work. 'That is our difference between our view and the orthodox point of view.' Streeter wanted to quote the work of Cannon (see below), but Dawson responded: 'We need not waste the time of the Committee on that.' Thorpe defended Streeter's right to quote from a textbook.

Streeter was asked: 'Are they (lesions) the cause of typhoid?' He replied, 'I think so'. He was then questioned on typhus, tetanus and bilharzia and the chief symptom of bilharzia. Streeter: 'I would not like to answer the question.' Jowitt: 'Diphtheria, anthrax, pneumonia? How does the treatment of pneumonia differ from orthodox treatment.' Streeter replied that, 'With every treatment we give we liberate a certain amount of toxins that are generated in the body as a result of bacterial invasion.... We appeal to the natural immunity of the body. We manipulate the spinal column for one thing and attempt to establish a free nerve and blood supply to the whole body mechanism.'

Jowitt: 'Now we are getting to it are we?...An osteopath would rub the spine. Is that putting it fairly?...What part would you rub?' Streeter explained he would manipulate it. He established that manipulation would be used in treating diphtheria. He agreed that when pneumonia and diphtheria end fatally, it is overstrain on the heart. 'May not manipulation put even greater strain on the heart?' Streeter replied, 'We are less likely to place a strain on the heart than if artificial remedies are used'.

Jowitt summed up that in osteopathic treatment manipulation is given and subject to exceptions, osteopaths do not give drugs. Streeter agreed that broadly speaking the statement was right. Surgery and medicine are common to the two schools and Osteopathy accepts bacteriology, radiology and toxicology.

Streeter quoted Cannon's *'Wisdom of the Body'*. "Only when the skin is broken or cut or the mucous membranes weakened or damaged does invasion occur", and Sir James Mackenzie in *'The Future of Medicine'*, that in those who suffer tuberculosis there must be factors that favour the growth of the bacillus (the soil) that has a distinct influence.

Jowitt argued that Streeter had departed from Still's theory and quoted Yale Castlio's 'The *Principles of Osteopathy'*. "There are a host of serums and vaccines on the market, most of which are without value, some of which are dangerous....Osteopathy in the beginning was a revolt against drug therapy....It had grown and flourished as drug therapy has declined. Drugs with few exceptions are without curative value....Among the classes of chemical agents that the osteopathic physician will find useful or indispensable are the antiseptics, anaesthetics, stimulants, sedatives, anodynes, cathartics and narcotics."

Jowitt asked, 'What is there in the Materia Medica that does not come within one or other of these categories?' Streeter argued these are emergency cases. Jowitt quoted further from Castlio the drugs and substances used in diagnosis that may be used. 'I see osteopaths do in practice use from time to time a list of drugs which seems both to you and to me to be pretty complete.' Streeter explained it was not for curative purposes, but for diagnostic and emergency cases. Jowitt: 'Assuming that there are occasions in practice when the use of these drugs is necessary, do you say that it is a right that the State should recognise as physicians competent and authorised to deal with every disease students who have no knowledge at all of the Materia Medica? Do you as a scientific man, ask their Lordships to pass a Bill under which the State is going to place on a Register, persons as being licensed and having the right to treat every disease, unless those persons have some knowledge of the Materia Medica?' Streeter agreed they ought to know something about drugs, poisons and their antidotes and a comparative knowledge of all therapeutics. They may need to know eight, ten, a dozen remedies that are beneficial, but not the entire Materia Medica.

Jowitt claimed an opinion on which drugs ought to be used would be entirely valueless unless founded on some knowledge of them. Streeter did not agree with this. He conceded to the value of a knowledge of the Materia Medica—but not as taught in medical schools.

Jowitt then quoted a BSO Prospectus that students were required to take a full year's course in pharmacology and therapeutics in order to be perfectly familiar with medicine and medicinal treatment in all its aspects. Streeter agreed it was appropriate for a student to receive this.

Jowitt argued that there were a large number of medical men who used manipulation, e.g. Sir Morton Smart and James Mennell and questioned the difference between what they were doing and what Streeter was doing. Streeter claimed that they do not apply manipulation to the cure of disease. Jowitt, however, considered they are working to restore complete integrity to the structure of the body. 'Would not a solution to the whole problem be this: Why should not you and the osteopaths start by passing these medical examinations and then develop your technique exactly on what lines you like?' Streeter considered that it would be just as reasonable to expect the Anglican or Non-Conformist clergy to train in Roman Catholic seminaries, or vice versa. Jowitt considered this a false analogy as medicine was based on reason. Thorpe and Streeter did nor accept this view. Jowitt argued if the State is going to take the responsibility of recognising any group or set of people as being fit or competent people to treat all disease, it is of fundamental importance that the State has the right to see that these people are well trained.

Jowitt: 'What you want to do in your Bill is to try to remove the present unhappy differences of opinion between the two professions? Do you think it is the least likely? I am afraid it is a completely false hope.'

Jowitt asked if in the curriculum which a medical student goes through there will be nothing which will not be useful to an osteopath. Streeter replied: 'If you had Osteopathy according to Dr Mennell in the medical schools, I would not object. If there were not osteopathic institutions in America he would not have got his knowledge. I think that anatomy as taught in the medical schools is not always useful as a different interpretation is put on anatomical facts and similarly therapeutics....I do not agree that that everything taught as regards Materia Medica is essential.' Jowitt responded: 'We are not going back on that. I have your answers. I can read them to their Lordships.' Streeter provided as examples of differences in anatomical interpretation the mobility of the sacro-iliac joints and the osteopathic spinal lesions.

Jowitt then claimed, 'So you expect a student to join up and adhere to the ranks of the osteopaths before he has any sufficient knowledge to enable him to form an opinion as to whether he is right or whether the doctors are right?' Streeter responded, 'That is just what he does when he goes into medicine'.

Jowitt sought clarification as to how entry onto the Register would be achieved. It was explained it would be by examination, or if a practitioner had been in practice for three years.

Streeter was then cross-examined by Radcliffe, who questioned a previous statement that Streeter had made that he, 'Never professed to cure anything.' Streeter argued, 'In the last resort nature does the curing. I try to help nature'. Radcliffe asked, 'Do you accept Osteopathy as a system of curing?' He quoted from Streeter's book regarding, 'Curing diseases without drugs'. Streeter explained, again, that it was to distinguish it from other manipulative therapies and in certain cases drugs and surgery are admitted. He had given a number of instances where drugs may be applied for curative purposes. He was then asked, 'How will you teach students in your school to apply the general principle of no drugs and how will you teach them to apply the particular case of the exception?' Streeter claimed that it was not part of the osteopathic concept never to use drugs under any condition.

Radcliffe: 'Where are drugs taught in your schedule?' Streeter replied, 'Poisons and antidotes'. Radcliffe responded, 'I did not say poisons, I said drugs'. Streeter explained, 'We are providing another year to give a chance to get in some of them....I think they need to know something about pharmacy, but not to the extent that it is taught in the medical schools.'

He was asked, 'In the case of typhoid what instruction will you give a student to enable them to know whether to apply drugs or not?' He replied, 'We do not think it necessary to administer drugs in typhoid. We rely on our own techniques....If an emergency arose and one felt it was necessary to consult with any other practitioner, I would like the privilege of doing that.' Radcliffe asked, 'How would your students know whether it was necessary or not to consult with another practitioner?' Streeter responded, 'How would any student at a medical school know whether it was necessary to have osteopathic treatment?' Radcliffe stated, 'I am afraid I cannot find any answer to my question in that'.

Radcliffe quoted McConnell and Teal regarding the treatment of diphtheria and typhoid. "Diphtheria concerns obstruction to circulation as a predisposing course. Stasis of blood favours growth of the bacillus." Streeter agreed it might be a very potent cause.

Radcliffe: I did not ask you that. You can answer yes or no. I think you should. Are you capable of answering yes or no to a question out of your own books?'
(Thorpe indicated it was not his book.)
Streeter: I think it is the most important single cause.
Radcliffe: Can you say whether you accept that dislocation is the predisposing cause?

Streeter: Yes I think it is—I do.

Radcliffe: A number of gentlemen are going to come here...to say that that statement is the purest nonsense, to quote their words.

Streeter: They may. They have said that all along about everything osteopathic, but that does not make it true.

Radcliffe claimed: 'You believe in all cases of typhoid fever there are lesions in the dorsal or lumbar spine. Have those lesions been traced in all cases by any known method of science?'...'I would not say in all cases. I believe there are evidences.'

...'Is the statement that you make based on scientific knowledge?'... 'We think so. We are demonstrating those facts in our research institutes.'...'Can you refer me to any of your publications containing for instance radiograms showing the presence of these lesions?' The request was repeated by Dawson. Streeter: 'Not in the case of typhoid.'... 'Why not?'...'We are a young profession yet we have not established all the facts.'...He admitted he did not have X-ray photographs....'Do you know they exist?'...'No.'...'Either in the United States or here?... Why is it that you cannot produce X-rays either in the US or here to demonstrate those facts in the same way as other scientific people demonstrate those facts?'...'There are many lesions which you could not X-ray. I do not think you can always show on the X-ray many or all of the maladjustments of the spinal column.' Thorpe interjected, 'If there is such evidence it shall be produced' and questioned whether it had anything to do with the Bill being passed.

Thorpe: 'If I am to pursue the line that my evidence must now be diverted as to whether the osteopathic theory of the causation of disease is right then I must get entirely new evidence. I did hope...that this matter would be conducted on the basis that osteopaths were giving benefit to the public...and that being so it was desirable and expedient that they should be put under some form of registration.' The Chairman claimed, 'You are in charge of the Bill and must conduct your case in your own way'. Lord Esher asked, 'Would Lord Dawson say if the medical profession had a theory about the cure of cancer that they have to prove that theory to be true before they are recognised?' The Chairman replied, 'With respect I think these abstract questions are rather besides the point', but Lord Elibank remarked, 'It is the same question that is being asked now' and was supported by Lord Esher. 'We are now not investigating whether the Bill should be passed or not...the whole of the theory and practice of Osteopathy...that is not the object for which this Committee has been set up.'

Radcliffe confirmed the relevance of his questions and stated, 'As far as you yourself know, you have no proof by radio-photography of the lesions in the case of typhoid. Is your answer the same with regards to the lesions in dysentery?' Streeter affirmed this.

He then asked who supported the Bill and was told that it was roughly 70 members of the BOA and 96 graduates of the BSO. Questions then centred on whether BSO graduates were recognised by the BOA.

Streeter claimed he did not know anything about the BSO. There were two graduates of the BSO who were members of the BOA. He was asked why so few. Streeter explained that there had been some differences between the two Associations in the past, but he did not know what the differences were. Streeter was then asked why he opposed the petition to Privy Council for a Charter in 1931. Streeter replied, 'If they were given the Charter there would be only three qualified osteopaths in England according to the standards they wanted to enforce'.

Radcliffe claimed he was anxious to discover what was meant by 'qualified osteopath'. In the BSO they devoted the last two years to purely osteopathic subjects and that was the only basis of qualification. The School was not recognised by the BOA or AOA, but Streeter indicated that it was recognised by the Province of Alberta. 'I think you will find it will be recognised by the AOA very soon.' Thorpe: 'Would you ask the witness if we have ever asked for recognition?' Radcliffe: 'No. I will not put your questions for you.'

Sir John Raikes then cross-examined on behalf of the chiropractors. Streeter confirmed he knew of the British Chiropractic Association and that his objection to Chiropractic was that it was founded on wrong principles. 'I think they have adopted one element of the osteopathic concept in a crude fashion.' He did not think they had sufficient course of instruction.

Raikes claimed, 'If it is reasonable for you to oppose us (the chiropractors) on those grounds, it is reasonable for the medical profession here to oppose you on the same grounds'. Streeter considered that they are not at all parallel. 'We are not opposing the Chiropractors' application for any Bill.'

Raikes emphasised the importance of interpretation of the Bill by the courts and referred to the amendment that no person should hold himself out whether directly or indirectly as an osteopath. Chiropractic treatment was similar. It was agreed to include a clause to relieve their concerns.

Jones then cross-examined Streeter on the proposed definition of Osteopathy. 'As a definition of Osteopathy it is sheer nonsense. Where is there in the definition a statement of the theory and practice of Osteopathy? There is not a word about spinal lesions.' Streeter explained that Osteopathy was not confined to spinal lesions. Jones persisted, 'I suggest to you there is not a word...that shows Osteopathy to be concerned with spinal or other osteopathic lesions'.

Jones referred to Edythe Ashmore's 'Osteopathic Mechanics' (1915). He could find nothing in it to suggest that Osteopathy is anything but the treatment of lesions. Streeter explained that book was devoted purely to osteopathic mechanics. His explanation was rudely interrupted by Jones: 'Have you finished?'...Streeter: 'It does not say so far as I remember that it is a textbook of Osteopathy.' Jones: 'It is at any rate a textbook of Osteopathy. In this book we do not find anything at all about operative surgery and that leads to me to suggest that operative surgery forms no part of osteopathic technique....When you finger the Eustachian tube I suggest to you are not doing anything osteopathic at all but are in fact performing a surgical operation.' Streeter replied, 'I differ from you entirely. That is a very good example of an osteopathic lesion in soft tissue'. Jones continued, 'When you deal with tennis elbow you are dealing with the condition not as osteopaths, but as manipulative surgeons. Is that true?'...'No, we differ.'...'You cease to be an osteopath and you become a bone-setter? When you treat say influenza you are ceasing in that particular to be an osteopath and you become a general practitioner of medicine, would you agree?'...'No.'...'A branch of the healing art not entirely self sufficient....'I do not think anybody is ever self sufficient.'...'That is not an answer....The truth is that after the Bill is passed you will be free to practise small amounts of medicine and surgery.'...'We are excluding major surgery.'

Jones then asked, 'What gives you, Mr Streeter and those associated with you a copyright on the word 'Osteopathy'?' Thorpe stated: 'We do not have a copyright.'

Jones argued that there were a number of other people belonging to other Associations, who were equally well qualified to practise Osteopathy, who would be frozen out by this Bill.

Streeter was then asked if he knew of the Nature Cure Association and Stanley Lief and Harry Clements, who had qualified as DOs from one of nine recognised colleges in the US. 'Do you know that they practise Osteopathy as part of the therapy?'

Jones then launched a further attack: 'Let me put it to you that Osteopathy pure and simple—the theory and the technique of Osteopathy—should not as a matter of fact take more than four or five months?' Streeter replied, 'I presume that is the basis on which your friends (i.e. the naturopaths) are qualified now'.

Jones asked, if they (the NCA) practised Osteopathy, were they entitled to go on practising it? Streeter replied, 'If they can satisfy the Board that their qualifications are satisfactory'. Jones responded, 'If they can satisfy your Board? Though having no representation on the Board and though having taken the degree of DO in colleges in America ?'

Jones claimed Nature Cure was a system of healing that did not rely on drugs or surgery and therefore, 'Conforms more closely than Osteopathy to the original teaching of Dr Still'. Streeter did not agree.

Thorpe asked, 'Dr Streeter, after a cross-examination, which at any rate in my experience, has no precedent for severity....Do you remember Sir William Jowitt suggesting Dr Mennell and Sir Morton Smart were doing in effect what you are doing today? If that which you practise is 'pure nonsense' have you any reason to believe that if the Bill does not meet with their Lordships' approval these doctrines will cease to be practised?' Streeter replied, 'I have not the slightest fear of such a thing'.

Thorpe ascertained from Streeter that neither he nor osteopathic students would divert their training and study medicine. If the Bill was not passed the position would be the same, with confusion in the public mind as to who is qualified and who is not qualified and this might increase.

He asked Streeter if Dr Still was a devout man and whether he appeared practical when he was dealing with patients. Streeter replied, 'Always'. The relevance of what Still believed to the acceptance of the Bill was explored by Thorpe through his questioning of Streeter.

Thorpe then returned to the boys who catch measles and those who don't. Streeter replied, 'We feel that there must be some predisposing cause and those that caught it lacked some immunity. The boys who escaped had some form of lesional integrity—some sort of structural immunity.' Thorpe asked, 'Supposing my learned friend called 100 doctors, you would still believe it?'...'Yes.'

On questioning Streeter explained that he would use drugs for diagnosis and extreme cases, but would not accept them primarily as curative agencies. He would never use drugs alone in any case. He agreed that it was desirable that future osteopaths should have some instruction in the use of drugs like insulin. Streeter agreed with Thorpe that, 'If the study of particular drugs is part of the curriculum the student would be better equipped at any rate to know when those drugs are desirable than he is today'.

The definition of Osteopathy and the distinction between osteopaths and other therapists and major and minor surgery were considered. Thorpe stated, 'It is very easy to criticise, but if my learned friend can offer a definition which is true to fact and is more helpful in making that distinction, you would be the first to consider it'.

They then considered why the BOA did not admit BSO graduates. Streeter had heard it suggested that the curriculum of the BSO was not of a sufficiently high standard. The whole purpose of the Bill was to raise the standard. If they laid down the standard and it was not acceptable to the BOA, 'That is the funeral of the British Association'.

Thorpe ascertained that the decision not to press for powers to sign death certificates and birth certificates was because it would be a direct invasion into the field of orthodox medicine.

He was then asked, 'If you employed an unqualified medical practitioner as an anaesthetist and the patient dies, do you think you stand as high in the opinion of the coroner's jury as you would if the anaesthetist had been registered? You are prepared to give up powers that you have today—not to give anaesthetics, not to practise major surgery? You are paying that price as the price of putting your profession on a proper basis?' Streeter answered, 'Absolutely so'.

Dawson confirmed that Streeter considered that boys who did not get measles had some structural advantage—they did not have osteopathic lesions. He then stated, 'I am quite sure that no responsible body of people would put that view forward unless they were able to base that opinion on a systematic investigation. What investigations in the past have been made to establish that view?' Streeter replied that they are carrying on quite a large number of investigations at the A. T. Still Research Institute....'What is the nature of those investigations?'... 'The relationship between spinal lesions generally and changes that go on in the viscera as a result of these lesions.'...'Do they include X-ray examination?'...'Yes, they include X-ray examination and animal experiments.'

He was then asked whether such investigations were made to substantiate the statements regarding osteopaths' views on measles. 'Will there be put before us the same kind of steady systematic investigation?'...'I think we should be able to submit quite a mass of information along that line.'...'I cannot submit any X-ray evidence of any osteopathic lesion, the correction of which would prevent one from getting measles.'...'Can you give us any evidence of a pathological or chemical character?'...'We can give you quite a lot of evidence to prove that osteopathic spinal lesions do affect the nerve and blood supply to all viscera.'...'No I am dealing with measles. I understood from you just now that the evidence exists—objective evidence.'...'I misunderstood you.'

Thorpe explained that it was one of the deductions that osteopaths drew from their general field of practice. Lord Dawson responded, 'Is the theory of osteopaths the result of long patient investigation and research, or is it something that comes out of a man's brain out of the blue?'...'There is no evidence of any investigation of a scientific character on which that theory is based.'...'I will take that as an answer.' Thorpe interceded, 'That was not the answer, with great respect. The answer was that the witness did not know it and your Lordship then said, that means there is no evidence'. Lord Dawson persisted, 'I am anxious to get evidence of systematic and careful enquiry in the way that Pasteur and Lister did their work'. Lord Elibank confirmed that research was undertaken at the A. T. Still Research Institute and established data would be provided.

Lord Esher asked, 'Suppose your theory of immunity turned out to be wrong. Would you still consider you ought to be registered?' Streeter replied, 'Yes'.

The cross examination of Kelman MacDonald

Dr William Kelman MacDonald, representing the BOA, graduated in 1907 with a Bachelor of Medicine, later qualifying in surgery and became resident physician at Edinburgh Royal Infirmary, then at the Royal Maternity and Simpson Memorial Hospitals. He undertook research for 18 months at the laboratory of the Royal College of Physicians before gaining an MD with First Class Honours, receiving the Gold Medal and Syme Surgical Fellowship. He obtained a Carnegie Scholarship for research on sensory nerve endings in muscle. He had originally planned to be a neurologist, but was influenced by his superior at the Royal Infirmary, Alexander Bruce, who used massage (based on the Swedish school of medical gymnastics and Ling's treatment) and high frequency electricity and did not have much use for drugs.

MacDonald's father had cerebro-arteriosclerosis and following recommendation from friends was treated by an osteopath, after which he was able to continue work. MacDonald did not approve at first. However, when young he had an accident playing rugby at school and because of crouching over a microscope, he developed abdominal problems. Under protest he received treatment from Streeter. As a consequence MacDonald then became interested in 'framework abnormalities', but went to America to prove there was nothing in Osteopathy. He was at Kirksville from 1910-1912 and met Still. He did only two years of the three year course in Osteopathy as he was a medical graduate.

MacDonald was questioned by Thorpe about Still. MacDonald claimed Still likened himself to a frontiersman, but he was practical and 'not a complete dreamer'. He was a great admirer of the works of Nature. They went on walks together, but Still initially rather ignored MacDonald. After six months, however, Still asked him to live with him and taught him personally, although Still had generally given up teaching students. MacDonald had started as Professor of Comparative Therapeutics, but Still then made him Professor of Principles of Osteopathy. Since then MacDonald had treated nearly 4,000 patients.

MacDonald explained that Osteopathy was, 'A system of healing and not a collection of methods. A system of practice which was based on a Principle. The body contains within itself power needed to heal, making Osteopathy not a mere system of healing, but almost a philosophy. I think that Osteopathy is still an art. I think that medicine is still an art.'

MacDonald was asked for a definition of Osteopathy. He replied, 'The osteopath stands for the physical make-up of man. I think the medical man stands for the chemical value of things.' He explained that they were not necessarily in competition, but functioned along parallel lines. Osteopathy was not limited to manipulation, but included diet, hygiene, sanitation and psychology. Structural integrity determined normal function. There was more than one factor in the production of disease. The deranged mechanism could be normalised by manual adjustment. He had a friendly feeling to non-drug giving natural methods of healing.

MacDonald explained the relationship between structural integrity and viscera, via the sympathetic nervous system, and how cells depend on a good blood and nerve supply and removal of poisonous products.

He described lesions as the complete or partial fixation of a joint within its normal range of motion. Primary ones were direct by injury, or indirect by posture and secondary ones were due to nerve reflexes. He considered that they were demonstrable by X-ray but were usually missed by radiologists as they were considered to be in the range of normal variation.

He argued that research in Osteopathy was still in its infancy, though important. There was a lack of research institutions and research workers. 'Yet if it is poor, we stand by its poverty.' He confirmed that if the professional position was regularised facilities for research would increase, but, 'We cannot prove all our contentions by the results of research'.

Jowitt asked where the research was recorded. 'Could I get some books about it?' MacDonald referred to the seven Bulletins of the A. T. Still Research Institute. 'Of the Bulletins, 1 and two were not worth reading and 3 was on the ear; only 4 — 7 were good, but not as good as medical research.' Jowitt asked, 'What about 4 — getting good — like the curate's egg?'

Discussion focused on the value of Osteopathy in treating acute diseases and the role of lesions in the susceptibility, and in the course and recovery from disease. Statistics were provided on the value of Osteopathy in the great influenza epidemic (1918-1922). Fatalities from influenza treated medically were 6%, but those with Osteopathy 0.25%. With pneumonia the medical casualties were not less than 30%, but with Osteopathy 10%. The figures were produced by the AOA and it was agreed there was no proof. The value of Osteopathy in reducing post-operative pneumonia was discussed.

MacDonald stated, 'I do not claim that Osteopathy can cure all diseases, but I do claim that there is no disease, acute or chronic, in which osteopathic treatment has not some all-important and irreplaceable part to play; all diseases have osteopathic manifestations and structure and function will ever go hand in hand'. He acknowledged curing disease might need medical intervention, but osteopathic treatment could assist. In certain emergency cases, there was a value in hormonal and serum therapy. Thorpe encouraged him to confirm that Osteopathy recognised that medicine has its own field, but the universal giving of drugs as a therapy was wrong.

MacDonald gave an account of patients he treated in one week: 30 women and 29 men, 6 — 91 years old, including three mental cases, two for deafness, one diabetic and one epileptic. He had never treated any case medically since 1912, though he performed surgery during the war. He only used drugs to treat a drug addict.

He acknowledged the value of insulin to treat diabetes, but he worked by making its use redundant as he considered insulin led to atrophy of the islets.

He ended the need for drugs (bromide) for an epileptic child. He treated one or two cervical vertebrae and two or three dorsal vertebrae where structural abnormality occurred. The child got better. There were records of 300 similar cases treated by members of the BOA.

He did not like the term 'manipulative surgeon' and the term 'bone-setter' should be reserved for unregistered persons. He admired Barker and had sent him cases—especially knee cases. 'All of bone-setting is included in Osteopathy, but the whole of bone-setting does not include the whole of Osteopathy.'

Discussion followed regarding the BOA. There were 71 British qualified osteopaths trained in the USA registered with it. Since 1927 the BOA clinic had seen 5,000 patients, and 60,000 treatments had been provided. There was a full time osteopath. In addition, the majority of London osteopaths gave their time free on a part-time basis. Poor people were treated free.

In addition, a College Committee was formed to establish a college in London. An informal meeting had occurred between six members of the Committee and six members of the BMA to carry out Neville Chamberlain's recommendation to start colleges. The value of the Bill was that it would enable students to gain a diploma which would carry a registered osteopathic hallmark. The college would enable medical practitioners to study Osteopathy, which would take at least 18 months.

There were people outside the Association, over whom they had no control and membership was voluntary. If a member was expelled, they could still practise. The public had no way of knowing this. They printed a Directory of BOA members for the public. Members of the BOA who were registered doctors were: Kelman MacDonald; George MacDonald, (his younger brother); Norman MacDonald, (his cousin); Dr Hope Robertson, who also went to Kirksville and another Edinburgh doctor, whose girlfriend MacDonald treated. Although qualified in medicine, MacDonald confirmed he had not been disciplined by the GMC for practising Osteopathy.

Viscount Elibank asked if passing the Bill would allow absolute freedom to professional men to do what they like as long as they had their degrees and acted properly. Medical practitioners and anaesthetist could not be associated with osteopaths. MacDonald had no problems as he was medically qualified. Lord Carnock acknowledged that if he (MacDonald) were not a registered medical practitioner the situation would be different. Even MacDonald had had some problems gaining a vaccine.

MacDonald considered that there were three reasons why osteopaths should be recognised: it was in the interest of the public. He estimated there must have been over 2,000 persons with little or no qualification holding themselves out as osteopaths. There were five or six within 300 yards of his practice. He related a story of how one attempted to acquire a patient from his doorstep.

Secondly, that there were cases dangerous for an unqualified manipulator to handle, e.g. with TB of the spine, or an aneurysm. Thirdly, osteopaths would have less difficulty obtaining the services of medical practitioners. He claimed, 'Our general guiding principle and our form of treatment are at complete variance with those of the medical school.' Elibank claimed MacDonald used drugs. MacDonald denied this, but that he passed patients to a person qualified to do so. Lord Dawson challenged him based on a previous statement that he used morphia and adrenaline. MacDonald claimed that if he used morphia it was not as a form of treatment. He considered that it would have no effect upon the disease.

In the schedule of the Bill there was only reference to toxins. Still taught about morphia and strychnine, as they were the prevalent drugs in his day. In the US osteopathic schools 162 hours were spent on Materia Medica—more than in half the medical schools. MacDonald agreed that students should know medicine that was not strictly in the armoury of osteopaths.

He claimed that if the Bill did go through it would not affect him personally. He had no axe to grind. An additional year in the course of 1,000 hours to teach Materia Medica was not needed. It would take at most 280 hours.

Jowitt referred to the schedule of teaching in Osteopathy and the minimum number of hours per subject and claimed, 'Putting any sort of educational system into a strait-waistcoat like this is as far as I know quite without precedence in this country'. MacDonald disagreed and cited Edinburgh University. It was agreed there was a need for an Educational Board and a schedule of minimum hours. 'What if a new discovery comes along, would the schedule have to change?' 'If there were a satisfactory Council of Education it should be left to it.'

He was asked, 'You would agree with this would you not, that there is not in this Country today and never has been any satisfactory educational body dealing with Osteopathy and there is no place here in this country where you can get a training in Osteopathy which would satisfy you?' MacDonald confirmed he was speaking only for the BOA. 'There is no English college whose degrees or diplomas...you would consider in any sort of way as satisfactory?'...He replied that, 'The British School of Osteopathy has been conducted by Dr Littlejohn and we all admire his effort. It is an individual effort and it has not yet been enabled to bring its educational standard up to the level at which we would like it. Dr Littlejohn has never applied to the BOA for recognition of his School so I myself know nothing whatever as a member of the BOA about it. Dr Littlejohn's School is the only School in England. There are correspondence schools. It is the only reputable School in England.' Jowitt: 'As far as you and your Association are concerned, you do not regard the diploma obtained by the study at that School as a satisfactory standard?'...'We do not.'

The Dentists Bill was discussed, which permitted a large number of unqualified people to be taken on to a Register, yet that was what the Osteopaths Bill was trying to avoid. 'There was a clause enabling a person who was practising Osteopathy for three years to go on the register. If the Association had its way you do not want any unqualified person on the register as they may do great harm. The potential for disaster is much greater than for dentists as a wider field is covered. An untrained man may come across conditions he has not seen. Putting qualified and unqualified people together is not protecting the public.' MacDonald replied that it was, 'An, unfortunate necessary preliminary step'.

He was asked, 'Are de facto practitioners going to be subject to an examination of the sort which you went through?...Unless you are going to have some very searching sort of examination the immediate effects of the Bill will not protect the public, but just the reverse.' MacDonald disagreed. He was asked, 'When the State takes upon itself to register people it rather gives it a cachet or hall mark?' It was agreed that it would be inappropriate to have a State Register for a good many healing cults. The only justification of a State Register is if the particular healing body...had scientifically justified itself. 'And unless you can make that good you would agree with me that you are premature in asking for a Bill.' MacDonald agreed.

'Would you accept as the test the opinion of unprejudiced scientific men, or would you make good your claim merely by the vox populi?'... 'We have the vox populi already. It would be difficult to get a scientific body of men who would be unprejudiced.'

'There is no doubt is there that the great bulk of scientific opinion in this county is against the claims of the osteopaths.'...'It seems so, yes.' Jowitt then produced a statement on behalf of 800 professors and lecturers in biological and medical sciences. It included 30 members of the Royal Society, including Joseph Barcroft, Professor of Physiology at Cambridge. Neither Thorpe, nor MacDonald, nor their Lordships had seen this statement before. Thorpe objected that such a petition had never before been produced for a Select Committee. He would accept it if they were called as witnesses. He considered, 'This a new procedure signed by people not here'.

Jowitt: 'Your Lordships might desire to know what is the trend of scientific opinion. Is it not the fact that the vast bulk of scientific opinion, not merely of medical men, but of scientifically trained people in the country is against the Bill?' MacDonald replied that, 'I submit they have not taken the slightest trouble to find out what scientific work has been done in evidence of Osteopathy....They have not investigated our claims and the names on a cursory examination are those...who are teaching Zoology, Botany and Embryology in a medical school—the non-vocational part of medicine.'

Lord Elibank claimed that it was not a petition but, 'A statement which could not be put before them without the witnesses appearing.' Jowitt said that he would not want 800 people called.

Jowitt: 'Are you suggesting (these famous scientists) have never heard of Osteopathy?...Do you suppose that these people do not keep themselves in touch with every sort of scientific development.' MacDonald replied, 'No they do not. They have set it aside as beneath their contempt'....'Apart from yourself and five other doctors the osteopathic concept has never been accepted ?'...'The concept has never been delivered to them.'

Jowitt considered that the medical profession supported progress. MacDonald stated, 'I think I can produce more evidence to prove that the attitude of the medical profession on new ideas is ultra-conservative and retarding of general progress than you could produce evidence to the contrary. Even their beloved Lister was scorned. And Pasteur too.' Jowitt responded, 'Yet his ideas were accepted'. MacDonald replied, 'We are not claiming registration on grounds that we have proved to the scientific world that our contentions are true. It is for the protection of the public.' MacDonald would not admit that the scientific claim should be made good before Osteopathy was recognised. 'I think that Osteopathy is here; the public want osteopathic treatment.'

He was asked about the claim of osteopaths to treat all diseases. He seldom saw acute cases, 'As one would need to see a person with pneumonia five to six times a day. This is impossible with 20-30 patients booked.' Jowitt stated that in the Bill osteopaths were asking to be recognised as persons competent to treat acute cases. MacDonald explained that they did not make a practice of it. Jowitt asked, 'Is it not illogical after five years' training that a man should be allowed to sign death certificates, if they are competent to diagnose and treat all diseases?' MacDonald agreed he should be allowed to sign death certificates and that any medical man should learn major surgery even though he was not going to practise it.

MacDonald argued that just because you qualify in medicine you are not immediately competent to be a surgeon. Jowitt considered it advisable that a medical man learnt major surgery as he needed to know when to advise his patients to go to a surgeon.

MacDonald had to agree that students should be taught major surgery as in medical school and gynaecology and obstetrics. 'It is only with great reluctance that we gave up the right to do obstetric work.'... 'Materia Medica?'...'I think a three month course is adequate.' Jowitt responded, 'Drink deep or not at all.' MacDonald disagreed. 'There is no advantage to an osteopath of knowing how to make up mixtures which he will never prescribe.'

Jowitt considered this was biasing students' education. 'Is it not better that the student should not take sides ?' MacDonald responded that, 'We only want to train those who are anxious to become osteopaths....We are not setting up a rival school of healing.'

He was then asked, 'What subjects of the medical curriculum would you leave out—Materia Medica, pharmacology, therapeutics, practical bacteriology?'...'We deal with the soil not with the seed....It is a waste of time spending so much time on bacteriology. We do not attribute to the organism the great importance attributed by the medical profession. The practice of medicine would be substituted by the practice of Osteopathy. Disease would not be left out but taught from an osteopathic viewpoint.'

The osteopath Jocelyn Proby was then quoted, 'The Principle is that the body contains within itself the power needed to heal the body of its ills'. MacDonald explained, 'We cannot hold and do not hold that diseases cannot originate from outside'.

Jowitt argued that in the vast majority of cases the function of the ordinary doctor was to assist Nature. It was unfair to represent doctors as not believing that the body would not heal itself. It was only regarding certain diseases and treatments that Osteopathy was different. MacDonald disagreed.

Discussion then focused on the difference between Medicine and Osteopathy regarding the diagnosis, cause and treatment of disease. It was agreed that the diagnosis of disease was the same for Osteopathy as for Medicine. MacDonald insisted, 'But to the picture of the diagnosis we add the physical framework abnormalities'. He claimed that, 'The profession of medicine has been very much retarded by over-emphasis on the importance of diagnosis—waiting for an exact diagnosis has

often not been in the best interest of the patient. It is the evidence of
'disharmony' which we look for'. MacDonald agreed that diagnosis of
acute diseases was of first importance and that diagnosis by osteopaths
and medical methods did not differ. They then moved on to causes.
Jowitt focused on typhoid. MacDonald was forced to admit, 'We have
no evidence that people who escape the ravages were osteopathically
sound, it is merely our idea'. Similarly with malaria, measles, and
tonsillitis. 'Again, no evidence we can produce. How can we get evidence
of that?' Jowitt then suggested a methodology. 'You must have treated
in your hospitals (in America) hundreds of cases of tonsillitis, have you
no statistics?'...'We have never found a case of tonsillitis that has not
osteopathic trouble.'

'What is the difference between you and medical men regarding
disease?' MacDonald explained that, 'Medical men look upon disease as
a thing that is conferred'. Jowitt replied, 'So do you. You have just told
me how all these diseases are caused.' MacDonald claimed Jowitt had
chosen exceptions. Jowitt said he was taking the common or garden
diseases. MacDonald insisted, 'You have chosen diseases which are
the best examples of the germ diseases'. Jowitt replied, 'So far as the
germ diseases are concerned there is no difference (between you and
a medical man)?' MacDonald explained that there was the invasion by
the germ. The effect of the fight was the actual disease. 'We are told
that there are many germ diseases which would not occur if the body
were kept in perfect osteopathic order.' He was asked for examples....
Measles, influenza, pneumonia, tonsillitis'. He was again asked for
evidence....'Contentions are not proofs....The osteopaths have not a
title of evidence of any sort or kind.' MacDonald claimed, 'We have
only our individual clinical experience. The justification I have for my
opinion is my own?'...'Are there osteopathically sound people?'...'No'.

Jowitt quoted a US Medical Committee that 80% of children and
young adults exhibited grades of poor body mechanisms and stated,
'As we get older it is almost certain that all of us are osteopathically
unsound....Can you really suggest that the question as to whether you are
or are not osteopathically sound has anything to do with the causation of
disease?' MacDonald: 'I do.'...'What diseases have you which you have
evidence of them being produced by an osteopathic abnormality?'...'In
all cases of asthma we find osteopathic abnormalities.' He agreed there
were successes and failures with respect to treating osteopathic lesions
and curing asthma as with orthodox medicine. 'We succeed where they
fail. Osteopathy has won its reputation by treating the failures of the
medical profession.'

He was then asked whether he had cause for complaint regarding how he was treated by his 'brothers' in the medical profession. MacDonald said, 'I have gone through a very bad time'. He agreed he had been sent patients by doctors and treated doctors and their relatives. 'There is no denying that all doctors admit that "in certain cases" Osteopathy has done good. It is these three words to which we object.'

Jowitt claimed that, 'There is wide opinion in medicine and controversy about indiscriminate drugging'. He quoted Oliver Wendell Holmes and stated, 'This theory about the revolt against drug therapy is much older than Dr Still. The battle against indiscriminate drugging has been fought and won.' MacDonald contended that this is very largely thanks to osteopaths. 'We have won that battle.' Jowitt responded, 'I will not grudge you your little halo for a moment', and then, 'It is ridiculous to say because I am not going to use drugs indiscriminately I am not going to use them at all.' MacDonald replied, 'I have never contended that'....'Dr Still did....Did Dr Still say never under any circumstances must I use drugs?'...'I never heard him say so.' MacDonald agreed he himself never administered drugs. Jowitt suggested if he used a drug he would have breached his theory. Jowitt: 'You are wanting to have the best of both worlds. You are wanting to adhere to Dr Still's theory and to use drugs.' MacDonald replied, 'No, I think I said many times that we do not want to use drugs. We admit that there are diseases which can only be cured by drugs and we hand them over'. Jowitt responded, 'You do not. That is the whole trouble of this Bill. You are asking in the Bill for permission to treat...those very patients. You realise that in this Bill you osteopaths ask to be recognised as being fit to treat all diseases. You recognise that there are a lot of diseases with which your treatment cannot cope?'...'I recognise that there are a few diseases that we cannot cope with so successfully as can be treated by medical methods.'

Lord Carnock enquired regarding the difference between Osteopathy and Chiropractic. MacDonald explained. Jowitt quoted Streeter on Chiropractic, 'That it rests on nothing more than a crude and ignorant misunderstanding of one of the principles of Osteopathy'. MacDonald agreed. Jowitt then quoted Still (1907). 'Anybody who uses drugs forfeits the respect of this School and its teaching'. Jowitt claimed, 'You are much too intelligent and scientific a man to accept any such limitation as that?' MacDonald replied, 'No, I am not'. Jowitt: 'But you have told us there are whole groups of diseases in that the best chance of cure involves the use of drugs.'...'It is the only chance.'...'You must see that the use of drugs therefore involves forfeiting the respect of the School and its teaching.'...'I submit that Dr Still's teachings is the ideal.'

MacDonald explained that, 'It is disharmony that we as osteopaths look for—which we remove before disease develops'....'There is no circumstances in the case of any disease would you ever give drugs?'... 'No, I did not say so, I have never said so. The principle of Osteopathy holds—even those diseases which do call for the immediate use of drugs.' MacDonald argued that no intelligent man engaged in the healing arts would never use drugs.

MacDonald acknowledged that, 'A few (of the medical profession) are alive to it (manipulation)'. Jowitt claimed there were medical postgraduate courses dealing with it. It was acknowledged that insufficiently trained persons might do grievous harm by manipulation.

MacDonald was asked, 'Do not you put your finger into the Eustachian tube?' He explained it was only into the ampulla and he did not currently practise it as it was a highly evolved technique. Jowitt asked, 'You are agreed that finger surgery unless it is done by a highly skilled person may have very bad results?'...'It is a specialist's job.'

Jowitt established that manipulative medicine had not been substantially practised in this country other than by osteopaths, all doing 'office business' and none attending hospitals. Jowitt raised again the case of acute diseases. MacDonald argued that manipulative medicine is not acute disease work only. Jowitt established, 'So far as acute diseases are concerned manipulative medicine is not practised in this country?'...'We have no opportunity of doing so.'

Viscount Elibank questioned the lack of opportunity. MacDonald explained he was debarred from treating patients in hospital. Jowitt asked, 'How do you know?'...'Because I have suffered in this respect.' Jowitt asked for the names of the hospitals but MacDonald requested not to provide them. Jowitt claimed that if an MD was an osteopath as well as a medical man it should not affect his rights. MacDonald said that they were affected. Lord Dawson asked, 'By the Law?'...'Not by the Law, no.' He was asked, 'Have you brought the matter up before some authoritative body in the medical world: the GMC, Ministry of Health, Governors of the Hospital (some of whom MacDonald treated)?'...'It is hopeless, majority rule.' Viscount Elibank referred to an annual meeting of a hospital in Edinburgh in which suggestions were made that an osteopath should be employed, but the Chairman of Governors declined to allow the subject to be discussed or to be pursued at all, although it was ascertained the osteopath was qualified and a qualified medical man.

The subject of pernicious anaemia was raised. MacDonald claimed he had known cases of pernicious anaemia cured by osteopathic treatment. 'We can by osteopathic methods increase hydrochloric acid secretion.' Jowitt then quoted McConnell and Teal that it was nearly always possible to obtain transient improvement, but death usually occurred within two years.

Lord Dawson quoted Minot, an authority on pernicious anaemia, that it was a deficiency disease of the liver. Jowitt claimed MacDonald was taking an opposite view that he could cure pernicious anaemia. MacDonald explained osteopathy was not the cure. He would advise liver treatment. Jowitt challenged him that this was giving a drug. 'It is not a drug. Osteopaths value the products of ductless glands.'

MacDonald saw a value in treating the liver by manipulation. Jowitt then asked for the statistics to substantiate this claim. MacDonald argued that he had personal experience and experimental evidence that osteopathic manipulation can induce all organs to function better. Jowitt: 'Do you or do you not say osteopathic manipulation cured a case of anaemia?'...'No one has cured pernicious anaemia.'...'Have you prolonged life? Have you evidence to produce to me?'...'I have merely my own personal experience.'

Lord Marley clarified. 'There are two ways of treatment—liver treatment or encouraging the liver. Can one not do both?'...'This is in fact what we do.'

Thyrotoxin was discussed in that once it could be manufactured chemically it became a drug. MacDonald argued he did not accept as a definition of a drug as anything that could be made in a chemical laboratory. Lord Redesdale asked, 'What is a drug? Liver has something to do with diet'. Thorpe asked, 'I wonder whether my learned friend would tell me if roast beef is a drug?' Lord Marley: 'Or liver and bacon?'

Jowitt asked, 'Have you any evidence that persons who have liver and manipulative treatment make better recoveries than people who had liver without manipulation?'

MacDonald said, 'No, but there is experimental evidence that manipulation increases secretion of bile. It has not been put to the test.' Jowitt asked, 'Why not?'...'We have not the opportunity, we have not the time, we have not the hospitals, and we have not the money.'... Jowitt: 'You have hospitals in America.'

...'I hold that in deficiency diseases we have more to hold out, or as much...as the practice of medicine has.'...'Although you are not prepared to put a single title of evidence before the Committee to justify that claim.'

Jowitt then moved on to diabetes and confirmed that MacDonald agreed it was due to insulin deficiency. 'Do you say that by manipulating the spinal column you can increase the supply of insulin ?' Bulletin No. two of the A. T. Still Research Institute was quoted as evidence. Jowitt recollected he claimed it to be one of the bad ones and asked, 'Was, the evidence like the Bulletin—bad too ?' MacDonald argued, 'Our osteopathic research is young. You keep asking me what evidence I have. Now when I have a little piece of evidence on the question I am told I am wasting time.' Jowitt responded, 'On the last occasion you turned to me and said (Bulletins) No. 1 and two are not worth reading. You have changed your mind?'

Tuberculosis was next considered. Jowitt established that in America osteopaths in hospitals must have had many patients suffering from TB. Jowitt asked for figures to show that manipulative treatment was beneficial. Lord Elibank asked if the medical profession had any cure. MacDonald replied, 'They have not and they should have'. Jowitt asked if there was evidence that the number of people cured by manipulation was greater than those cured not subject to it. MacDonald stated that there were no statistics. Elibank interceded, arguing that he knew of few cases cured by the medical profession.

It was acknowledged that in cancer there was no cure in many cases. MacDonald was asked to show that (manipulative) treatment rates were better than for doctors and that cases in America were treated by manipulation?'...'I do not know. I never do.'

Jowitt asked if the 2,000 people placed on the register who were not qualified were all going to be recognised as being physicians fit to treat all diseases. 'Before anybody can be qualified and treat disease it is perfectly certain he must have a long time in a hospital, is it not?'... 'Yes'....'What hospital are these fellows going to get into.'...'None'....'If they are not, how can they be qualified to treat disease?'...'We can only be qualified to treat disease if and when the Bill becomes law and we get access to hospitals.'...'Just observe how illogical the whole thing is. Osteopaths are not allowed to sign death certificates, give anaesthetics, attend confinement cases, do major surgery and not go to medical school.' MacDonald considered that it was an undesirable necessity that students would study anatomy and physiology for two years in a medical school and probably also pathology. They would go into hospitals. Jowitt asked why should they not qualify as doctors and then take a postgraduate course as osteopaths. MacDonald replied, 'It is unfair to ask a man who wants to practise Osteopathy to spend seven or eight years to do that'.

Jowitt questioned him that after one year at Kirksville he became Professor of the Principles of Osteopathy. 'Does it not occur to you that if you are able after a year's training to become a Professor of the Principles of Osteopathy at the most important osteopathic college in the world, it would be a very good thing for a medical student?...He might use his own knowledge...as to what method to adopt and what method not to adopt. He can do what doctors are doing with respect to manipulative surgery. It would avoid having 200 unqualified people on the Register.' MacDonald explained that the objection was a very practical one. 'The person wants to study Osteopathy and not become a medical doctor. He is advised to see Dr Littlejohn, but all he gets is the Diploma of an unrecognised, unofficial college. That is why we want this Bill on the Statute.'...'If this Bill is not passed for some time to come men will do what you have done?'...'Yes and men will do the other alternative and in greater numbers; they will go to the osteopathic college only.'... 'Then finally you will be able to start osteopathic hospitals in our big cities.'...'Will we? Not without the Bill.'...'Let us have this plain. You are asking this Committee to pass this Bill on the strength of the claims which osteopathic medicine has made in America?'...'We have 25 years experience of osteopaths working here.'...'Though we have had all this discussion today about not being allowed into hospitals?'...'I submit that what the osteopaths have done in this country justifies our asking for the privileges for which we are asking.'...'Although the osteopaths have not had any real opportunity for dealing in this country with any acute diseases?'...'We take every opportunity of treating acute diseases in the homes of our patients.'...'I thought you never did.'...'Not never.'... 'Your real fear at present is this: You are frightened lest the medical profession should take the osteopathic principles and popularise them for themselves.'...'I do not think we are frightened of anything. It is actually happening, that the medical profession will pick out of Osteopathy what they consider to be useful, but they will not adopt our principles. To get the highest result of the practice of that art you must have a guiding principle.'...'My suggestion to you is this, that that is exactly what you have been doing and that you have wisely and properly put on one side the guiding principle which Dr Still elaborated for the simple reason that no intelligent man today could possibly accept that guiding principle.'...'I most definitely have not done so. I found that medicine contained no basic guiding principle. I went to America and I saw that Osteopathy had a guiding principle and had a practical method of putting that guiding principle into practice.'

Jowitt: 'I can put what I want to say in two questions: Do you adhere to Dr Still's principle?'...'I do.'...'Was Dr Still's principle that anybody who used drugs forfeited the respect of the school and its teachings?'... 'Dr Still said so.'...'Was that his principle?'...'No. The early osteopaths did not want to be interested in drugs. They were forced to do so if they wanted to become competent physicians. They are lazy people in all professions—it was easier to give morphia than to investigate the body and find out what was causing the pain.'...'Was his principle that the body contained within itself everything that was necessary for the cure of diseases?'...'That was his principle.'...'Do you accept that principle today?'...'I do.'...'You have never put anything in the body to assist the body to cure disease?'...'We do.'...'Then if you do that, what I suggest to you is this—you are not accepting the principle, you are paying lip service to the principle, and, in practice, you are departing from it.'...'I most strongly protest.'...'Will you explain how you reconcile these?'... 'Because in the powers of healing art there can be nothing absolute. It is not a question of Science. I have said so. Medicine is not a Science. Osteopathy is not a Science. I protest most strongly that my sincere effort along osteopathic lines has anything to do whatever with lip service.'

Radcliffe then cross examined MacDonald. He returned to the figures for influenza and pneumonia. 'You said they were put before the committee for what they were worth. What do you think they were worth? What were the osteopathic figures obtained from?' MacDonald explained that questionnaires were sent out by the AOA. 2,245 were returned of some 5,000 members. Many of them were not doing acute work at all. Nobody knows what the results from the other half would have been.'

MacDonald was asked about Osteopathy on the continent. There were three osteopaths in Paris. He explained it was unknown there because of the language difficulty.

He was asked, 'There is nothing revolutionary of course to the medical idea that the body contains great curative forces in itself, is there?'...'Yes, there is a great revolutionary idea there.' Radcliffe claimed that Dr Bruce was teaching on much the same line....'No, he used physical methods mostly....Physical science as applied to the investigation of disease has not received from the medical profession the attention it deserves.'...'That is not the same thing as saying that it is revolutionary, is it?'...'I am not saying that Osteopathy as a practice is revolutionary.'

He explained that six-sevenths was common to osteopathic and medical training and agreed that even in osteopathic training some attention would have to be paid to Pharmacology, Pharmacy and Materia Medica.

The benefits of his previous medical training were discussed in relation to his gaining a Professorship at Kirksville. MacDonald explained, 'I carried nothing of my previous medical training as far as treatment was concerned which has been of the slightest benefit to me....I had to rid myself of many doctrines which were false.'...'You were made a Professor over all the heads in one year.' Radcliffe tried to argue it was because of his medical training. MacDonald explained it was because he got his training direct from Still.

Discussion followed regarding the teaching hours for a course. 'We have first of all a very excellent beginning made by Dr Littlejohn in the BSO and if the Bill becomes an Act, it will enable him and enable the BOA, all to work enthusiastically together to make the college worthy of Osteopathy.' Radcliffe asked, 'Is it your intention that the BSO should be the nucleus of the teaching in the future?'...'Most assuredly, but there may be other colleges'. The BSO had, 'Made to my mind a most commendable effort. The wonder is not that the college is in such a state, but the wonder is that it exists at all. I want to make that point very strongly. The BOA has, rightly or wrongly, gone on the idea that they suddenly want a full-blown college to come into existence, all of a sudden with hospitals, five years training and everything, but they will under this Bill meet and make in the first instance the BSO an institution worthy of our practice. We are not going to take students into this college who have not passed the necessary medical educational standards.'

He mentioned that the BOA had a College Committee and Pheils could answer all the questions regarding a college.

Questions then centred on whether it was part of the osteopathic teaching that the osteopathic lesion was responsible for all diseases. 'No. We do not claim that it is a primary cause of disease.'...'Do the osteopaths claim that it is possible to have many diseases without an osteopathic lesion being present at all?' Radcliffe then referred to typhoid and cited a book in which it was claimed to be present in all cases. MacDonald explained, 'We hold that a person is more liable to typhoid fever if he has in his spinal column structural abnormalities which will interfere with the normal function of the bowel. If there were no pre-existing abnormality the fight between the bowel and the *Bacillus typhosus* reflexly produces in a previously normal spinal column abnormalities which we regard as being lesions—they play a part in the maintenance of the condition.' Radcliffe asked if in all cases of typhoid fever an osteopathic lesion is present. 'In all cases...you would find reflexly produced abnormalities which we pay attention to.'...'You said you found in all cases. Is that based on the universal experience of osteopaths.'...'Yes.' 'You postulate that the unhealthy bowel is produced by osteopathic abnormalities.'...'We have found by experience.'...'Do you mean by that that there are records of that experience.'...'No. Because how could there be records? We do not know who is going to make himself liable to an attack of typhoid fever.'...'I am right, am I not, that it is a pure postulate?'...'We find definitely that there are these abnormalities and they are in nervous relationship to the bowel.'

Lord Dawson asked, 'In an epidemic of typhoid, what proportion of people stricken have lesions and what proportion have not. Has there been such a scientific enquiry?'...'No.'...'Therefore it is an assumption as far as typhoid fever is concerned.'...'Yes.'...'What evidence that cases aborted if treated osteopathically in the first week?'...'The statement is founded on my experience.'...'You would agree in a large proportion of cases we cannot say whether it is typhoid at all until the first week is over?'...'I quite agree.'...'Therefore we cannot demonstrate the statement, but we can think they are probabilities.'...'We can just think they are probabilities. It is very broad-minded of you, if I may say so, to admit that it is even a probability, because it is quite impossible to make that diagnosis.'

Radcliffe moved to the predisposing cause of diphtheria and bacteria....'I would guarantee to examine necks and tell which one is more likely to be prone to diphtheria than the others...but if you allow me to treat one of these necks and make them normal, I would be more confident that that person would not pick up diphtheria.'...'Then it is this, that there must be a reason for these things happening and you think your reason is the best.'

Lord Dawson cross-questioned. MacDonald explained that the medical profession was inclined to look upon each disease as a separate entity. He looked upon diseases as the effects of previous disharmony in the body. He claimed he would be willing to research this claim if there was a diphtheria outbreak. Dawson stated, 'May I put it to you: I take it this is a very important statement about the predisposing cause. I take it you would not have made that statement without making sure that there is objective evidence in support of it?'...'Yes, I believe there is.'...'Where could we find that?'...'I have not got the evidence to give to you. I am merely in all sincerity holding it out to you as a practical test

(as a practical proposition) and such is our confidence in our belief.'...
'Surely you would agree that a belief in science has to be based on data
and you would deduce your theory from data.'...'I am asking, has not it
been done already before such a serious statement such as this has been
made?'...'I submit it is a rather unfair idea. Jenner went on for 30 years
before there was any scientific proof of his contentions. Why should we
be asked?'...'I am sure there must have been some objective evidence',
some such experiments before such a statement was made and I want to
know what they are.'...'I cannot give you figures relative to diphtheria
alone.'

Lord Esher asked if the medical profession investigated this claim,
if they were interested in scientific investigation? MacDonald said it
was not for him to answer. 'In all cases of diphtheria which have come
your way have you found on examination these subluxations of the
cervical vertebrae existing?'...'Yes.'

In the discussion that followed, MacDonald explained that in an
intact mucosa without a subluxation, the diphtheria would not develop.
Radcliffe asked, 'Osteopaths do not themselves administer serum do
they?...Would you hand a case over?'...'No, as the giving of a serum is a
perfectly simple matter.'...'What were the cases you would hand over
to doctors?'...'If we had our way we would hand over none....If we were
getting the five year course we would train our students to be complete
physicians.'...'Is it your view then that after this five year course they
could and should deal with all diseases? What hospital experience will
they get?'...'All we can get.'...'How much will that be?'...'I cannot tell
you.'...'You do not propose to teach them as I understand more about
drugs and bacilli.'...'The Board will decide what education they think
it is necessary for an osteopathic physician to have. I would not waste
the osteopath's time by teaching him methods that he will not practise.
We will have in schedule two a course in Comparative Therapeutics
and after all men can read the *British Medical Journal* and *The Lancet*, a
compliment that you do not pay in return to us.'...'But he will be taught,
will he not, to be suspicious of drugs?' MacDonald agreed. 'He will be
taught this, that there are two main divisions of things you take into
your body: foods and poisons. If it is not a food, it is a poison.' (Radcliffe
pursued this). 'He will not be interested in the developments of drug
therapy after he has passed your course?'...'My Lord Chairman I do not
think because we are teaching a student our methods...his critical faculty
will be lowered.' Radcliffe persisted: 'It goes further than that, does it
not? You are going to teach him the great basic principle?'...'Yes.'...'How
do you think he will be able to keep abreast of developments in drug

therapy? After his student days are over will he be interested in the developments of drug therapy?'...'I think he will.'

Jones took up the cross-examination. 'Earlier in your evidence you expressed a friendly feeling, did you not, towards the non-drug healing school including the nature cure practitioners?...May I take it you have informed yourself of the principles and their practice?'...'I know a little about their practice. I do not know anything about the principle.'...'Do you know that as part of their principle and their practice they practise Osteopathy?'...'No. I will not admit that Osteopathy as practised by the Nature Cure practitioner is the Osteopathy of a qualified osteopath.' Thorpe asked, 'Does that mean to infer that they hold themselves out as osteopaths?' Jones claimed they hold themselves out as osteopaths and they were qualified in Osteopathy as he was going to prove. 'You would agree with me would you not that Osteopathy... forms a natural part of nature cure practice?'...'Yes, certainly it is a natural therapy.'...'And should it be a part of the equipment of every nature cure practitioner?'...'Yes.'...'With a view I take it of reducing the amount of drug giving and...surgery?'...'Yes, but I am not at all in favour of mixing them. I do not think you can be a good drug physician and a good osteopath at the same time.'...'I thought you told us just now that you wanted your students to be trained to be complete physicians?' MacDonald agreed, but stated, 'I think you will be better osteopaths if you are doing Osteopathy all the time than if you are jack-of-all-trades'. Jones got MacDonald to agree that medicine and surgery had a certain part to play in the treatment of disease—and hydrotherapy, diathermy, sera, vaccines, antibiotics and all kinds of surgery. Jones stated, 'There has been a strange hesitancy shall we say...to give an exact definition of what Osteopathy is. I am going to suggest that we did not have it from you and we certainly did not have it from Dr Streeter.'

Thorpe interceded, 'He told my Lords that he gave the best definition he could....We are not satisfied with it ourselves; it is the best we can produce.' A definition was in the Bill. Jones asked, 'Could the man in the street reading that definition get a clear view in his mind of what Osteopathy is?'...'Yes.'...'I may be strangely dull, but I personally cannot.'

Jones then proposed a definition. MacDonald objected, 'I am not here to accept any other definition of Osteopathy than the one that we put forward'. He was asked if it was a fair definition. Thorpe and MacDonald indicated that they would have to give it a great deal of thought. The Chairman interceded that it was perhaps not fair to put a definition to a witness at a moment's notice and ask him to accept it. Jones claimed it was rather important to his case that they should get a clear definition of some kind different from the one in the Bill. 'The one in the Bill means nothing at all and it means nothing to those instructing me.' MacDonald stated, 'I really think it is almost a waste of time to consider a definition which we did not put forward. We are not here discussing Osteopathy through the nature cure glasses.' Jones replied, ' I am not asking about nature cure or anything else; I am asking for a definition of what Osteopathy is'. MacDonald emphasised, 'It is in the Bill'. Thorpe asked if he would be prepared to consider Jones's definition. 'Will my friend withdraw from the room if he gets the definition he asks for?' Jones said, ' Not for a moment'. Thorpe: 'There does not seem to be much point in getting it.' Jones: 'It is essential to my argument to get it.' The Chairman brought the matter to a close: 'You have argued that enough Mr Jones.'

Jones continued along another track. 'You have claimed have you not that bone-setting forms an essential part of Osteopathy?'...'No, I said that there is nothing in bone-setting which is not included in Osteopathy.'...'Is orthopaedic surgery a part of Osteopathy too?'... 'Yes.'

'The fact remains that Orthopaedic Surgery and Osteopathy are two entirely different arts....Osteopathy is only a part; it is a thing that has a useful part to play in the treatment of disease.' MacDonald would not admit that osteopath is only a part....'We mean to make Osteopathy a complete system of healing.' Jones re-established there were many diseases that Osteopathy could not treat at all. There were some diseases which could not be cured by Osteopathy except along with other treatments. 'I agree there are certain diseases which only medicine can cure.'...'In which Osteopathy does not play any part at all.'...'I did not say that. Osteopathy always helps a sick man.'...Jones stated, 'It seems to me that an osteopath is being called an osteopath and being trained to do many other things besides Osteopathy (hydrotherapy, dietetics). Is that true?'...'No. It is in so far as Osteopathy embraces all natural methods of healing.' Jones claimed MacDonald said they were an essential part of Osteopathy. He denied this and stated that, 'It is most unfair that anybody here should suggest that I did say that they were essential parts of Osteopathy when I did not say that'. Jones commented, 'It is very simple...'. MacDonald said, 'It is not very simple and I refuse to have these words put into my mouth'. Jones: 'An osteopath is a man who is taught and practises Osteopathy in addition to a number of other therapies.'...'I do not agree.' Jones continued: 'And I suggest that the Nature Cure Association when they call themselves osteopaths are in a much more logical position than the osteopath because...they call themselves nature cure practitioners which properly includes Osteopathy.' MacDonald did not agree. A five year course in Osteopathy had been proposed. 'I would like to point out to you (My Lord Chairman) that the Nature Cure system must think that they can learn all about Osteopathy in a few months. I took two years after having first studied medicine.'

Jones asked, 'One reason you put forward this Bill is that you have got the vox populi behind you?'...'Yes.'...'A large proportion of that large number might be found to be approving of Osteopathy in compete ignorance of what it is.'...'I do not think anybody could come for treatment, unless he had heard that his friends had benefited from treatment.'...'But I have to keep on putting it to you that an osteopath does not merely practise Osteopathy, he practises a number of other things as well.'...'You cannot put such a proposition to me.'...'Does not he practise as a surgeon?'...'Not in this country.'...Jones cited operations on the orifice of the Eustachian tube. MacDonald denied it was surgery, as no surgical instrument was used.

'If this Bill goes through is not the effect going to be to detach osteopaths from the Nature Cure movement, an art to which they properly belong?'...'I am not concerned with that. But if it does become law one result will be that the medical profession will look a little more kindly on us all.'...'I do not see that as an answer to my question.' Lord Elibank said, 'I thought you would be able to answer that, not the witness'. Jones replied, 'Provided that we can prove that Nature Cure practitioners are qualified to practise Osteopathy'. MacDonald said, 'I submit they are not. There is nothing in the Bill which interferes in any way with the activities of the Nature Cure practitioners. It only says he cannot hold himself out to be a fully trained osteopath.'

Thorpe returned to cross examine MacDonald. 'Did you know that the nature curers called themselves osteopaths and hold themselves out to practise Osteopathy?'...'Yes.'...'Had they in your view the slightest qualification for any such claim?'...'No.'...'It is suggested that the effect of this Bill will be to stop them practising as osteopaths, in your view will that be a good thing?'...'That will be a good thing.'

'Do you remember that Lord Dawson suggested that you should go somewhere where there is an epidemic and collect statistics. What chances would you have if you or three or four of you descended on that locality and said to the Medical Officer of Health we want to test the principle of Osteopathy on your sick people?'...'I do not think we would have any chance of getting our proposition taken up at all. A very definite attempt was made five years ago and one a few months ago. We always met with deadlock.'...'You have volunteered that if that occasion should arise and you were invited by the medical practitioners, you would gladly go and demonstrate your beliefs?'...'Certainly.'...'It amounts to this does it not, that until you get the invitation it will be quite impossible in this country at any rate to produce the evidence that seems so desirable?'...'Yes that is so.'...'Have you any reason to believe that the invitation will be extended to you?'...'I do not think so....It is an absolute dead end as far as we are concerned.'

Discussion of Los Angeles County Hospital took place. It had 1,666 beds in two units: a medical unit and an osteopathic unit that worked side by side for four and a half years. 196 beds were in the osteopathic unit. Patients were allocated alternately, i.e. there was no difference in the type of patient seen. Deaths were less in the osteopathic unit.

'Has there been any serious attempt on the part of orthodox medical practitioners to investigate either the claims or the results you have achieved?'...'Absolutely not as far as I can find out.' Until he handed over to the BMA Council the A. T. Still Research Bulletins on Osteopathy, a few days previously, he was unaware of any attempt whatsoever on behalf of the medical profession, 'to investigate Osteopathy.'....'May I recall, gratefully, that it was a noble Lord on the Committee who asked for those seven books of wisdom?'...'Am I right in this, that any satisfactory result must really have the co-operation of the medical men?'...'I think so.'...'And as the world is today, you are never likely to get that?...'No.'

Thorpe: 'Am I right in this that the standard for which the BOA have always stood is this, that there should be an effective college of a certain standard, or no college?'...'Yes.'...'There was another school of thought, was there not, represented by Littlejohn?...Was it not better to have some college than no college?...If this Bill should be passed and the college is automatically brought up to the standard laid down by this Bill, will that be acceptable as far as you know, to the BOA?'...'Most assuredly.'...'If the Bill passes will the result be that the School authorities and the Association will be in complete agreement and willing to accept the standard set down by the Bill?'...'Yes.'

They then discussed the curriculum. 'Do you think it would improve the curriculum to add pharmacology and comparative therapeutics?' He agreed....'And minor surgery? So if we struck out the word minor, that would meet the criticisms?'...'Yes.'

'I think you hold by the basic principle that you do not wish to use drugs for curative purposes?'...'That is so.'...'There are exceptions?'...

'Yes.'...'The exceptions are cases where, for choice, you would accept
drug therapy but always in conjunction with your own principles?'...
'That is so.'

Lord Redesdale asked, 'Are osteopathic lesions in any way
catching?'...'No.'...'Are they always the result of some shock?'...'They
are purely individually acquired. We have evidence in both animals and
in humans that the tendency to them can be hereditarily acquired.'...'Is
the sole reason why osteopaths do not deal with the very acute cases,
the scarcity of osteopaths?'...'Yes.'

Lord Dawson asked for objective evidence of the effectiveness of
osteopathic treatment of epilepsy: X-rays, experiment, or post mortems.
MacDonald agreed that there was no post-mortem evidence. When
ligaments of a joint were cut the essential vital characteristics of the
lesion disappear. Lord Dawson asked for X-ray evidence....'I have no
such evidence I can put before you....We cannot bring evidence up here
of every disease or condition.'...'Is it available anywhere?...Something
comparable to what I can get in the proceedings of the Royal Society
for example?'...'No. It is only available in the Journal of the American
Osteopathic Association.'...'Perhaps we might have the evidence
produced.'...'X-ray plates show localised oedema and fibrosis and joint
distortion.'...'Is the evidence forth-coming? Can I find it anywhere? It
is to be had? Absolutely, systematically, serially arranged?'...'No.'...'Laid
out as I would lay it out if I was going to a medical meeting?'

Lord Dawson referred to the press coverage regarding MacDonald
not being allowed to treat a patient in hospital and argued if he (Lord
Dawson) sent a patient to a hospital he would not expect to be allowed
to interfere. MacDonald agreed and was sorry to see the press had taken
it up. Thorpe interceded, 'If a patient is sent to hospital he will continue
to be treated from a medical standpoint, whereas for a patient treated
osteopathically that kind of treatment would cease'.

Regarding osteopaths' claim to be complete physicians, 'If
Osteopathy claims that wide embrace it would carry a corresponding
responsibility for all diseases?'...'Certainly.'...'Whether they be acute or
chronic, or medical or surgical?'...'Yes.'...'If that is the case would you
be willing to abandon the right to sign death certificates, would that be
consistent with your professional self respect and would it be for the
public good?'...'I take it that until such time as we have a college running
where our education of osteopathic students can be actually inspected,
we cannot expect to have the privilege of signing death certificates.'...
'You are including in your embrace the really dangerous diseases of the
human body, which carry with them a definite mortality?'...'Yes.'...'What

would happen if there was a death? Every time there would have to be an inquest. That cannot be in the public interest? I put it to you as one professional man to another, I should see red if anybody asked me not to have the responsibility of signing a death certificate?'...'We cannot go to Parliament and say we want all these privileges until we have proved to Parliament that we have educational colleges where our students can get the necessary education for these privileges. We are willing to give way on many points merely for the granting to us of a recognised professional legalised existence.'...'If you are fit to treat people you are fit to sign the death certificates. If you are going to treat these grave diseases you ought to be allowed to sign the death certificate.' Thorpe indicated he was responsible for that clause not being pressed.

Lord Dawson then concentrated on the difference between Osteopathy and Medicine. In osteopathic treatment the human body contains within itself all the means necessary for the curing of disease. MacDonald objected that he always corrected it to, 'Contains all the power'. 'I cannot substantiate the fact that it contains all the means. I cannot maintain it holds substances like emertine as you rightly pointed out.'...'One of the real difficulties that makes me most despair of this enquiry is that I cannot nail a single thing to the counter. I cannot get an answer to a question. I want to show that in those 20 examples here for which I have collected the evidence you would use external remedies if you were up against it.' Esher: 'The difference between Lord Dawson and the witness is the definition of what is a drug.' Lord Dawson corrected him. I said, 'An external remedy'. MacDonald indicated, 'We are not up against external remedies, we are up against drugs'. 'Homeopaths are able to join in the orthodox curriculum and teach its tenets. They run a hospital and it co-operates increasingly with the orthodox medical profession.' MacDonald agreed. 'Homeopaths manage to get along with the ordinary medical curriculum as regards the treatment of disease.'

'You claim that (the osteopathic lesion) is the outstanding single cause—the most important single factor....That is what is new; that is what is original, that is what is revolutionary. Does that theory more than any other lead you to claim to set up something which has never been set up before in this country, or on the continent....A system of medicine, with a separate education, separate curriculum, separate examination and separate registration? It is a tremendous claim to set up a parallel system of medicine...productive of a large amount of administrative inconvenience, because of it the army, navy, Ministry of Health, should have osteopathic and orthodox doctors. We should in fairness, have to have duplication in all branches of the profession. It makes it doubly and trebly important that the case should be made out to the hilt to justify such a revolutionary change.'...'I agree with that.'...'I mean something which will go through the tests before scientific bodies on the lines I have mentioned, not mere odd collections of personal experience; however valuable they may be, they do not go very far.'...'What more can I do? We have worked, or I would rather say I have worked for 20 years with the self same special lesion as the only factor in ill-health to which I paid attention as far as treatment was concerned....I am more than satisfied that the medical profession have missed a great truth. I produced to the Council for the BMA and to yourself not all the research work that was available, but I produced the seven Bulletins of osteopathic research....I would point out that I have not been asked one single question on the research question, on the scientific basis of Osteopathy.'

Discussion took place regarding the statement signed by the 480 members of the medical profession. Lord Esher asked, 'Have they examined the osteopathic theory?'...'That is my first question.' Lord Dawson asked, 'It is a rule in scientific life that a person who puts a new theory forward has to prove it, is it not?'...'We are here pushed in front of your Lordships by public opinion because of the results of our work upon sick people. We have what we consider to be abundant scientific proof that our contentions are at least worthy of scientific investigation and we think further, that the osteopathic lesion has been proved on the scientific basis, not adequately enough for absolute acceptance by a critical let us say supercritical and rightly supercritical medical profession, but more than enough to justify our presence here. We welcome any tribunal that will go into the scientific aspect of it, but we deny them the right to make any such statement as that Osteopathy is incapable of scientific investigation.'

Lord Dawson claimed, 'I have no antipathy to this at all. I am showing no bias at all. I put it to you that it is necessary that the case should be proved according to the recognised standards of all scientific inquiry, that goes back to the days of Bacon and Newton.'...'I definitely submit that we have...the scientific proof of Osteopathy and I also submit that this is the first hour in this country that the evidence has ever been asked for.' MacDonald offered articles from the *Journal of the American Osteopathic Association*....'Then I should have the case before me?'...'You will give me a week.' Lord Marley said, 'I think you would want about six months at the present rate we are going'. He then drew an analogy between the services of different chaplains in the army and navy and did not think there would be any administrative difficulties of two medical services. But Lord Dawson indicated, 'You would have to have separate hospitals'. Lord Marley referred to the two hospitals in Los Angeles. 'Does any difficulty arise there?'...'None whatsoever.'

He questioned why Streeter's name was not on the list of BOA members. When the BOA formed he was not a member. MacDonald explained that he later joined, but then he was not in favour of a certain small policy and resigned.

Lord Esher claimed the medical profession was much richer than Osteopathy, had more facilities for scientific investigation, that more cases came before them, but they had never investigated the osteopathic theory....'May I assert they have not? If they have I challenge them to produce it. Do osteopaths want to certify lunatics?'...'I do not think we have ever gone into the question.' Thorpe stated, 'I think I am right in saying in law we should not have that right under this Bill'.

The Chairman asked, 'What do you consider to be a drug from the osteopathic point of view?'...'A drug is a chemical which is given for therapeutic purposes in order to alter the quality of the body reaction.... That is the drug that we do not wish to administer.' Lord Dawson got MacDonald to agree that if he were up against it with full responsibility he would use drugs. Lord Marley asked, 'If you got the case at an early stage you would be able to prove that they would never reach the stage when the giving of a drug would be necessary?'...'Most essentially so.'

Lord Dawson referred to the 20 diseases that were discussed. 'Are not there amongst those a large number of acute invasions of which we get no warning at all, e.g. acute dysentery, typhoid? If you are going to save that life, you have to give emertine as soon as you can get it in?'...'Yes.'

Discussion centred on the proposed School. No student would be allowed to enter until he had first passed the medical preliminary matriculation examination and then pathology in a medical school and had clinical experience in hospital.

He was asked about accepting qualifications of foreign schools. If the course was less than five years then American trained osteopaths could not practise in the UK.

Half the BOA members were American, some were British subjects. 'You propose that this Association, which consists partly of non-naturalised British subjects should have the power of appointing members of the Board?' He was asked if all those qualified in America had passed the State Examination. 'I could not tell you. They all hold diplomas from a reputable school other than two members.' The Chairman asked, 'It may well be that members would be admitted to be registered who would not be allowed to practise Osteopathy in America?'...'I could not tell you, My Lord. I can only tell you that I never took a State Board Examination. I could not practise either medicine or Osteopathy in America.' He was questioned on membership of the Incorporated Society. 'They were all graduates of the BSO, 98 in all. The Osteopathic Defence League was a lay body with thousands of members.'

MacDonald's final statement was, 'I want particularly to thank Lord Dawson of Penn because he has shown great willingness to understand us in all our apparent heresies and I would like him to appreciate the fact that we know he has done so'.

MacDonald wrote a book in eight days on, *'The Scientific Basis of Osteopathy'*. It reproduced the seven original A. T. Still Bulletins, inspired by Lord Dawson's invitation to produce any scientific evidence available.

Chapter 6

The Select Committee — Other Witnesses

A number of witnesses were called additional to Streeter, MacDonald and Littlejohn. There then followed a final statement by Thorpe on behalf of the defence. The final summary is also provided below.

Sir E Farquhar Buzzard Bart KCVO MD FRCS

Buzzard, Professor of Medicine at Oxford, produced a statement opposing the Bill signed by 800 medical persons and biologists, of whom 23 had an FRS, 75 a DSc and 40 a PhD. 'Their objections to the Bill are based, in the first place, on its menace to the interests of the public, and, secondly, on its menace to the prestige of scientific medicine in this country in the eyes of the world.' The statement was unacceptable to the Select Committee as each signatory would have to be called to speak.

Buzzard indicated that they were concerned about the lack of medical training, the lack of research and that the theory of Osteopathy with 'the osteopathic lesion' as the primary cause of disease was unsupported by scientific evidence. Buzzard considered that, 'No biologist, anatomist, physiologist or pathologist of a British University had observed this 'osteopathic lesion' and no evidence capable of verification has been bought forward....There can be no compromise; the theories of medical science and of Osteopathy are incompatible and contradictory....Official recognition of Osteopathy as a theory of Medicine is completely opposed to the teaching in British universities....It would create far-reaching and revolutionary changes in scientific, medical and biological education.'

He then went on to claim, 'The doctrine of Osteopathy is dying in the country of its birth'. This claim was based on talking to people in the US during a visit. He considered that the testimonials of cured patients were worthless; that the medical profession anyway had long ceased to regard the use of drugs as the most important single factor combating disease (i.e. they were no different in this respect from osteopaths) and he claimed that Osteopathy was being replaced by Chiropractic. Thorpe challenged, 'This most material allegation. A distinguished gentleman comes and says Osteopathy is on the decline.' Buzzard considered that adding to the Registration Board a medical practitioner appointed by the GMC, 'Adds enormously to the danger of the Bill, sanctioning it in the eyes of the public. I cannot believe that the medical profession would lend itself to a step so retrograde and so dangerous to the interests of the public.' He produced a photograph from the A. T. Still Institute Bulletin No. 1, which he stated, 'Exhibits a complete ignorance both of the anatomy and of the pathology of the spinal cord'. He was later asked by the defence why this criticism was not communicated to Dr MacDonald. 'It might be that he would agree with you.'

He was later recalled and initially cross-examined by Radcliffe on the scientific evidence for Osteopathy. 'Every medical man of repute in the country...repudiates the osteopathic creed and is ashamed that his country is the happy hunting ground of these cults. There is no evidence of osteopathic lesions on pathological examination. There is not a single museum specimen at the British School of Osteopathy, nor among their 10,000 slides.' He was opposed to osteopathic education as it was based on one theory.

Thorpe questioned him on the signed statement and how the signatures were obtained and argued that the majority of academics had not signed. Buzzard claimed this was quite wrong, but admitted the signatures were obtained in a great hurry.

The statement claimed, 'In the Universities, workers are constantly engaged in the examination of current doctrines and theories'. Thorpe asked if any University research laboratory had researched Osteopathy, being a 'current doctrine'. Buzzard claimed there was not the prima facie evidence making it worthy of prolonged investigation. Thorpe responded, 'No prima facie evidence when hundreds of your patients go to an osteopath. What would be the minimum prima facie evidence that would be necessary to set in motion the great machinery, which is always waiting to consider current theories or current doctrines ?' Buzzard considered Osteopathy has been before scientific bodies for 50 years in the US and still there was no evidence. Thorpe asked, 'Has not British research a duty to the public to investigate it?'

The statement referred to the idea that the osteopathic lesion, was the primary cause of disease was unsupported by scientific evidence.

Thorpe asked, 'Where did you get that from?'...'From reading.'...'Can you refer to any textbook?...Did it not occur to you that in an important document like this it would be desirable to get from some apparently official source what the official theory of Osteopathy is?'...'No biologist, anatomist, physiologist or pathologist has observed the lesion.'...'Have any of those gentleman looked for one? Did you know what you were looking for?' He was reminded that MacDonald had claimed they would not be obvious at post-mortem. Buzzard responded, 'That is very convenient'.

It was claimed that theories of medical science and Osteopathy were incompatible and contradictory, but other witnesses, Morton, Smart, Mennell and Brackenbury, had indicated they had something in common.

Buzzard explained that his claim that Osteopathy was dying in the land of its birth was based on a six year old publication. Lord Esher elicited that when in America, Buzzard had not talked to osteopaths. 'It would not strike you as scientific to take their view?'...'No. I don't think so.'...'Is that your idea of Science. To have a talk with only one side?'

Buzzard had claimed that medical science could produce as many grateful patients as MacDonald, however, MacDonald had not produced any! Buzzard's objection to the Bill, that it was, 'A menace to the prestige of scientific medicine' was discussed. 'Is it not in the public interest that a man like Dr MacDonald should be allowed to continue these fallacious theories and practice?'...'No.' Buzzard had referred to a book by Yale Castlio, but it was established that he had not asked British osteopaths if they accepted it as an authority. He had seen a demonstration of Osteopathy that had not convinced him that the claims could be substantiated, but it was an after dinner presentation and no patient was used. He only became interested in it again in 1931, because someone (the BOA) was asking for a Royal Charter.

Brackenbury (who was cross-questioned both before and after Buzzard) had stated that he would like to give Osteopathy every credit. Buzzard's comment on this was, 'I will give them all the credit due to them'....He was asked, 'Is any credit due to them?' He agreed that some hundreds of patients went to osteopaths and a great number benefited.

He described a situation when a doctor saw a patient after being treated by an osteopath, the osteopath having made a wrong diagnosis. He was asked, 'But don't some go to osteopaths after seeing a doctor?' He was obliged to admit that sometimes doctors get the diagnosis wrong and that they vary in their diagnosis and treatment.

Buzzard considered that it would be wrong for any medical men to sit on a Board that recognised osteopaths. It would give a cachet of medical approval. Radcliffe asked, 'Would you think a theory as in Castlio's book is incapable of being a scientific theory?' (I.e. subject to research)...'Absolutely. It is the business of the people putting forward a theory to supply the scientific evidence of its value.' Lord Esher said that MacDonald claimed he had submitted evidence but the medical research people refused to examine it.

Lord Elibank asked, 'Is it not wrong that the Medical Council should take no notice in spite of the fact that osteopaths are practising all over the country and the public are going to them?' Buzzard could not understand why this was wrong. Elibank explained the need for research to protect the community.

Lord Esher asked, 'I suppose you think that medicine is securely based on science? When did medicine become scientific?' Buzzard agreed that there was a time when medicine was not based on science at all. 'At that time do you consider it was a danger to the public?'...'Yes.'... 'Would it not have been a pity if it had then been discouraged? Yet that is what you are proposing to do with Osteopathy. You do not think it is the duty of unbiased scientists to examine a new idea?...Suppose a man had been curing cancer, you would think it the business of well endowed research institutions to examine the theory?' Buzzard agreed if his statements and those of his patients were marshalled together.

Redesdale considered the demonstration of Osteopathy was equivalent to looking down a microscope at bacteria taking good care they only had an empty slide to look at. Buzzard claimed that osteopaths were welcome to put up their scientific case. Lord Elibank asked him, 'Is not their case prejudiced by the 1,600 signatories of his statement? In fact, with all respect, it seems to me that you are prejudiced against Osteopathy in all your evidence.' Buzzard denied this.

Jowitt's speech

He summarised that at that time there were 2,000-3,000 practising osteopaths, amongst which some 179 stood in a somewhat different category (having some form of qualification), of whom 96 were 'old boys, if I may call them such, of the BSO' and the other 83 had some American qualification of whom roughly half were Americans. American medical degrees were not acceptable in the UK. There were fears that the unqualified osteopaths would be put on a register as were the dentists. 'Are we certain after that that everybody who practises will be properly trained? I think that the cart has been put before the horse.

The first thing to be done was for the osteopaths to get some proper school (as Neville Chamberlain suggested). The divergence between Dr Kelman MacDonald on the one hand and Dr Littlejohn on the other is about as great as the divergence between the North Pole and the South Pole. The BSO cannot be regarded as in any way satisfactory or I regret to say a reputable school. Of the 96 old boys, some 15 are Looker students. Spencer's certificate claiming he attended the four year course...is not an honest certificate, and Dr Littlejohn, I will say quite plainly, is not an honest man. If you are going to have a satisfactory education hereafter in Osteopathy (I will say quite frankly what I mean) the less Dr Littlejohn has to do with it the better.'

He asked, 'You are expecting people to submit to an examination that may prevent them earning a living?'

He considered that there were a number of healing cults that needed to be scientifically proven otherwise it was premature to have a State Register. 'They want to put on a register people who treat all disease—There is no evidence that an osteopath in England treats acute diseases. MacDonald and Streeter both have office practices. If put on the register it implies that they are fit to treat all diseases—but not to sign death certificates. If they can diagnose a disease from which a man is suffering, should they not be able to diagnose the disease from which he has died? Why do they bar themselves from using anaesthetics and obstetrics?...The distinction between major and minor surgery is an wholly unworkable one. If a person is going to refer to surgery he must learn something about major surgery....The value of education is not imparting knowledge, but to enable a man to think for himself. It is inappropriate to start an education with a prejudicial point of view. You are never going to use drugs or anything of that sort. When a man passes his degrees his education has just begun. Therefore it seems to me it would be lamentable to start these young men from a sectarian point of view.'

He was flattering of MacDonald. 'If there is anything in manipulative theory, then it is better to do what Kelman MacDonald did and do it as a postgraduate course.'

Sir Henry Britten Brackenbury

He was a registered medical practitioner on the GMC, and was Vice-President of the BMA.

Elibank raised the issue of MacDonald's ostracism and the difficulty Streeter had finding an anaesthetist. Brackenbury claimed there was considerable freedom to consult with MacDonald. That he could not follow a case to a fever hospital, 'Applies to all of us'. Following further questioning from Elibank, he argued he would not deprecate any ostracism of osteopaths. Lord Elibank then asked why Axham was struck off. (See Chapter 1). Brackenbury explained that the GMC only investigates a situation if there is a complaint. Later Lord Redesdale ascertained that the anaesthetist would examine a patient and therefore assume responsibility.

Brackenbury referred to the large number of GPs in colliery areas who practised manipulative skills and that the medical curriculum was revised in 1926 and the importance of manipulation had increased. 'There were 'many hundreds' of doctors capable of doing the osteopathic work, the manipulative work, certainly more than the osteopaths…who were almost all concentrated in the wealthier districts.'

The difficulty of distinguishing between major and minor surgery was discussed. In rural areas it was necessary to do a wider range of surgical operations, i.e. it was difficult for someone to be permitted to perform minor surgery alone.

He considered diagnosis important in medicine, but an osteopath's diagnosis was really directed to the location of a spinal osteopathic lesion. Having diagnosed, there were other classes of persons to whom he (Brackenbury) could turn to: the Chartered Society of Masseurs, 'biophysical assistants', who had a voluntary register and had to pass examinations, but they could not treat without a patient going through a doctor, as they could not diagnose.

He considered that there would be a problem administering more than one Register under two different government departments. There would be even greater difficulties in establishing a criterion of incapacity for work under the National Health Insurance Act, with a different body of persons looking at health questions from a different angle. Osteopaths would have had to be represented at maternity and Child Welfare Centres. Every child would need to have its spine examined if the incidence of infectious diseases was related to an osteopathic lesion. two sets of Medical Officers of Health would have been needed. It might also lead to a recrudescence of agitation against inoculation for smallpox.

He quoted Louis Reed regarding Osteopathy in America: 'Following the development of Chiropractic the growth of Osteopathy has practically stopped and also due to Osteopathy approaching medicine and taking over its therapeutic agents. With the rise in osteopathic standards the sect ceased to attract those who wanted to become healing practitioners on short order....Osteopaths dilute the quality of medical care available....A group of substandard medical practitioners.'

Harold Murphy raised a formal objection that while Streeter, Littlejohn and MacDonald had experience of Osteopathy all over the US, not a single question was put to them on matters elicited from someone who admitted quite candidly that he had only just visited there.

The claim that in the US Osteopathy had ceased to grow, Jowitt argued, was a result of the Basic Sciences Laws and that Streeter had the opportunity to provide figures, but had been unable to do so. (Streeter shook his head, but Jowitt argued he had).

Brackenbury was asked why he made enquiries regarding Osteopathy in Canada....'For no reason except that I wanted to.' Elibank pushed the matter....'Because he thought there was or was not something in Osteopathy?' Brackenbury claimed he was interested, 'In the sociological point of view—social welfare and public health developments'.

On questioning on the alleged decline in Osteopathy in the US, he replied that Osteopathy had approached so nearly the medical standard that those who wished to go in for healing took the full medical course. Those who did not went over to Chiropractic. Lord Esher argued that, 'Not having been to America, of course, you have not studied the psychology of the American people? They are people who get tired of one thing more quickly than any nation in the world and move across to the latest fashion.'

Murphy ascertained it was not a Government Committee that he had quoted and Reed was simply an individual member of the Committee expressing his own views. Nothing indicated in his report had received the approval of the Committee as a whole. Murphy argued that Reed's report indicated that (osteopathic) educational standards had risen. He was asked if there were official figures indicating that Osteopathy was, 'Dying in the country of its birth'....Brackenbury replied, 'Yes', but he did not have them with him. Murphy considered that, 'Not much inference could be drawn from the fact that the figures were rising for ten years and were now stationary'.

Murphy had figures from the Office of Education of the US Department of the Interior showing an increase in osteopaths from 1930-32. He claimed, 'The figures that you have given for Nebraska and Washington have nothing on earth to do with the fortunes of people possessed of a Diploma in Osteopathy who have passed a Basic Sciences

Examination'. The view was later stated that the decline in the number of schools could be due to a desire to raise standards of education.

Brackenbury claimed the BMA did not oppose a Register, only a State Register, which would, 'Give a cachet of authority to theories and beliefs which are unaccepted by almost the whole scientific world and imply to the public some sort of State guarantee that there is a scientific foundation. Once there is a State Register then the State is obliged to see that those people who need Osteopathy receive it: maternity and child welfare clinics, Poor Law persons, National Health Insurance, in hospitals.' He agreed that he was not advancing the inconvenience to the State as an argument against the Bill....'Not if it can be scientifically proven, then there would be only one Register.'

Brackenbury claimed he was not condemning manipulative treatment. 'The value has been increasingly recognised of later years.' He gave osteopaths credit for having brought the matter forward. 'I have no doubt whatever that there has been much drugging and too little manipulation....I should like to give the osteopaths every credit for having enhanced those points.'

He objected to the claims of osteopaths, 'To deal with all diseases and theories of causation, which as far as I can see have no foundation whatever. It seemed illogical to give a right to treat all diseases, which presupposes an ability to diagnose and at the same time to withhold a right to sign death certificates. The Medical Register would have to be wiped out if the osteopathic theory were true as the basic principles of medicine would have been proved false.' Other objections he had to the Bill were that it would set an inferior medical education with regard to duration and there was a compulsory bias of the teachers in one direction.

The Chairman argued that medical education was biased. Brackenbury claimed that medical education is based on basic sciences. 'Those who believe the world to be round are biased against those who believe the world to be flat.' Dickens asked, 'What sort of bias does a student get, if any, at a medical school?...Brackenbury replied, 'No bias....In fact nothing is taught as a fact which has not been accepted as a fact by the general body of the scientific world'. Lord Redesdale asked him to confirm that medical students in their training are taught to keep an open mind.

Jowitt asked if osteopaths would feel themselves to be pariahs by the medical profession if the Bill was passed. 'They would be like the lion and the lamb lying down together.'

Brackenbury claimed that the Register would not lead to closer collaboration with those with biased education and fixed ideas. Anybody on the Register would be somebody he had no use for.

Lord Elibank asked how collaboration could be brought about. Brackenbury had claimed that some osteopaths were doing good work. Jowitt suggested that, like MacDonald, osteopaths should first become medically qualified, or have a register like the Chartered Society of Masseurs, so that cases were referred to them by doctors.

Lord Esher asked, 'You said in your evidence that the osteopathic theory had been repudiated by the scientific world, but MacDonald said he made continual efforts to get the scientific world to examine his theories?' Brackenbury disputed this.

Lord Dawson confirmed that the main difficulty the medical profession had was the osteopath's claim to cover the whole field of disease, including constitutional diseases. However, of the many thousands of patients treated by osteopaths, there had never been a death.

St John Raikes took exception to Buzzard's statement that Osteopathy was the forerunner of Chiropractic and Chiropractic, 'was an old form of faith cure', and to Brackenbury that, 'the less scientific become chiropractors'. 'If the knowledge of Osteopathy by those who are opposing this Bill is on par with their knowledge of Chiropractic, I am afraid they will not carry you very far in arriving at a just conclusion.'

James Beaver Mennell

He was Medical Officer of the Physico-therapeutic Department at St Thomas's Hospital and had spent 30 years in orthopaedic surgery. He started joint manipulation in 1907 and wrote a book on 'Back-ache'. He explained what he meant by manipulation.

MacDonald had claimed that Mennell's book (*Physical Treatment by Movement, Manipulation and Massage*) read like an osteopathic textbook and was, 'Inspired by our teachings'. Mennell, however, claimed that he did not hold with the osteopathic theory or any part of it, that he learnt treatment by mobilisation from Lucas-Championniere in Paris and he never encountered Osteopathy before 1919. He had seen an osteopath (who was also a qualified practitioner) treat two patients and he had read 'Osteopathic Mechanics' and read Tasker and several osteopathic journals, but by that time he had already gone far with his own work. If he stole from osteopaths, then they had stolen from bone-setters.

He could not accept that childhood diseases were due to an osteopathic lesion. He considered that standards of training must be of the highest before it was safe to practise and warned against accepting training lower than that of a medical school.

He claimed patients may be led to believe that they have a definite lesion of the spine from which they have not recovered, and presumably never will recover. 'The psychological injury of that infliction is incalculable.' He was critical of those who claim, 'A bone is out of place'.

He considered it important to have a foundation in every branch of medicine before specialisation, i.e. it is not wasting time for an osteopathic student to study all the matters studied by a medical student. 'He ought to have an adequate knowledge to know when he himself is ignorant.'

Mennell considered the theory of Osteopathy to be founded on fallacy. He agreed that there are certain types of cases in which properly qualified osteopaths could undoubtedly bring benefit. 'The thing that has kept back the whole of this particular branch of physical treatment is the theory.'

He admitted he had met osteopaths (e.g. Pheils, the Chairman of the Education Committee of the BOA) to discuss the standard of education that orthodox medicine would consider acceptable. No conclusions were reached.

He agreed with Thorpe that he had a tremendous amount in common with osteopaths, 'Except their creed'. Thorpe questioned him regarding a confidential letter he had written to one of his pupils, Dr Ousdel in April 1931 claiming that A.T. Still was his 'great master' and stating, 'I know quite well the truth of your statement that every figure and every page is a corroboration of the teaching of Dr Andrew Taylor Still.' Mennell claimed it was the creed that was the heresy. It was manipulation he had in mind when he wrote that. He also wrote in the letter, 'The great point gained is that I have been able to produce an osteopathic textbook.' Mennell was grieved at these quotations as the letter was written in confidence.

He supported manipulation, but it was not appropriate for pneumonia and meningitis and was practised by orthodox practitioners. Mennell's work was to establish manipulation on a sound, scientific foundation.

He could not think of a single situation in which manipulation was preventative. He insisted that manipulation was founded on science not a craft.

Viscount Elibank asked, 'Because medicine had certain beliefs 50 years ago which are not held today, that would not stop you practising medicine? Surely that is rather belittling the whole subject if you say, I am not going to admit Osteopathy because of the theory on which it is founded. At the same time I am going to admit the practice of Osteopathy is all right.' Mennell denied this was a contradiction as to accept Osteopathy is to accept the creed regarding the primacy of the cause of all disease.

Sir Morton Smart

He worked at 40 Park Lane. Since 1896 he had practised and studied manipulation and written a textbook and articles on the subject. He considered that manipulative surgery required a sound knowledge of medical science. Osteopaths were of value, but under the direction of a medical practitioner.

He had studied osteopathic literature for a long time and lectured on the subject, both in the UK and in the US. He considered Osteopathy was based on a theory which was unsound and unscientific. The Bill if passed would give approval to the Principles of Osteopathy in spite of the overwhelming evidence that the medical profession disagreed.

He acknowledged the practice was valuable in some cases — but not universally so and 'Osteopathy had now wandered far from the original theory and now embraced practically every method of treatment known to scientific medicine'. Osteopaths themselves had realised that the original theory could not possibly be the cause of all diseases and they had taken every other method that they could lay their hands on to get a result. Osteopaths were adopting the Materia Medica in the States. He quoted Still's plea for, 'Simon Pure'.

He considered that while the vox populi — public opinion — was in favour of Osteopathy, there was also a large number of people who had been to osteopaths and not successfully treated and were not keen to have osteopaths on a Register. Viscount Elibank asked, 'Would you not apply that to doctors as well?' Smart argued that successes are not evidence that the treatment is scientifically sound. He considered that cures in Osteopathy are isolated cases. There are temporary cures, coincidences, or cures in spite of treatment, actual cures, failures and causes of harm. He considered that there was indisputable evidence that harm has been caused by osteopathic manipulation, bad manipulation, or manipulation of wrong cases, e.g. treating a tumour of the brain. There was also the danger of psychological effects on the patient. He described the case of a girl who was told that due to contracture of the pelvic outlet she would be in danger if she had children, but this was not substantiated by X-ray.

'If registration is based on public use it would be impossible to decline registration to any and every cult which can prove popularity with the public, e.g. chiropractic and nature-healers command as large a support as osteopaths.'

'I think it would be intolerable that diplomates of the BSO should be placed on a State Register after what we have heard. Little is known of the standard of education in the American colleges. No (American) college should be recognised for the purposes of the British State Register. Half the membership of the BOA is American therefore there would be a powerful American influence on the Board. I have never been able to understand from anything I have read what an osteopathic lesion is; the basis of their theory.' He was not opposed to the Bill because of fears of competition.

He considered that the majority of patients get better in spite of osteopathic treatment. He admitted there are cases where patients had gone from a medical man to an osteopath. Cases had been presented of cures. 'It is almost pathetic how inaccurate they are....They are extraordinarily exaggerated.'

There had been widespread acceptance of manipulative surgery since Sir Robert Jones. (See Chapter 1.) Smart had treated nine riders of the Grand National and personally examined thousands of spines. His interest in manipulation came from bone-setters, as with Jones.

Smart acknowledged Osteopathy would have advantages if osteopaths were trained to a minimal standard and they ignored the theory. The five years' training of osteopaths depended on a standard assured by the Board. The response was that in America, in spite of a Board, it was not controllable. 'It will be impossible to bring them to the standard of Universities.' He was opposed to a Register as it would open the door for every cult. 'The Bill would not protect the public. People would still practise, but not call themselves osteopaths.'

Sir Norman Walker

He was 28 years on the GMC and President of it for over three of these. He claimed there was no monopoly on medicine, but Thorpe challenged that.

He considered, 'The Bill would create confusion in the mind of the public'. A Register would contain the names of people whose standards of education varied from that of the GMC. Not everyone would be able to differentiate between one Register and another.

He favoured a Royal Commission to investigate Osteopathy. But who would sit on it? Who could be impartial? Buzzard had indicated that the theories of Osteopathy and medical science were incompatible and contradictory. Lord Esher claimed, 'You are the first medical witness we have heard who has not shown a prejudice against Osteopathy'....'My business here is neither to oppose nor to favour.'

He confirmed that it was not illegal to give anaesthetics. The ruling of administration of anaesthetics for an unqualified practitioner applied to dentists. Before the 1921 Dentists' Act, medical men were enabling unqualified dentists to practice. From 1898-1912 there were only si9x charges, all but one referred to dentists. four cases were proved, but the names were not erased. Only Axham's name was erased. (See Chapter 1). He could not understand why Streeter should have difficulty finding an anaesthetist. There was no problem with anaesthetists assisting osteopaths, providing the anaesthetist made the diagnosis.

George Ernest Gask

He was Professor of Surgery in the University of London and worked at St Bartholomew's Hospital. He had no objections to a Register if osteopaths had a thorough instruction in surgery as he believed there was no hard and fast line between major and minor surgery.

He had signed Buzzard's statement. Thorpe asked him, 'Would you sign a statement without hearing a prisoner's defence? How far did he call on the prisoner for his defence?...How had the statement come to you?'...'On the table at the staff common room.' Not all had signed.

Jenkins then cross-questioned him. 'Had he experienced malformations of the spine to be associated with disease?'...'No.'... 'Would he be able to detect an osteopathic lesion?'...'We do not think that there is one chief cause of disease.' He agreed that if research was submitted it would be given careful consideration.

Lord Esher asked him if he had he actually looked for an osteopathic lesion. 'You have not been really making what we could call a scientific examination of the osteopathic theory?'

Gask argued that osteopaths should be just as capable of making a diagnosis as a medical practitioner, but agreed that qualified medical practitioners made mistakes.

Gask admitted not having read the Bill carefully, despite the fact that he signed the statement. Jenkins argued that the statement was against Osteopathy, not the Bill, but Elibank challenged that. The statement was to the Select Committee considering the Bill.

Sir Arthur Robinson

He had been Permanent Secretary to the Ministry of Health for almost 15 years. He considered there should be a full enquiry into the theory before recognising the Bill, to test the validity of the claims of Osteopathy, conducted by the Medical Research Council. He considered that pending an enquiry there should be no State Register, but a voluntary Register. The Register would also be a cachet for the soundness of the sect.

There would be no right to put an osteopath on the panel. Robinson considered that it would be difficult to refuse access to osteopaths to children with infectious diseases and the whole state services connected with health matters would have to be duplicated.

S. P. Vivian

He was Registrar General. Discussion centred on whether osteopaths should be allowed to sign death certificates. The Bill had since been modified to exclude this.

Reginald Cheyne Elmsie

He was an orthopaedic surgeon at St Bartholomew's Hospital and appeared on behalf of the Royal College of Surgeons. He objected to the Bill on three points. Firstly, it was impossible within any reasonable time to establish a system of education of the quality of a medical student. Secondly, manipulative surgery was already available. Thirdly, there were risks of manipulative surgery undertaken by osteopaths inadequately trained. He considered that the existence of spinal lesions had not been proven. He was also concerned about the influence on the 'massage profession'.

In Britain there were only five osteopaths with medical qualifications. Others were British (BSO), or American-trained osteopaths, but only some American colleges were recognised by the BOA. His hospital, however, required 25 Departments to teach medicine and had a complex curriculum.

He considered that the ordinary methods of diagnosis used in scientific medicine are to a large extent ignored by osteopaths. He saw six to eight patients a week who had seen an osteopath. 'I have no hesitation in saying that the average osteopath does not take the steps to arrive at an accurate diagnosis that would be taken by a responsible medical man.'

He considered that, 'Either Osteopathy is a complete system of healing in which case the training, qualification and experience should be equivalent to that of a medical man, or it is simply a system of manipulation, then it should be ancillary to medical practice, as is massage. If osteopaths have unique techniques then either there should be postgraduate instruction of medical practitioners, or they should practise under the direction of medical practitioners.' He believed that there were risks involved in Osteopathy, e.g. forcible manipulation under anaesthesia. Backache may be due to sinister causes requiring accurate diagnosis without delay. Osteopathy leads a patient to presume something is seriously wrong with their spines.

He was Chairman of the Council of the Chartered Society of Massage and Medical Gymnastics, who were opposed to osteopaths. The Ling system (on which its system of therapeutics was based) dated from 1812. The Society was founded in 1894 with the object of safeguarding the profession and furthering the study and practice of massage by establishing an examining body. In 1900 it was incorporated by licence of the Board of Trade. During the First World War the Almeric Paget Corps undertook massage work. In 1920 it was granted a Royal Charter. There were 9,000-10,000 members in 1935.

Henry Sessions Souttar

He was a surgeon and emphasised the importance of the clinical side of training, such as a medical person receives, if an osteopath is to treat every kind of disease. He quoted a pamphlet and also from McConnell and Teal's textbook of Osteopathy regarding the predisposition for diphtheria. He considered it was 'fraudulent'. five years of training would make no difference.

Interruption

Thorpe interrupted the proceedings as he considered that the desirability that the osteopaths should prove the scientific justification for their theories before such a Register was granted was a new issue being pursued during the enquiry. He recommended an enquiry in the form of a Royal Commission, or some equally constituted or responsible body, to consider the scientific justification for the theory and practice of Osteopathy.

Horace Bramwell Bennett

He was an accountant whose family had been treated by osteopaths for six years. His wife had a long period of discomfort and pain after the birth of their first child. After the birth of the second, she saw osteopaths (Barrow and Oxenham). She required only three weeks confinement instead of 15 months. His sister had valvular disease of the heart and she could have died. Barrow, in consultation with Littlejohn, treated her, which was a complete success. She became an enthusiastic folk dancer. He was treated for a liver disorder, but he could not explain to Lord Dawson what it was.

Florence MacNaught

When living in Dublin she had a swelling in the neck diagnosed as Grave's disease. She saw a specialist in London. It was considered incurable, but she could not have an operation because of her heart. She was treated in Dublin by an osteopath for three to four months and the symptoms disappeared. She then went to Siam with her husband and lived in the jungle. Her husband was treated for neuritis by Harvey Foote.

Walter William Hughes

He was station foreman at Enfield. He hurt his leg and hip through jumping on the line. The pain got worse and it was diagnosed as rheumatism. He lost weight and his leg shrunk. His Doctor claimed that arthritis had set in and he would be crippled for life. He was treated by Harvey Foote. His weight and leg returned to normal.

Colonel Henry Cecil Lloyd Howard

Three years previously his wife had neuritis in her arm. Medical treatment did not do her much good. She saw Streeter who, 'Cured her completely'. Howard was sceptical of osteopaths. He had a stiff back, shoulders and legs. He had broken bones in both his legs in the past. His GP advised shoe inserts. His father suffered from arthritis and Parkinson's disease and he was concerned he might develop them. Streeter treated him under anaesthesia and he was then able to play squash every night. He had been treated 82 times since 1932 and was still under treatment.

He was a Trustee to his nephew, Lord Kenyon, who was short-sighted. Two eminent oculists advised Kenyon to leave Eton at once. Kenyon then saw Streeter, but his mother was sceptical. In a fortnight the boy could dispense with his spectacles. Previously he could not read the top letter of the opticians card at one foot. After treatment he could read the bottom line at five feet.

Lord Dawson wanted reports from the oculist. Thorpe suggested the reports should be obtained by an official.

Sir Hereward Wake

He had a riding fall and injured his spine. It got worse. He saw several therapists. He was recommended to rest for a year on his back. He did so for three months and still he was no better. He received Osteopathy for 20 years from Prat, a partner of Streeter, in Glasgow. He had since sent a number of family and friends to Streeter. Treatment was always successful. He considered that in some cases the diagnosis was correct, when it had previously not been so with other therapists. He was volunteering evidence to protect the public against unqualified osteopaths and to make treatments available in hospital. 'I never have a cold so long as I have a little osteopathic treatment.'

He admitted he sent his boys to Streeter when their tonsils were bad, but despite treatment one boy had to have them out. When a horse kicked him in the shin, however, he went to an ordinary medical man.

Dr Harold K. G. Hodgson

He was radiologist at the Middlesex Hospital. He examined MacDonald's X-rays: seven plates of three cases, allegedly showing curvature of the spine, before and after treatment, but Hodgson did not consider the cases novel and believed that they were treatable by orthodox means. MacDonald claimed that one plate showed an osteopathic lesion at a particular location but Hodgson claimed there was nothing unusual there. Hodgson claimed the reason why a joint can and cannot be seen is due to the angle of the tube. two of the X-rays differed, as one was a poor X-ray. He agreed that bony maladjustments may be absent on film, but palpable, but that is because oedema or fibrosis are present. What MacDonald described was the ordinary adolescent curvature of the spine.

To prove that soft tissue changes are not evident on X-ray, Hodgson had undertaken some experiments with Porterhouse steak—cutting it in two and water-logging one piece and then X-raying them on a young man's abdomen. No difference was found. He took radiograms of his butler's spine before and after the butler drank a pint of beer. No difference could be discerned. He injected 40 teaspoonfuls of fluid into a corpse inside and along the spine. No difference was seen. A patient had seven major operations and was covered in scars but none were seen on X-ray. An Achilles tendon is not evident on X-ray. Thorpe argued that the experiment with the steak and butler were not real oedema. Hodgson claimed the effect would be the same. It is impossible to show oedema and fibrosis in an osteopathic lesion. MacDonald had referred to fibrosis of the 'lateral ligaments'. Hodgson denied there were any as at that location the nerves and vessels were located.

Hodgson once had difficulty in understanding what was meant by an 'osteopathic lesion', but he had since read MacDonald's book. He considered that there was no evidence of the relationship between lesions of the spine and abdominal disease. He had often looked for such, but never found it.

Thorpe considered his interpretation may not be that of another medical person. Hodgson considered that there was not one radiologist in this country who would agree with what MacDonald had said.

Regarding an X-ray of a girl with an alleged pelvic twist, MacDonald claimed it was a single curvature, whereas Hodgson claimed it was double. Hodgson was critical in that the hip joint was not included. The person may not have been standing correctly. MacDonald said he took care to see that the child was standing straight. Thorpe considered that the only thing that emerged was that the witness and MacDonald did not agree.

Sir Henry Halett Dale FRS

He was Director of the Central Research Institute for the Medical Research Council. He inspected the A. T. Still Research Bulletins 2, 3, 5, 6, 7, especially Bulletin No. 2. and considered, 'They do not seem to me to have the first qualification of a real scientific investigation. Experiments were carried out in order to provide what might look like evidence for a theory already accepted.'

He was asked, 'Did you find throughout the Bulletins you looked at any evidence that justified the attribution of particular diseases to particular osteopathic lesions?'...'I found none that would convince me at all.'...'Would Osteopathy be worthy of enquiry?'...'There is no scientific basis to enquire about.'

It emerged that he had the Bulletins for less than a week. He had only read No. two and the others hurriedly. 'Approaching them from a scientific point of view, I find then entirely unconvincing. If I were called upon to make a detailed critical examination of the evidence...I think it would take several months.' He would not do so as he considered the evidence largely repetition and unconvincing. Lord Esher stated, 'Once again we come back then to the fact that the medical profession will never admit that the fact that people are cured by a thing is prima facie evidence of its value'. Dale did not think that the evidence tendered for the scientific basis of Osteopathy would justify the expenditure of public money.

Final Statement for the Case

Thorpe summed up:

'In the course of the enquiry it became inevitable that a different issue should be presented. That issue, as I understand it, took this form, that it was desirable before such Register was granted that the osteopaths should prove scientific justification for their theory.

The Bill requires for its main structure the existence and continuance of the British School of Osteopathy. You will remember that Dr MacDonald in his evidence said he himself was not satisfied with the standard taught at that school...and my clients do not feel justified, in asking your Lordships to pass the Bill with the School as it is at present constituted occupying that position in the new organisation. That being so my clients say that we should not be justified in asking your Lordships to pass this particular Bill. He would not try to induce their Lordships to pass something which we believe to be fundamentally unsatisfactory.

I am instructed to say that immediately a voluntary register of osteopaths will be formed and as soon as possible a school of Osteopathy, qualified in the view of the osteopaths to give a proper training, will be constituted....It is not for me to do more than urge respectfully upon the Committee that an enquiry in the form of a Royal Commission or some equally responsible body should be asked to consider the scientific justification for the theory and practice of Osteopathy.'

The four supporting parties intimated that if an enquiry were set up then none of those who signed the statement from teachers in the universities and medical schools should be appointed to serve on it. To appoint medical men would be inappropriate as Osteopathy and medicine are based on different principles. Any findings by osteopaths were considered unacceptable to the opposition.[6]

Summary of Outcome

Before the evidence of those opposing the Bill had been concluded, the supporters of the Bill decided not to proceed as they desired that the scientific basis of Osteopathy be further explored. Furthermore, 'They could not properly ask for a measure which required for its full operation the granting of powers to the British School of Osteopathy, the present constitution of which the principal supporters did not approve'.

The principal object of the Bill was to protect the public against the practice of Osteopathy by incompetent or unqualified persons. The Counsel, in opening the case for the Bill, put it that it would be sufficient for him to establish (a) that Osteopathy was extensively practised, and (b) that the public in large and increasing numbers were desirous of being treated by it. He asked that Parliament should authorise the establishment of a state register for osteopaths, with a prescribed qualifying education and standard of proficiency.

'In all comparable cases for which a Statutory Register has been authorised, three conditions have been fulfilled: (i) The sphere or territory within which the vocation operates has been clearly defined; (ii) The vocation has long been in general use; (iii) There has been already in existence a well established and efficient system of voluntary examination and registration.

The establishment of a State Register also gives the guarantee of Parliament that persons...registered are within their own sphere worthy, and the only persons worthy, of the public confidence.

In the case of the Osteopathy none of these conditions were considered to be fulfilled:

(i)   No definition of Osteopathy was included in the Bill as introduced, and although one was subsequently proposed for inclusion in the Bill, and others suggested, none emerged which satisfactorily differentiated the osteopathic sphere of activity.

(ii)   The practice of Osteopathy...is carried on in the United Kingdom by no more than 2,000-3,000 practitioners, of whom only about 170 can claim to be "qualified".

(iii) The only existing establishment in this country for the education and examination of osteopaths was exposed, in the course of evidence before us, as being of negligible importance, inefficient for its purpose, and above all in thoroughly dishonest hands. Pending the setting up of any adequate machinery in this country, therefore, the only training ground would be North America, and it is alien to recognise qualifications which have been conferred by foreign educational institutions. Moreover the Committee had no evidence before them as to the standard of education of osteopaths in North America.

In view of the fact that the establishment of a Statutory Register would give something in the nature of a 'hallmark' to Osteopathy, the Committee felt it their duty to enquire at some length into the nature and value of osteopathic treatment. It emerged clearly that Osteopathy is not—as popularly supposed—a craft or art limited to the treatment of maladies or defects of the bones etc. by manipulation; in this sphere the Committee has no doubt that qualified osteopaths perform valuable services. They may even possibly be regarded as having at one time developed a technique in advance of medical science, which has to some extent been accepted by members of the medical profession who practise what is called "manipulative surgery". Osteopathy, however, claims to be a method of healing which is suitable for the treatment of *all diseases of any description.* 'We claim', said Dr. Streeter in evidence, 'We have a different school of healing, and we want provision made for it, and an orthodox curriculum. We want to develop along our own lines; we feel we are just as competent as any physician to act as a family physician and General Practitioner.'

As the law stands, anyone is entitled to practise the art of healing, but only registered medical practitioners are entitled to hold themselves out as duly qualified to treat all diseases. Were the present Bill to pass, registered osteopaths would be entitled to make a like claim. It is true that, on no logical principle, provisions were proposed for insertion in the Bill, excluding osteopaths from the right to perform 'major surgery', to practice midwifery, to administer anaesthetics and to give certificates of the cause of death; but neither of the distinguished practising osteopaths who gave evidence before us would recede in any way from the full claim of Osteopathy to treat all disease.

It is hardly necessary to point out the far reaching nature of this claim, involving as it does the statutory recognition of two alternative, and to a great extent conflicting, theories of healing. Dr. Kelman MacDonald explained his views as to the scientific basis upon which the osteopathic theory reposes, and the Committee would wish to pay tribute to the ability and sincerity of this witness; but Dr. MacDonald is actually a registered medical practitioner, and, whilst he clung to the formulae on which Osteopathy is based, it was clear that in actual practice he would not deny his patients, where necessary, the benefit of appropriate medical or surgical treatment.

On the other hand, in answer to a question whether the Bill would, 'Provide a bridge over which one will be able to pass and meet the other in the middle', he answered, 'I think so, but on the other hand, you must remember that our views on the actual causation of disease, and our general guiding principles, and our form of treatment are all at complete variance with those of the medical school'.

The Committee accept the claim that cures are frequently effected by osteopathic methods. On the other hand there have been some failures. The same may be said of other methods of healing. The Committee have not been in any considerable degree influenced by evidence either of cures or failures.

The Committee find on the evidence before them that the claim of the osteopaths to be able to treat all diseases has not been established, and that it would not be safe or proper for Parliament to recognise osteopathic practitioners as qualified, on a similar footing to that of registered medical practitioners.

Further, the Committee are of the opinion that the question of establishing a Register of qualified osteopaths by Act of Parliament should be deferred until the sphere of Osteopathy has been defined, and a system of education in the principles and practice of Osteopathy has been developed in one or more well equipped and properly conducted institutions.

A question was raised in the course of the hearing as to whether there should be what was described as 'scientific' enquiry into the merits of the principles and practice of Osteopathy. The President of the General Medical Council said he had no objection to such an enquiry. The Minister of Health considered that before any Register was authorised by statute the theory and practice of Osteopathy should be established by such an enquiry.

The Committee recommend that the Bill proceed no further. It was withdrawn by its sponsors on 12 April 1935.[1,6]

References

1. Report from the Select Committee of the House of Lords appointed to consider the Registration and Regulation of Osteopaths Bill [H.L.] together with the proceedings of the committee and minutes of evidence. (1935). (London:HMSO).
2. British Medical Association (1935). The Osteopaths Bill. A report of the proceedings before a select committee of the House of Lords. (1935). (London: BMA).
3. *The British Osteopathic Review*. (1935). May.
4. Dutton, C. Personal communication.
5. *The Journal of Osteopathy*. (1935). June-August, VI(3 & 4): 3.
6. McKeon, L. C. Floyd (1938). Osteopathic Polemics, pp. 97-104. (London: C. W. Daniel Co. Ltd).

Chapter 7

Following the Bill—The Formation of the GCRO

The outcome of the Select Committee of the House of Lords was the recommendation of a voluntary Register. Before that could be effectively achieved wounds had to be healed and a greater trust and respect developed between rival factions.

Littlejohn's response

Littlejohn (and senior Faculty at the BSO) were particularly angered by the personal criticism that he and the School had received at the Select Committee.

His response was published in the *Journal of Osteopathy*.[1] As he was editor of the Journal it is probable it was actually written by him. Some key points were as follows. They have been included in detail as they indicate the strength of feeling:

'(1) It is stated, 'The claim of the osteopaths to be able to treat all diseases has not been established.' The British School of Osteopathy made and makes no such claim.

(2) "The Committee accepts the claim that cures are frequently effected by osteopathic methods. On the other hand there have been some failures." The same may be said of other methods of healing. This we all accept.

(3) "The Committee is of the opinion that the establishing a Register of qualified osteopaths by Act of Parliament should be deferred until Osteopathy has been defined and a system of education in the principles and practice of Osteopathy has been developed in one or more well-equipped and properly conducted institutions." This means, postponing the recognition and regulation until Osteopathy is fully established. Attempts have been made to do this by the BSO for the past 18 years against all sorts of prejudice and opposition....Its demonstration depends upon clinical results. The British School of Osteopathy is now assisting in the development of an Institute of Osteopathic Research to attain this ideal.

(4) ...It is stated that only about 170 can claim to be qualified. Of these about 70 are American-trained osteopaths, the remaining 100 being BSO graduates, whom the Committee, therefore, recognise and acknowledge as entitled to claim to be qualified. This was admitted by Dr MacDonald. The hands of the British School of Osteopathy are said to be dishonest. Were they dishonest hands that treated and taught how to treat gratuitously the 24,000 cases which passed through the clinic last year, without casualty, some of the poorest people with beneficial results? Were they dishonest hands that taught pure Osteopathy and never once trod on the heels of medical or surgical practitioners? Was Dr Mennell dishonest when he told one story in America and another in England regarding Osteopathy?'

'Osteopathy is too big a science to be destroyed by prejudice or to be handicapped by epithets of dishonour from whatever source these come. The people know, will judge and in due time will see to it that Osteopathy receives its proper recognition in the field of healing. Meantime, we pursue, as our American predecessors did when called dishonest, our course undisturbed. We appeal to the people, as every great movement had done.'

'Many misstatements have been published in the press. It was definitely stated that the British School of Osteopathy was the chief prop on which the Bill was built as originally introduced. Everyone connected with Osteopathy knows that this Bill was prepared by one man, Dr W. A. Streeter, without any consultation with the British School of Osteopathy or any of its representatives. Dr J. J. Dunning has stated that the Bill was prepared by two practising osteopaths, neither of them members of the British Osteopathic Association, and that the BOA stepped in to save Osteopathy. The *"Osteopathic Review"* says that the British School of Osteopathy was discredited. How? Only by insinuation and statements presented in cross-examination. The truth is, Osteopathy was discredited; Dr A. T. Still was discredited; Dr MacDonald's idea of Osteopathy and the Osteopathic lesion and even his X-rays were all discredited by the Medical witnesses. All of this, however, was personal opinion based on prejudice and ignorance.'

'The *"Journal of Osteopathy,"* Kirksville, says that the British School of Osteopathy was not satisfactory and could not be included in its present form. The counsel for the supporters of the Bill kept saying repeatedly that Dr MacDonald was dissatisfied with the teaching of the British School of Osteopathy. The only true statement is that given by the British Medical Council in its report in the BMA Journal, that Sir Wm. Jowitt *suggested* that the British School of Osteopathy graduates were not worthy of consideration. By a process of quibbling, bullying and insinuation, counsel tried to make out that the Dean of the School had taken in the Looker students on six months' credit; and that the statement of the Dean of the School that the students were attending medical schools for the pre-medical work and the second year work in anatomy, physiology and dissection were untrue. Both of these statements (*i.e. the criticisms*) were proved untrue by the evidence submitted in writing giving proof that the Looker School had a three year course, and that all students taken in had, not only three years' credit of work done, but also special studies for three years under their own association and 12 months' accredited work under the BSO, passing the final examination satisfactorily. In addition the names of the 1st and 2nd year students of the British School of Osteopathy and the Medical Schools they had attended or were attending were also furnished, giving a complete answer to the challenge of counsel.'

'The BSO did not claim perfection. It stated what had been done in face of difficulties and obstacles presented by the medical profession and the medical authorities and existing regulations and conditions of educational institutions. The British School of Osteopathy expressed its readiness to adopt the five year course. As a matter of fact the BSO passed a resolution by its Board of Directors in June 1934, before the present Bill was introduced, setting forth the five year course as the standard of education and expressed the hope that facilities would be offered for the full training in Osteopathy, not in Medicine and Surgery, as the policy of the School. What was there under those conditions to prevent Parliament from passing a Bill granting a certificate to practise Osteopathy "without the use of Drugs and Major Surgery" as in the laws in active existence in the majority of States of the US? To comply with this the teaching and the facilities for full qualification were absolutely adequate in the BSO.'

'We do not criticise the curriculum in our Schools of Medicine.... We do not profess to teach Medicine, so called, or Major Surgery, because these belong to the fields of specialism which we have found by experience to be non-essential in the equipment of the ordinary osteopathic practitioner. (BSO Annual Prospectus 1934-1935).'

'When counsel for the supporters kept stating that Dr MacDonald did not acknowledge the BSO he forgot or seemed to forget that Dr MacDonald stated: "The BSO has been conducted by Dr Littlejohn and we all admire his effort. It is an individual effort and it has not yet been enabled to bring its educational standard up to the level at which we would like it....It is the only reputable school in England." This admits the effort to build up a School towards the point of recognition. Later Dr MacDonald states that the difficulties in the way of the building up of a School had been the reason for no "proper" School being in England. The same conditions existed in the United States in the early years of Osteopathy and in the early history of medical schools both in this country and in the United States. The building up process is a gradual one and the evolution must be slow, especially when every obstacle is put in the way of progress by those who antagonise the idea of osteopathic therapy. The same is found in the evolution of any science or system of education.'

'When the Select Committee was appointed by the House of Lords, all parties were invited to co-operate, which seemed to be the case up to the point of the statement made by Dr MacDonald that he, speaking for the BOA, the first time disunion was projected, said he did not recognise the teaching of the BSO. How and in what way no one can tell, because neither he nor any of his colleagues ever entered the BSO much less knew what it was teaching or how it was teaching. Dr Streeter had previously said he did not know and the BSO could speak for itself. This opened the door for all the insinuations presented in the cross-examination by Counsel for the British Medical Association. The purview of this is best expressed in the language of the BMA supplement to the BMA Journal, June 2nd, 1935, page 272, in the supplementary report of the Council. "Counsel for the Bill indicated in his opening speech that the principal argument of the supporters of the Bill was that the public was going in large numbers to osteopaths for treatment, and that therefore whether Osteopathy had a sound or scientific basis or not, it was in the interests of the public to enable it to distinguish the osteopath who had received some training from the osteopath who had received none. It was no part of his case, he said, that Osteopathy was founded on scientific truth, and he submitted that the Committee was not concerned with this aspect". This in short compass is a true statement of fact and of the basis of united support of the supporters of the Bill. In fact, the Committee of the House of Lords was not instructed or empowered to investigate under the Bill, either the scientific basis of Osteopathy or the Schools to be recognised. After the Bill was passed, if successful, a Board of Control was to be established which was to determine the standard of education and then determine the School or Schools to be recognised. The British School of Osteopathy was not mentioned in the body of the Bill, but *a* British school of osteopathy. Hence when the BSO was black-balled it was *ultra vires* and it was done on the principle of bullying and blustering to defeat the Bill by side-ventures.'

'This is confirmed by the later sections of the BMA Council Report. In opening the case for the Association, Sir W. Jowitt pointed out that, although the purpose of the Bill was to enable the public to distinguish the qualified from the unqualified, it proposed to place 2,000 unqualified persons on the Register. That was a matter for the Board to determine, not Counsel, or even the Select Committee. "Of the 160 qualified persons that remained, 90 were 'old boys' of the British School of Osteopathy" who he *ventured to suggest* were not worthy of consideration. That was the sneer and personal opinion and statement of Counsel. "Old boys." What about the old girls? They were in reality old boys and girls, who, not in their teens, but with fully developed minds, found out that Osteopathy had benefited thousands, gave up professional and business occupations to study Osteopathy; then studied it with a seriousness and earnestness and as a result in the past 10 years had treated with success thousands of patients whose gratitude repaid all the sacrifices of these old boys and girls to enter a profession they loved because it helped suffering humanity. Counsel's jeers will fall *flat* when the public realise this, especially when they know that many benefited by Osteopathy were helped after the medical profession that now flouted and sniffed at their work and their honesty had failed to help them. To flout and bully in such manner makes one feel that when serious argument fails scoffing takes its place...'

Littlejohn quoted an article in the *Journal of Osteopathy*, Kirksville, May 1931 (pp. 259-60), which referred to the Bill introduced by Adamson, "Regarding the recognition of irregulars", It said, "This might be distasteful to the legitimate osteopaths but it is something that must be done whenever initial legislation is adopted....It is hoped that the forces may be unified to win the fight for Osteopathy, *Personalities should be forgotten....*" 'What about the "old boys" of 1858, who, though they had never been inside a medical school, were slated on the first Medical Register as fully qualified physicians and surgeons? Was the King dishonest in signing the Bill? Were the Members of Parliament dishonest when they passed that Bill and made it the starting point of the legal recognition and status of the present medical profession? Has the British Medical Association and its Counsel forgotten these facts?'

He then reflected that history repeats itself as the ASO had a similar history. He explained how Osteopathy was discredited by the BMA. 'In cross-examination of the witnesses for the Bill, the Association's Council...secured from the principal witness for the osteopaths (Dr MacDonald) the admission that he could not and did not ask for State Registration of a body of practitioners without proof of the scientific basis of their claims. His questions secured the repeated statement, that osteopaths claim to treat by osteopathic methods all varieties of disease, was in conflict with those of scientific medicine; that osteopathic theory did not appear to give a reasonable explanation of well-known diseases; and that osteopaths in practice conflicted with Osteopathy in theory and that the osteopath uses not only osteopathic methods but those of the medical sciences that he condemns.'

'In other words, it was not "the old boys" who were discredited, because it was admitted amid the thousands of cases treated in the BSO clinic no casualties existed. Osteopathy itself was discredited, it methods repudiated, its scientific value disowned; and in addition, that the American section of osteopaths who have been so loud in denouncing everyone else as unqualified, not only practises Osteopathy but Medicine, that is, were untrue to the Science they professed to follow. Counsel got no such statement from the British osteopaths, because time and again he was told that, as publicly stated in the Journals of the BSO, the BSO recognises Medicine and Surgery and its practitioners, and that its practice is definitely limited to osteopathic methods. Here the BSO definitely repudiates the idea that British osteopaths practise or want to practise Medicine. If the BSO falls short of the much boasted American Schools, it is this, that the BSO and its graduates desire to cultivate the friendship of the genuine Medical practitioner, adhering to the osteopathic lines of diagnosis and treatment. Thus the aim is co-operation with all who are genuinely qualified to practise the Healing Art, that all may unite in helping suffering humanity.'

'That this idea, however prejudiced, was in the minds of the BMA, is brought out by another statement, "of the remaining 90, half are American citizens". Was it proposed to set up a State Register—a step involving a change in the basis of English Law—which would be the virtual monopoly of a group of American citizens?" This is what the Right Hon. Neville Chamberlain had said in 1925. It was this that stimulated the B. S. O. to persist in its efforts despite obstacles and difficulties, to build up Osteopathy, pure and simple A. T. Still Osteopathy, in this country...leaving Medicine and Surgery to the fully qualified medical and surgical practitioners. If the medical profession as a whole realised this then, 'A better understanding could be established that would lay the foundation for co-operation among those equally concerned with the health and well being of the people.'

Littlejohn reflected on the statement he made as spokesman and President of the BOA to Neville Chamberlain, Minister of Health on 9 June, 1925 and the response and what preceded the Select Committee, when he agreed his support and how there was unity among the four interested parties.

'Valuable contributions were made to the osteopathic cause, although many insinuations were made detrimental to Osteopathy, its founder and its principles. All of a sudden the united front was broken when Dr MacDonald stated that he did not accept the teaching standard of the BSO and formulated the idea from the BOA of a "proper" College of Osteopathy. This was never broached at any of the conferences either together or with Counsel and hence it was entirely outside both the basis of united support and the instructions to Counsel. It was a distinct violation of the unity of interest in Osteopathy that had prevailed up to the moment.'

'The BSO was not set down as a standard or the standard in the Bill. Like the others interested in the Bill its graduates were to be admitted on the passage of the Bill on the same basis as the graduates of a college of Osteopathy outside Britain and those who had been in practice for three years with no necessary collegiate education or qualification. After the Bill was passed, if it were successful, a board of Control was to be appointed by the Crown to administer the Bill. It rested with the Board to lay down the standard and to enforce it as in the Schedules. It also rested with the Board to determine the College or Colleges coming up to this standard. It was definitely stated in evidence that the BSO accepted the proposed amendment of the standard course to cover five years to be adopted as the future policy of Osteopathy so as to make Osteopathy of high standing in qualification. Hence the statement that the BSO was below standard was a breach of faith among the supporters of the Bill. It was stated by the Dean and confirmed by Dr MacDonald that the School had done its best, with the facilities offered and with the obstacles in its way, to build up the standard of education. It was also stated that it was expected that the passage of the Bill would open up better facilities and thus lay the foundation for coming up to the standard. And according to the Bill 12 months were allowed to permit the School to attain its ideal. It was stated that since 1917 the School had set out to establish the same standards of pre-medical, anatomical and physiological education as was required of medical students and that difficulties had arisen in trying to reach this, which made it impossible, at first, but that during the past two years the students of the BSO were required to take this course and the names of the students and the Schools they were attending were furnished to the Select Committee as promised in reply to the challenge to the contrary of Counsel for the BMA. This of itself was proof that the BSO had reached its ideal and it was definitely stated that during the past two years over 50 students prospective had been turned down because of their refusal or failure to comply with this requirement.'

'...It was 1931 before the Kirksville School was accepted as up to the standard for acceptance by the State of New York. And yet in the interval the Kirksville School was not discredited...'

'In the evidence given on behalf of the BSO the cross-examination consisted of insinuations and personal attacks on the qualifications, integrity and honesty of the Dean of the School and the sincerity of those working with him in the School. The leading Counsel for the supporters of the Bill never gave a helping hand although all the information was available. Everything could have been completely adjusted on re-examination following cross-examination. When the cross-examining Counsel suggested "I have been told" (with respect to the Looker school having a six month course) he introduced an element into examination contrary to legal procedure, quoting Mr Justice Swift on the Revelstoke case in the *Daily Mail* for 15 May, page 4, "Let us observe the bounds of propriety. We do not know and do not care, and we ought not to be told what you have been told." No proof was offered or suggested.'

Littlejohn criticised J. J. Dunning. 'Attacking the School in an underhand way he plays into the hands and plans of the enemies of Osteopathy....It was in the same spirit that the Dean of the BSO was attacked and his honesty and sincerity questioned after 38 years of devoted service to Osteopathy....'

Littlejohn then provided a biography, followed by a history of Osteopathy in Britain and the Foundation of the BSO.

Support for Littlejohn

Following the criticisms of the Dean, the Faculty Representative of the Students' Union, James Canning and the Honorary Secretary to the Faculty of the BSO, Edward Hall, sent a letter to all graduates, enclosing verification of Littlejohn's qualifications:

'Dear-
You have doubtless read some of the very biased and incomplete press reports of Dr Littlejohn's evidence and cross-examination before the House of Lords Committee which appears to indicate that Dr Littlejohn is falsely claiming to possess a PhD Diploma and that he had dishonestly issued Diplomas of the BSO.

The undersigned in company with Dr Harvey R. Foote, have personally examined and verified all Dr Littlejohn's Diplomas and Degrees and the appended chronological list should make it evident that his qualifications as Dean of the BSO are beyond adverse criticism.

The origin of this false impression has a very simple explanation and will, we hope, even be turned to advantage in the final summing-up by our Counsel.

The misunderstanding arose over the method of cross-examination by opposing Counsel who asked, "Have you a PhD of Columbia University?" On the Dean attempting to explain that the PhD was conferred by Chicago National University and not Columbia, he was demanded to give a straight "Yes" or "No". The apparently unreasonable demand by Counsel provoked in the Dean that characteristic trait of which we are all aware—that of retiring within himself and refusing further explanation. While admitting that this was a decidedly mistaken attitude, in the vital interest of the profession we can only assume that the Dean failed to realise fully the dangerously false impression this might create in the minds of the public and how prejudicial the issue might be to the value and status of the BSO Diploma.

Re Looker Graduates. You, as graduate of the BSO, are aware of the reason for, and the condition under which members of this Association were absorbed.

This letter is an appeal for your wholehearted loyalty and support, for your school and its Dean at a time when Osteopathy in this country is passing through a critical period in its history.'

The BOA and a 'College' of Osteopaths

The animosity to and criticism of the BSO did not end with the Select Committee. On 5 April 1935 Kelman MacDonald asked the BOA Council for absolute secrecy in regard to a long talk he had had with Viscount Elibank. Assuming that the Bill in its present form would not pass, they would like to put a very strong recommendation for, 'The creation of a voluntary register with high standards; The establishment of a first class, trustworthy School of Osteopathy (i.e. a BOA School); graduates of certain osteopathic colleges with a 4 year course, to undertake postgraduate work at the BOA college in order to satisfy a Board in all respects. This would not apply to those who have already started and an agreed plan of education to include a number of years at ordinary medical schools, pending the establishment of a full course at the Osteopathic School.'

Pheils moved that in view of the disclosures at the Select Committee regarding Littlejohn and the BSO, they continue to dissociate themselves from the BSO.

The BOA intended to control the voluntary register. There would be an independently appointed Board of the Register, under control of the Board of Trade that should be composed of two men of Science appointed by the Board of Trade, two medical men appointed by the BMA, three osteopaths, of whom two would be appointed by the BOA, and one by the Osteopathic Defence League.

MacDonald proposed the Council should be, 'The General Council of British Osteopaths', but then felt that the General Council of Great Britain and Northern Ireland would be more appropriate. Its duties would include the establishment of a Register and examination of those desiring admission onto it. Osteopaths whose names appeared on the Register would be known as 'Registered Osteopaths'.

MacDonald thought that it seemed a little unfair that graduates of the Littlejohn School would not go on the Register. It was thought that the best plan would be for the Board to examine the credentials and training of every applicant individually and state what further study must be taken at the new college to qualify for the Register.

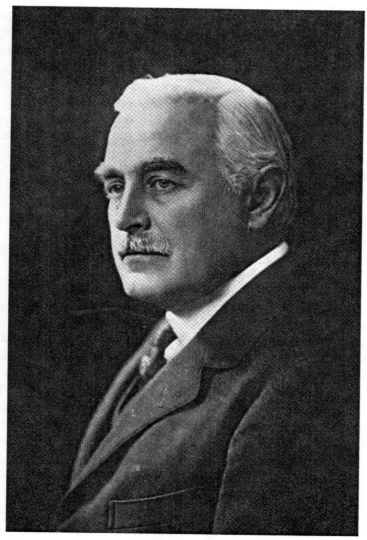

Viscount Elibank

By December 1936, Osteopathic Trusts Ltd was recognised as the official Educational Committee of the Association in attempting to establish a BOA College.

A J. B. P. Alvarez of 12 Baron's Court Road, London W14, stated he was taking steps to establish the London College of Osteopaths and to set up a Register. Cooper received a letter from him in September 1935 regarding a 'Council of Physical Medicine' which was establishing a 'Register of Physical Medicine'.

The General Council and Register of Osteopaths (GCRO)

Thorpe was instructed not to press the Bill, but to say that a voluntary register of osteopaths would be formed. On 8 April 1935, a Memorandum from the Ministry of Health stated that it appeared that a sufficiently strong case had not been made for the proposals in the Bill. Those who were practising Osteopathy would have the choice of either qualifying themselves for admission to the Medical Register, or of constituting a voluntary register and establishing effective training institutions for the qualification of persons who might desire to be admitted to the register in the future.

At that time there were three professional bodies representing 'those practising Osteopathy':

a) The BOA, whose members were one of the six approved osteopathic colleges in the US:

b) The Incorporated Association of Osteopaths Ltd., whose members were graduates of the BSO.

c) The National Society of Osteopaths Ltd., whose members held diplomas from other training establishments, or had acquired their proficiency by apprenticeship.

On 22 July 1936, the GCRO was incorporated as a company limited by guarantee, and not having a share capital, with Viscount Elibank, who had sat on the Select Committee of the House of Lords, as President. He remained so until 1944. Elibank was a Scottish MP in the First World War and went up to the House of Lords in 1927 as the 11th Viscount. He introduced the Bill into the Lords and when the GCRO was formed he helped frame its Constitution and its Articles of Association and he helped reconcile opposing points of view. In August 1950 he retired to Cape Town where he died on 12 March 1951. Wilfrid Streeter wrote a tribute to him in the summer issue of *The Osteopathic Quarterly* for that year.

A Memorandum of Association was produced and in June 1937 a code of ethics drawn up.

There was provision for several grades of membership, but only two were used: Full Membership and Associate Membership.[2] Full Membership was permitted to graduates of approved American colleges, and after some amendment to the course, to those of the BSO. Associate Membership was permitted for those lacking specific academic qualifications, but who were, 'Practising for a reasonable amount of time'. Associate Members could upgrade to Full Membership by satisfying an Examination Board, but no time limit was set on this and there was no compulsion to upgrade.[3] Not all Associates were prepared to do this and of those that did so, not all satisfied the examiners.[2] Membership was initially small. In the first Register, published in 1939, there were 130 Full Members and 21 Associate Members.[4]

The Functions of the Register

R. F. Miller, who was Registrar of the GCRO, published in *The Osteopathic Quarterly* a summary of the functions of the Register:

> 'The two chief functions of the Register of Osteopaths have been defined as:
>
> (a) To regulate the standard of qualification and professional conduct, and
>
> (b) To protect the public by supplying them with the names of those who are so qualified both from a technical and professional point of view.'
>
> These have also been summed up rather neatly by one who, differentiating between the Register and the Osteopathic Association of Great Britain, said: "The purpose of the Register is to protect the public from the osteopath; the purpose of the Association is to protect the osteopath from the public."
>
> The machinery for carrying out the first of these functions is quite simple. The General Council of the Register has laid down a standard of qualifications and competence to which all members must conform before they are admitted. Whether an applicant has the necessary qualifications and skill is decided by an Examining Board....In view of the fact that admission is on a purely voluntary basis, it is obvious that the applicant is willing to abide by the Code of Ethics which the Register had prepared to govern professional conduct.
>
> All this is done with the object of safeguarding the public, who, when they see that a practitioner is registered will know that he is fully qualified, both technically and professionally and as such, guaranteed to be in all respects competent to practise Osteopathy in all its aspects. Conversely, they will appreciate that the practitioner who is not on the Register may not be qualified and competent.
>
> ...A. T. Still, the founder of Osteopathy, realised quite early that a danger existed in permitting the semi-trained to practise in the name of the new science. In an address which he delivered on June 22nd, 1895, he said, in his customary

forthright manner, "One objection to Osteopathy is that it may make thieves and scoundrels. Some men come here for a little while and go away and say, 'I have been in Kirksville; I am an osteopath', and so on. They steal from the people wherever they can until found out. So far it is dangerous. The medical doctors have said it was dangerous because with a few cures in a neighbourhood, Osteopathy is liable to become the grandest system of robbery in the world."

Merely to record the names of registered practitioners is however, only a passive way of protecting the public. The Register has gone further than this by obtaining the co-operation of a large section of the press in stamping out the undesirable practice of advertising by so-called osteopaths. The Members of the Register have voluntarily agreed not to advertise in any shape or form. Indeed, it can be said that they do not need to do so. But there are still to be found in various publications advertisements and announcements (some masquerading as news items) inserted by persons calling themselves osteopaths and usually displaying a formidable array of letters, including D.O., after their names.

The Register has, at present, no legal grounds for objecting to these advertisements; but it has usually been found that the proprietors of the publications containing these advertisements have been quick to appreciate that it would be no great service to the public to repeat them.

It is of the first importance that the public should be educated to understand that they can look to the Register of Osteopaths to protect them against charlatans and the semi-trained. This will not be done easily or quickly; but there is every indication that even now the knowledge is spreading gradually through the best channels. One method formally adopted was the publication of carefully worded announcements in the national and leading provincial newspapers; but it is not believed that the results were good—although it is extremely difficult to assess how good they were.

Probably the best publicity for the Register is that which is spread by word of mouth, when one person says to a friend who has decided to consult an osteopath: "Be sure that you go to an M.R.O." Distribution of the Directory of Members and particularly its being available in public libraries are other valuable ways of spreading information and are now undertaken on an increased scale by the office of the Registrar.

If the work of the Register is not yet widely known it is simply because the organisation was not set up until 1936 and had little chance to develop during the war years. In the near future, however, much more will be heard of it and its functions will appear of obvious benefit to the public.'⁵

The Osteopathic Association of Great Britain (OAGB) and the GCRO

The Incorporated Association of Osteopaths became the OAGB in 1936, as the professional body to which BSO graduates belonged. Not surprisingly, it wanted representation on the GCRO (in the early days often referred to as the General Osteopathic Council, the GOC) and registration for its members, although the BSO had not been officially recognised as an established institution for the teaching of Osteopathy. In 1937, a joint meeting was arranged between the GCRO and OAGB to discuss this.

Littlejohn suggested that before the OAGB Committee met the GCRO it should meet members of the BSO Board. It was decided that only if the School was recognised as an established institution for the teaching of osteopathy would the OAGB apply for membership of the GCRO. four points were agreed between the BSO and the OAGB:

1. That the BSO be recognised as an accredited school. It was willing to conform to any high standards provided that the facilities be made available. The GCRO should assist in providing these.

2. The School to have a representative on the GCRO following the precedent of the GMC with regard to medical schools.

3. That no graduates or professing graduates be accepted by the GCRO until they present their diplomas and confirmation be obtained from the BSO.

4. That the GCRO receive into full membership all graduates of the BSO recommended by the School.

An Extraordinary General Meeting of the OAGB was held in Manchester on 16 October 1937, because of considerable dissatisfaction by many members regarding 'certain transactions' that took place at the AGM on two October regarding the GCRO and the OAGB's policy to it, and because there had been an error in dealing with proxy votes. A further Meeting was held in December at the Mayfair Hotel, Berkeley Street, chaired by Herbert Milne, who stated, 'This meeting may alter the course of the history of Osteopathy a good deal in this country.' It was to decide the OAGB's attitude to the GCRO. The meeting lasted from 11.00 to 17.30 and the minutes run to 80 pages. 71 people voted.

Much discussion took place about the relationship between the OAGB and the GCRO and whether the resolution of two October (details unknown) could be overthrown. It was considered that as few people were present on that occasion and the majority of other members were unaware of the technicality, the resolution should be reconsidered.

It was agreed that the Resolution accepted by the Extraordinary General Meeting on 16 October be accepted to replace the Resolution at the AGM. It was agreed:

> 'That this meeting gives the Negotiating Committee a free hand to complete negotiations with the GCRO subject to their receiving official written confirmation that the BSO be recognized by the GOC as a reputable School.'

The Chairman of the OAGB (Milne) had written to Kelman MacDonald, who suggested the following:

a)   Three members of the OAGB nominated to the GCRO should make application for full membership of the Register. (The GCRO had originally agreed to one representative. Through negotiation that was raised to two and then to three). He would get their applications passed through the Examining Committee and the Council would place their names on the Register at the meeting in November.

b)   That he readily and sincerely promised a continuance of such goodwill as he was able to extend.

c)   That he would do in all his power at the next Register Council meeting to get an official recognition of the BSO passed by the GCRO.

d)   That all applications from members of the OAGB made by 31 December 1937 would be considered for full membership.

A resolution was passed by the GCRO regarding the BSO:

> 'That this council is very sympathetically disposed towards the BSO. It realizes the difficulties that it has had to contend with, and the Council appreciates the manner in which it is attempting to meet them. In so far as Dr Norman MacDonald is external examiner, we feel that until such time as this Council raises the standards in 1940, the BSO be invited to carry out immediate post-graduate and under-graduate teaching with our approval. But the Council retained the right to admit

or reject, by further examination if necessary, any individual applicant from the School to the Register.'

Milne had written to Kelman MacDonald asking if that meant official recognition of the BSO and noting that there was no mention of representation of the School on the GCRO, which he considered a necessity. He was informed by MacDonald's secretary that he would receive a reply in a day or two, but it was not forthcoming. On telephoning he was told that MacDonald was ill.

Canning challenged the appointments of the three OAGB representatives (Milne, Saul and van Straten, the Chairman, Vice-Chairman and Secretary of the OAGB, respectively), who were chosen by the Council of the OAGB and not the membership and proposed that full time graduates of the BSO should have stronger representation. It was stated that they were not appointed because of their office but because they were the best people to conduct the business. Canning responded: 'I feel that the position of the School is so vital in Osteopathy and I will ask you to remember that there is only one road to recognition, and that is through a School. I feel that as the School is beginning to right itself, that our three representatives have become impatient with the slow work, and they do not know enough about it.' Holditch commented that if they did not re-elect the same three people it meant that anything they had negotiated with the GCRO would collapse: 'It is going to put the whole thing in a most unholy mess.' Canning claimed that for years there had been a campaign of whisper and insinuation against one man and felt that the three representatives had already been subjected to that same campaign.

After much debate the three OAGB representatives were re-elected to serve on the GCRO.

Canning argued: 'The only avenue to recognition is through a School. That has been made clear to us on three approaches to the Government. They sound very pleasant (referring to letters from Kelman MacDonald) and I am quite willing to accept them, or would be if I had not an uneasy feeling in my mind from some private information that I cannot divulge to you that even quite recently there has been a change in policy—which has been discussed in letters—an intention not only to damn the School with faint praise, but a definite suggestion to give no help whatever in the hope that may give it a quietus. We have a long history here of a school that has struggled against extraordinary difficulties....A lot of mud, which on analysis is very harmless, was thrown forward (at the Select Committee). That had its origin in deliberate treachery on the part of certain osteopaths; and that treachery was based on a personal animosity to one man.'

'On several occasions members of the opposition body have offered to come and take part in the teaching of the School, but they have petered out.'

'It was considered that a sum of £575,000 was required for the BOA school that will never be realised. It had its origin chiefly in a desire to put on a better footing the clinic, which has failed through lack of voluntary service and was in debt.'

Banbury considered that the three representatives joining the GCRO was in direct contravention of the wishes of the Extraordinary General Meeting at Manchester.

The Chairman considered it was a tremendous danger to exclude themselves voluntarily from the GCRO. 'We as full members will have voting power on that body; in 1940 we shall be able to influence the course of policy drastically and it will mean very much to the BSO...and that we should be very observant of the development of negotiations with the National Society of Osteopaths.'

Hall reviewed the history. 'The GOC was formed originally without any knowledge of anybody else. It was formed to function for the BOA entirely. Why did they come after a little while to the OAGB? They came because they realized they could not exist as a body controlling Osteopathy. For the past three years I have been pointing out the danger of the National Society. While they (the GCRO) were negotiating with the OAGB they were also negotiating with the National Society. So they not only took in the OAGB but started to negotiate with a newly formed body which was not in existence when the Bill came out and a body which we should not have negotiated with.'

Despite personal letters there were no official negotiations with the BSO as the only training institution. They were inspected twice and had favourable reports. The four points (see above) had been ignored. The BSO could not expect help to bring it up to the stated required standard. 'If every member of this Association backs up this Register and by 1940 they will all be in that Register, the Register raises its standards to a pitch that it is impossible to comply with and after that no School graduate can be admitted to the Register....We will not be able to get students if we cannot even offer them membership of the Register....You are not getting recognition of your Diploma. You are getting recognition as members of the OAGB. It is only fair that the members should realize that that is just another sprat to catch a mackerel and it is the wickedest thing ever foisted on an unsuspecting public.'

He then referred to the proposed School of the BOA. They were asking for £575,000. They had received £20,000, but under £3,000 in cash. Members of the Osteopathic Trusts told him that they never hoped to get even as much as £50,000. On the asset side they had an income of £18,000 against an admitted deficit of £42,000 per year and would be reliant on endowments. 'It takes a lot of money to endow a deficit of £42,000 a year and that is putting it at their estimate....The School itself is a fantastic impossibility.'

The clinic was purchased and given to the BOA by Dudley Docker in 1927. 'It has been an absolute failure since then. Why is Dudley Docker not backing this scheme?...Because he is a little fed up. He has not even been paid the interest on that £10,000 he laid out on Dorset Square. On the other hand you have this other college, this British School of Osteopathy. You have the nucleus of a very good faculty. Within 18 months that School could be made the most perfect school under the existing laws in this country...If we go forward and join this GOC without having that college fully protected and recognised, then I can assure you your college will not get recognised. You must not do it. You must protect your own diploma. The GOC when you have all joined will raise its standards....The School will close and then your diploma will not have the prestige and value it should have. If you value your diploma, you must hold firm until such time as all these very nice, charming personal assurances are absolutely confirmed.' (Applause.)

Leary referred to Kelman MacDonald's 'ambiguous telegram'. 'I think it is actually insulting to us to say he "feels sure". It is an epitome of their feelings towards us, and I personally feel we should no longer tolerate that sort of thing.'

Hall: 'If you are going into the GOC as an Association then you are automatically backing the Osteopathic Trusts Ltd School....We are backing up a school that is non-existent and we are automatically thrusting our own school into the background....'

Leary indicated that at the last Extraordinary Meeting, it was felt that when they obtained recognition of the four points, including recognition of the School, then they should go forward.

Hall responded: 'This is what is tragic to me. Those four points embody everything we are asking and if those four points had been got, everything would have been fine and dandy.' He argued that the Association should have stayed out until the four points were accepted by the GOC.

Saul claimed that the four points had come from the School. 'We agreed on them as a basis of negotiation to back you, but we did not say we agreed on each point.' Saul asked why the School did not negotiate directly with the GOC. The meeting became very heated. Saul said to Hall: 'If you take umbrage at my inference may I not be permitted to take umbrage at your tone of voice?'

Saul then argued the importance of unity in the profession, of protecting the public by an organisation that governed osteopaths professionally and ethically. 'Let the BOA have their cranks. We are not frightened of meeting them. We want to fight and meet them in this general body which has that nucleus of unity....The School stands definitely protected on that point. At the present time the bickering going on shows that the individuals are being far too self-centred, and you are coming very near the point of being designated not men giving your services to the public for the public's good, but very near the border line of parasites who are living on the public for their own good.

I am rather proud of my diploma. I hope all the rest of you are. I hope we shall be prouder still in the passage of time. But it is not a reasonable thing to expect that a body of this kind should recognise diplomas of any school as an unconditional means of entry into that body....We have been told that in going forward and securing seats on the GOC we have impeded the progress of the BSO, but not a single shred of evidence has been adduced to support that assertion. At the present time the prestige of the BOA and of the GOC is, temporarily at least, rather in excess of our own. There is a real possibility that unless our arrangements are virtually completed, the GOC will cease to continue present relations with the Association and both the Association and the School may be ignored and the GOC proceed to compile a register of members.'

The Chairman emphasised that in 1940 the only School in existence would be the BSO and therefore no council of any kind that had a sense of responsibility could think of setting standards impossible for it to attain. The position of the school was strengthened by the existence of the Association.

The Secretary commented: 'If...the GOC really and sincerely are going to meet these points, why do they not say so? If they do not, there must be a reason. I am sorry but I cannot feel anything else.'

Hall asked: 'At what point , if they fail to give recognition to the School, you would realize that there has been bad faith and negotiations must break down ?'

The Chairman recommended that application forms for registration should be sent out after the meeting. 'If the Association is disrupted, the School will be tossed about. The GOC will have nothing to do with it.'

Saul: 'The three representatives...can demand an official statement from the Council...that the School is given official recognition...that the Council gets in touch with the School and settle their differences instantly.'

Leary was concerned about the Osteopathic Trusts. 'Money is going to the Dorset Square clinic to teach postgraduate courses to doctors and they will go on the market purporting to give osteopathic treatment....Osteopathy is a full time job. You cannot do Osteopathy and medical work at the same time.'

Tanguy said: 'I am surprised at the low grade of intelligence of some of the members. Unless we do something quickly the whole thing is going to tumble into pieces and we are going to put Osteopathy back for years. You agree with Dr Milne or disagree. If we disagree with him, then we are finished as an Association; we are going to split up.'

The Secretary pleaded that somehow or other they must try to avoid this split and that members should apply to the GOC. 'Once we had entered that body the GOC dare not, could not, would not allow us to depart. It would strengthen our argument.'

There were again concerns about the representatives. They could argue with the weight of the Association behind them but others were concerned that matters might go a little beyond their control.

Holditch summarised the difference: 'We do not come in until you recognise us, or we'll get in first and then try and get the recognition. Three determined men on that committee can do a tremendous amount of damage to the BOA itself. Let them go forward with this thing and let us not bind them down to any conditions.' (Applause). An amendment was made to a proposition of Webster-Jones: 'That this meeting authorises the Council to complete its negotiations with the GOC and to forward the members application forms to be completed.' Voting went 40 for and 31 against. The resolution was put forward endorsing the action of the Council in making the appointments.

The BOA and the BSO 1938-1939

By July 1938 negotiations were in progress between the GCRO and BSO regarding recognition of the latter. The BOA Council, however, suggested to members that they refrain from any active professional association with the School, until such time as the position between the two bodies was definitely established. An invitation was sent from the BSO to the BOA to attend their Annual Convention. The BOA decided that individual members could go as friends, but the BOA would not be officially represented. The BOA Council discussed whether the BSO should be sent an invitation to the BOA convention. It was agreed that only individuals should be invited and that no official invitation should be sent.

By November 1938, following approval of articles of the School, the GCRO recognised the BSO. four or five members of the BOA were to be on its Board. Pheils stated he was endeavouring to obtain something in writing from the BSO to present to Osteopathic Trusts, whereby the latter could feel justified in helping the School financially at some future date. At that time the School owed Littlejohn approximately £5,000. The position of Littlejohn was discussed. He was to continue as Dean, but not as the owner of the School. He would be one of three trustees.

At the BOA Council meeting in November, Pheils indicated that pressure had been brought to bear on the School to put their affairs in order and he stressed the importance of every effort being made to stop the fight between members of the BOA and the graduates of the BSO. 'Sooner or later we must recognise the BSO, however critical our feelings may have been in the past.' No diplomas were to be granted from the BSO until the students had been passed by an External Examiner as well as an Internal Examiner. Graduates of the BSO, after being passed by the Examining Committee of the GCRO, would be admitted to membership on the Register on the same footing as members of the BOA.

There was a correspondence with Webster-Jones regarding an exchange of directories between the BOA and OAGB. The BOA pointed out that if the OAGB wished for reciprocity between the two Associations, it might be better if the OAGB would allow the BOA to appoint a representative to edit their Journal. The letter was not favourably received. The BOA wrote to Webster-Jones: 'Since there is a move amongst all osteopathic bodies for greater harmony, the Council of the BOA recommend that two of our members meet two representatives of the OAGB and talk over the matter of the exchange of directories in the hope of a friendly and amicable settlement.'

Setting Educational Standards

The GCRO Council considered an initial task in supervising and elevating osteopathic educational standards was to investigate the curriculum and administration of the BSO.

In 1938, the BSO requested the GCRO to appoint a Negotiating Committee, to meet its representatives to discuss these standards and the means of attaining them. Meetings took place in May and November. The GCRO agreed to collect the names of persons willing to be External Examiners at the BSO (See below).

In 1939, the School was prepared to give additional instruction to Associate Members of the GCRO, to enable them to qualify for full membership. The standard of education laid down by the GCRO were not considered satisfactory by the BSO. The BSO Board invited the GCRO to nominate three persons to contribute a Joint Committee of Education with three persons nominated by the BSO Board, to consider details of the course, fees and examination standards required. The GCRO appointed four members to the Joint Committee, so the Board of the BSO decided to appoint a further member.

The Joint Committee of Standards met in May 1939 and considered the course of osteopathic training under three headings:

1. Membership Examination for osteopaths who had three to five years' practice to their credit.
The examination was to be conducted twice yearly until October 1940, after which date it was suggested the clause with reference to Associate Membership be deleted. It was to be conducted at the BSO, the Examining Board to be appointed by the Register in conjunction with the School. There were to be three written papers (general diagnosis; principles and diagnosis; practice and technique covering in addition hydrotherapy, physiotherapy and diet). Each paper was to consist of eight questions of which six were compulsory. There was to be a viva-voce examination taking the form of an interview, the examiners paying particular regard to diagnosis and technique of an essentially practical nature. The Examination was to be first held in July 1939.
For candidates referred, a course of training at the BSO was proposed of a minimum of three months on the subjects examined. Candidates would be allowed to take the course in separate monthly terms so that they could keep in touch with their practice.
2. Ordinary Undergraduate courses.
The course of study for osteopathic qualifications for those applying for membership on or before the first day of October 1945 was to be four years and for those applying for membership after that date, five years.
3. A course with credit for registered medical practitioners and other practitioners.
The Committee recommended that a registered medical practitioner may receive a Diploma after four terms' full time

study at the BSO with an additional nine weeks' clinic work in the long vacation. It further recommended that the School might, at its discretion, extend the course in time. In order to reduce the chance of medical practitioners discontinuing the course before completion, as had sometimes been the case in the past, the School could require them to pay full fees in advance.

It had been the practice in the past for the BSO to allow credit to other practitioners (chiropractors, chartered masseurs, naturopaths, chiropodists and practitioners holding diplomas of irregular osteopathic schools) on individual merit and qualification. The School sought guidance from Council on this.

The Committee asked the Council of the Register to empower it to investigate, where possible, those other schools issuing diplomas or certificates, in order to assess their value for the purpose of allowing credits.

A Dispute over Examiners

In May 1939, in accordance with the report of the Negotiating Committee of the previous year, five persons were recommended as Examiners for the year 1939-40: three internal (Littlejohn, Webster-Jones and Hall) and two external appointed by the GCRO (Watson and Goodall). The Council of Education of the BSO considered that the qualifications of the latter was inadequate for the post and protested. A letter was sent to Elibank, Streeter and MacDonald. Hall said that Goodall was only a member of the Register by virtue of representing the National Society of Osteopaths and would not have received a Diploma from the School. He said that the appointment would cause ill feeling among graduates of the Register and also among the candidates of the examination.

The President of the GCRO intimated that it was not possible for any alteration to be made. A letter of protest was sent from the Board of Directors of the BSO condemning the manner in which the appointment had been made and accepting it under protest. Arising out of this Hall resigned from the Board of Examiners and was replaced by Hope Robertson.

Changes to the Control of the BSO

The Articles of Association of the BSO had to be modified to vest shares in the hands of three trustees. Discussion regarding this was completed in October 1937. In November 1938, it was agreed that the

80 shares held by Littlejohn should be transferred to Trustees and the first should be Dr J. M. Littlejohn (Littlejohn's son) and M.B.U. Dewar. The third was Lord Hankey as a completely independent person. On Dewar's death, Seebohm Rowntree became trustee and after his death, Lord Semphill.

It was suggested that the loan by Littlejohn to the Company should be secured by means of a Debenture creating a floating charge on the assets of the company and should be repayable by instalments to commence during 1939.

Kenneth Brown Baker and Baker (Solicitors), wrote to Dewar in January 1939:

> Lord Elibank rang me up yesterday, and it appears that there is a small war going on—whether declared or not I do not know—between Mr Streeter and Dr Pheils, the former saying that Osteopathic Trusts are entirely useless and ought to be wound up, and the latter offering to find the money for the School, but only if Osteopathic Trusts get complete control. It seems to me that both are wrong. If Osteopathic Trusts put up all the money then they ought obviously to have a voice as to how the School is to be run, but I am dead against them having control. It seems to me the way they can achieve this is by putting a Director on the Board, and the Trustee position ought to be left where it is.'

In January 1939, the Board considered it could not take any action regarding the transfer of shares from J. M. Littlejohn, as it was unaware of a source of money to purchase them.

Osteopathic Trusts were asked to provide funds for a full time specialist teacher; a fully qualified pathologist and/or anatomist; equipment and accommodation for the School and clinic; and to establish a hospital for appropriate treatment of indoor cases, modelled on the plans of medical schools, which provide collegiate training in the academic subjects, with hospital training in the clinical aspects. 'In this way pathological, laboratory work and research can be made a necessary part of the standard course in osteopathic training.'

Osteopathic Trusts claimed they were unable to make any grants to the School at that time. They did not want to be associated with the BSO and could not help it unless 90% of the BOA were behind them. An Extraordinary General Meeting of the BOA was called to consider the whole situation. (The outcome is unknown).

The composition of the BSO Board was revised in November 1938, following recommendations from the President of the BOA, the President of the OAGB and the Negotiating Committee.

In January, 1939 the Chairman, J. M. Littlejohn, welcomed the new members to the Board, which then consisted of E. T. Pheils, R. Hope Robertson, T. Edward Hall, James Littlejohn, J. Canning, J. M. Ferguson, Frederic Davis and Jocelyn Proby. Pheils then resigned on the grounds that he was Vice-Chairman of Osteopathic Trusts. The Secretary informed him that so far as the School was concerned there had been no lack of toleration and co-operation, and further, that the Board hoped shortly to be in a position to put forward a scheme of development in which Osteopathic Trusts could co-operate. four months later Davis resigned, as the BOA refused to support the School. It was not possible for him to remain Secretary of the BOA and retain his Governing Directorship of the BSO. Proby and Hope Robertson also resigned, though Proby continued to work in the clinic. T. Mitchell-Fox, S. W. Ratcliffe, O. B. Deiter and E. Hollingshead Clark were then appointed as Directors. Deiter was an American and graduate of the Philadelphia College of Osteopathy. He visited London in 1927 for a year's work and stayed.

In February 1939, a BSO Committee reviewed student recruitment. A letter from R. Hope Robertson in February 1939 indicates he was a member of a Student Loan Fund Council.

The BOA and the GCRO (1939)

By February 1939, Canning and Webster Jones had joined the GCRO. In April,1939 there were five BOA members: Norman Macdonald, Elmer T. Pheils, William Cooper, Sutcliffe Lean and R. W. R. Watson.

The BOA were concerned regarding the membership of the GCRO. Pheils indicated that when the Register was formed it had not been realized that other osteopaths would be on the Council, or that members of the OAGB and BSO graduates would be in the same category as BOA members. Pheils had previously suggested that two OAGB members were sufficient but this was not accepted by the OAGB and the number was increased to three. He suggested when the BSO was recognised one representative would be sufficient, but the OAGB had insisted on 2, which would diminish the power of the BOA. He considered that the Memorandum and Articles of the GCRO were unfair to the BOA. By May, Norman MacDonald had died and Pheils and Cooper had resigned. The BOA President (Sikkenga) received a telegram from Lord Elibank regarding the resignations, 'Which will seriously injure your Association and the whole profession if the Register is wrecked'.

By a decision of the Council of the GCRO in February 1939 authority was given for the publication of a Register containing the names of those who were Members to date and who could use the post nominal letters MRO (Member of the Register) or ARO (Associate Member of the Register).

Despite the fact that in its early years the GCRO was dominated by BOA, American-trained osteopaths, it is perhaps not insignificant that of the 139 members of the Register in 1939, 75 were OAGB members (representing 95% of that organisation) and 48 were BOA members (representing only 46% of their body).[6]

References

1. *The Journal of Osteopathy* (1935). June-August, VI(3 & 4).
2. The Osteopathic Blue Book. (1958). <u>The Origin and Development of Osteopathy in Britain.</u> (London: General Council and Register of Osteopaths).
3. Handoll, N. (1986). <u>Osteopathy in Britain. Its development and practice</u>. (Hereford: Osteopathic Supplies Ltd).
4. Daniels, B. A. (1997). A Brief History of the GCRO. Annual Report for 1997 and News Bulletin. No 35, GCR 6/97, pp. 41-50. (Reading: The General Council and Register of Osteopaths).
5. Miller, R. F. (1949). The functions of the Register. *The Osteopathic Quarterly*, July, 2(1): 23-24.
6. Dove, C. (2000). Speech given at Osteopathy 2000. Historical development of the profession.

Chapter 8

The Rest of the 1930s

The 1930s was a decade of change for the profession. Following the Select Committee of the House of Lords in 1935, Osteopathy in Britain was never the same again. The consequent formation of the General Council and Register of Osteopaths in 1936 defined standards of education and therefore quality of practitionership. The largest School in existence, the BSO, and its Dean, Dr John Martin Littlejohn, had received scathing criticism in the House of Lords. The School entered a period of self-reflection and improved its standards, particularly by appointing external examiners and by having BOA members on its Board of Directors. The late 1930s saw a growing interest in research, partly in response to the criticisms of the osteopathic theory by the Select Committee. There were also attempts to set up osteopathic hospitals. Other schools and associations came into existence, but the outbreak of war in 1939 brought all these developments to a grinding halt.

The Register was not the first, nor the only list of British osteopaths. As early as 1930 the Membership Committee of the BOA printed a register of all 'qualified' osteopaths in the UK and the London Vegetarian Society published a list of 'qualified' osteopathic practitioners in the Food Reformers' Year Book. In 1937, T. E. Hall received a letter advertising, 'Who's Who in Natural-Therapeutics', that intended to incorporate the names, addresses and general particulars of all graduated practitioners in Naturopathy, Osteopathy, Chiropractic, Electro-therapeutics, Psycho-therapeutics, Manipulative Surgery, Botano-Therapy etc.

By 1930 inappropriate advertising was already a concern. The BOA expressed disapproval of Martisus's 'unethical' advertising. In 1932, he agreed to stop soliciting for patients in daily papers and to cease handing out books on Osteopathy with his name on them. Even in 1937, a Dr

Johnston had an advertisement in the *Evening Standard* offering expert tuition in Osteopathy at five shillings per session (evening classes).

In 1931 the Rev, Hugh C. Kinred, Vicar of Crowfield, who graduated from the BSO in 1929 and claimed he had experience (of manipulation ?) in Russia as far back as 1911, was obliged to appear before an inquest following the death of a diabetic girl that he had manipulated.[1]

The BOA

In the 1930s, the British Osteopathic Association was in its prime. By 1935 it had 75 members of whom 30% were American.[2] Criticism of the BSO by the BOA continued through most of the decade. In February 1930 Doctors Webb and Semple moved that the BOA Council recommend the Advisory Committee to investigate Littlejohn's School, with a view to taking action.

Littlejohn told the Advisory Committee that the BSO was a corporate body under trust control and that he was merely a member of the Board. He claimed to be collaborating with certain medical schools and referred the Committee to his printed announcement regarding requirements, curriculum etc. He did, however, express willingness to confer with the BOA Committee, if the BOA would reciprocate. On 14 March Littlejohn resigned as a member of the BOA, stating his unwillingness to subscribe to the Legislative Committee work. By September 1931 the resignation was accepted.

In 1930 the BOA instructed Sydney Vernon and Christmas Humphreys, its advisors, to prepare and formulate available evidence with respect to the BSO and to use this evidence as they saw fit. Docker considered the success of the new clinic and the launching of a Royal Charter would place the BOA in an unassailable position.

The following year Pheils suggested that if the BOA were to write to Ontario and explain the situation regarding the BSO, the recognition of the BSO by Ontario would be withdrawn. This happened in 1935.

By 1934, realising that taking over the BSO was an impossibility, the BOA discussed forming a separate school. A circular was sent to BOA members to find out what time/subjects they could offer. By the end of the year a College Committee had met several times. It was intended to teach medical students, as a stepping stone towards a School run on the lines of the US osteopathic colleges. There was concern regarding the possibility of turning out students of a lower standard than the existing medical standards. They agreed to ask the Deans of medical schools whether or not they would make it possible for their students to attend the osteopathic college.

In December 1934, the BOA decided to form a company, which became Osteopathic Trusts Ltd in 1935, an educational charity to further osteopathic research and education and to raise money to open an American-style college of Osteopathy in Britain. In 1936, Baron J. Davenport gave a gift of £2000 to launch the appeal for the college and by the end of the year Osteopathic Trusts was recognised as the official Educational Committee of the Association, in an effort to establish a college. The following year Cleghorn Thompson was appointed Director. Progress was hampered by the war, but the London College of Osteopathy came into existence in 1946.

In 1931 the BOA moved to 24-25 Dorset Square (Andrew Still House) and with the help of Dudley Docker a long lease was purchased.[3] A complete redecoration was carried out in the summer of 1935. The Ladies' Association had insisted on the need and, by means of entertainments and social functions, bore the entire cost. At an annual bazaar in November 1935, it raised nearly £208. HRH The Duchess of York gave a brass and enamel cigarette box. Queen Mary had given a glass vase the previous year.[4]

In 1930 the Board of Trade refused a request for the clinic to be registered as a charitable institution. In May 1932, Dunning was in touch with Dr Adrian Boult regarding a broadcast appeal for the clinic. By 1933, there was also a BOA clinic in the headquarters of the Christian Volunteer Force in Glasgow.

Records of the BOA clinic are as follows:[5]

	1934	1935
Total number of treatments	6,072	8,771
New patients	459	720
Discharged	76	74
Ceased to attend	291	14
Unfit for treatment	39	5
Clinic fees	£621	£660

Close links still existed between the BOA and AOA throughout the 1930s, with members of the former paying an additional subscription to the AOA and attending its meetings. A joint meeting was proposed with the AOA, to take place when its health cruise ship arrived at Monaco in 1932. In 1936 BOA members were present with AOA members at the Olympic Games in Berlin. (See below).

In 1933 the BOA decided that there should be more co-operation and friendliness among its members. Meetings and buffet lunches were arranged at the clinic. Relations with other groups of osteopaths, however, were respectfully cool. In the same year, the Incorporated Association invited the BOA to send a representative to the annual banquet at Liverpool. The BOA reciprocated with an invitation to their banquet. Streeter was also invited. By 1934, however, the BOA stated that discretion was needed in associating with non-members of the BOA, though the President of the Incorporated Association was invited to dinner at Claridge's.

Certain well-known names came up for discussion by the BOA Council. In 1933 there was mention of the 'W. Stanley Lief case' and Captain Lowry was asked to resign or appear before Council.

In 1934, a painting of Sir Herbert Barker was given to the BOA.

The IAO and the OAGB

The Incorporated Association of Osteopaths was initially founded by and for graduates of the Looker School, but from 1929 it became the Association for graduates of the BSO.

It arranged the first postgraduate course at the BSO in May 1931. A small committee was formed with Edward Hall as the Secretary. Harvey Foote described foot techniques, including the recently developed Bynum technique. Other subjects included bedside technique, enteroptosis, technique for the lymphatics, asthma and chest troubles, dietetics, skin troubles, catarrhal deafness, mechanics of the spine and differential diagnosis of the abdomen.

It held an annual dinner. In 1932 it was at the Trocadero in London W1 and the following year in the Adelphi Hotel. In 1934, a dinner and dance took place at the Mayfair Hotel, which was enjoyed by a larger and more distinguished attendance than ever before. In addition, there was a convention with lectures and demonstrations. The Mayfair Hotel became a popular venue for osteopathic meetings. The Annual Dinner of 1935, held in the Park Lane Hotel, Piccadilly, was the last before the Incorporated Association of Osteopaths became the Osteopathic Association of Great Britain (OAGB) in 1936.[6] All past Presidents of the OAGB are named on the presidential gold chain of office. Those for the 1930s were:

1936	Patrick Saul
1937	Herbert Milne
1938	T. Edward Hall
1939	T. Mitchell-Fox

The National Society of Osteopaths

This was founded in the 1930s for osteopaths who were neither

American-trained, nor graduates of the BSO. In a small, undated pamphlet, it claimed:

'For some considerable time past the need has been felt in osteopathic circles for a central organisation providing for the promotion and general advancement of Osteopathy, and which would bring into unity and mutual association all those professionally engaged in the application of osteopathic principles.

In the present day there is neither time nor place for small bodies or groups to attempt constitutional constructive work, but if qualified British osteopaths present a united and unanimous demand for the recognition which is justly their due, useful action can be taken to protect the public, and to give their own profession a satisfactory and recognised basis, as well as to secure such advantages and privileges as rightly belong to them in connection with public and other services.

It is with this purpose in mind that the National Society of Osteopaths has been established with Registered Offices at 75, Gloucester Place, London, W.1, and a cordial invitation is extended to each and every person of qualified osteopathic status to co-operate at a time when united representation on their part will be of the greatest importance and service to the profession.

The following are some of the objects of the Society:-

To organise and unite all duly qualified osteopaths and to compile and maintain a Register of Members of the Society.

To support and protect the character, status, rights and interests of osteopaths, to give advice and other assistance in all professional matters, to promote honourable practice, to repress malpractices, and to decide questions of professional usage and courtesy between and among osteopaths.

To obtain statutory recognition of all members of the Society or other legal acknowledgement for enabling the Society to carry any of its objects into effect and to oppose any proceedings or applications which may be considered to prejudice, either directly or indirectly, the interests of the Society and its membership body.

To provide for the delivery and holding of lectures, demonstrations, clinical research, public meetings, conferences, conventions, classes, and such other means calculated to promote the general advancement of Osteopathy and the cause of osteopathic education, whether general or professional.

To increase facilities for the training of students desirous of entering the profession by establishing a proper training school.

To provide or arrange for examination by a Board of competent examiners of all candidates for Membership of the Society, who as students have undergone a satisfactory course of training and instruction in the requirements of the profession.

To institute and maintain a library, and to publish a journal and other literature relative to Osteopathy and the Society.

To co-operate with osteopathic educational institutions and other professional osteopathic bodies throughout the world for the furtherance of professional protection and education in science and practice.'

The constitution then followed. Sessions and meetings of the society were held regularly and informal meetings and study circles held from time to time. An information bureau, professional service and legal defence and liability insurance were organised. The annual subscription was three Guineas.

There were three grades of membership:

Licentiate: For those who had been in practice for three years continuously and were generally recognised by other practitioners in the area;

Member: For those who had undergone the prescribed course of study at an approved osteopathic training institution and passed the Examinations;

Fellow: For those who passed the Honours Examination for fellowship.

The membership examination consisted of three parts:

Pre-osteopathic examination in chemistry and physics

First professional examination in biology, zoology, comparative anatomy, embryology, anatomy, histology, physiology and biochemistry.

Final Professional Examination in pathology and bacteriology, Osteopathy, principles and practice, including ethics.

Its Patrons were Sir George Hamilton MP, Sir Algernon Tudor-Craig and Sir Hubert A. Dowson. Its President was W. Skirving Rutherford DO MRO. Members of the Council were:

R. Cooper-Brown DO

T. Jackson Eyre DO

Donald N. Goodall DO MRO (Director of Studies)

Capt. C. S. Price MBE DO

Ronald C. Albino esq.

The Director of Examinations was Joseph S. Bridges MA LLD BSc, Barrister-at-Law.[7]

It was associated with the Salvation Army Goodwill and Slum Clinics, with branches at the Paddington Slum and Goodwill Centre and at Bristol, Glasgow, Liverpool, Everton and Manchester.

Rutherford and Goodall were eventually elected members of the GCRO. In 1938 members of the National Society of Osteopaths were circulated with application forms to enrol onto the GCRO. In 1939, when the GCRO appointed External Examiners for the BSO for the first time, the GCRO chose Goodall. (See Chapter 7).

The Osteopath was the National Society's Journal. In December 1937, there was an article on research, indicating that the National Society had a research department and a clinical records bureau.[8]

The United Association of Osteopaths, Chiropractors & Naturopaths of Great Britain and Ireland Ltd.

In an undated pamphlet, ten objects were listed, one of which was to register fully qualified Osteopaths, Chiropractors and Naturopaths and all others in similar practices and to examine and award Degrees and Diplomas to members satisfying the standards of the Company, as determined by the Bye-Laws of the Company. Its President was Norman Harris, who was also Principal of the Edinburgh College of Naturopathy, Osteopathy and Chiropractic. (See below).

The BSO (1935)

The proceedings of the Select Committee of the House of Lords reveal details of the school in 1935.[9] Its trustees then included Edgar Martin Littlejohn, G. R. Curzon Barrow (nephew of Herbert Barker) and Norman Warren (elected by the graduates for two years).

The course was of four years' duration, each year of nine months. Littlejohn told the Select Committee that he would welcome a five year course. 'We ourselves have considered that independently of this investigation.'

There were 45 students at that time. eleven received a Diploma the preceding year. In total there had been 98 graduates, of whom two had died and 96 were practising and two were medical men. Another 46 had given up the course.

Entry required a certificate of completion of a regular high school course, or a certificate of preliminary qualification to enter a medical school.

The first two years following matriculation (or its equivalent) required attendance at a premedical course in the regular medical colleges, covering: physics, biology, chemistry and anatomy, physiology, histology, embryology, biochemistry, dissection and histology. It was for the students to arrange this course with the medical schools. Students were required to present a certificate of having passed the pre-medical examination for entry into the third year. After 1934-35 they were also required to attend medical school and take the first professional examination. There was, however, difficulty in getting students into medical school. Before 1935 only nine or ten had done so. In September 1934, 50 applicants were turned down by the BSO as they could not or would not go to medical school. Only eight were accepted.

In addition students were required to attend courses in fundamental principles of Osteopathy, applied anatomy, and foundation principles of technique in diagnosis, manipulative science and clinical technique at the BSO for four hours a week in the first two years, i.e. they had a fuller curriculum than medical students. This was also difficult to accomplish and so they were required to undertake this work in the third and fourth year—an extra five hours a week.

Third and fourth year students were required to treat 700 patients under supervision of the two superintendent of clinics, John Martin Littlejohn Jr and Elsie Wareing, who were the only paid staff. 97 patients were treated daily in the clinic on average. 18, 000 patients were treated in 1934, equivalent to 24,000 treatments. Ten clinical assistants worked one or two hours. There were qualified demonstrators—Littlejohn and six others. There were nine demonstrations a week. Littlejohn taught 12 hours a week.

There were 13 other affiliated clinics in and around London, conducted by graduates for poorer people, but under supervision of the school. Difficult cases were sent to the main clinic.

Littlejohn was asked at the Select Committee the advantages of the Bill to the School. He explained that intending students would see that there is a proper field for osteopathic practice, it would improve facilities, there would be better co-operation with the medical schools providing the first two years of the course and it would enable them to have their own hospital, or access to public hospitals.

The BSO (1935-1939)

Records of Annual General Meetings and of Meetings of the Board of Governing Directors exist from 25 July 1935 and of the Council of Education from two February 1939. Present at the Annual General Meeting of the School in July 1935, were Harvey Foote (Chairman), J .M. Littlejohn (Dean), Canning, Hall, James and John Littlejohn, Minifie, Oxenham, van Straten, Waren and Elsie Wareing.

Darlison claimed that the clinic at Buckingham Gate was of great service to thousands of poor people, who were treated free, or who paid a small fee that they could afford.[10] The Radiological Department was opened on 14 March 1938. The X-ray apparatus was acquired at a cost of £846 4s 9d by hire purchase.

The Children's clinic commenced as a separate Department in September 1937 for children up to the age of ten, on Monday and Thursday mornings. Two rooms were set aside. It was run initially by Shilton Webster-Jones, assisted by Muriel Higham, and then by the latter on a honorary basis for two years. During the School year 1938-9 senior students attended, in addition to their regular clinic work. With the outbreak of war and the evacuation of children, the department closed and very few children were treated in the clinic until after the war ended.

From its inauguration until the end of April 1938 27 children had been treated. The largest group were various forms of paralysis, chiefly spastic paraplegia, hemiplegia and poliomyelitis. 'Definite improvement has been obtained in most of these cases. The little patients thoroughly enjoy having treatment and look forward to it eagerly.'

In 1938 a Department of Refraction and Orthoptics was established to deal with 'symptoms of the eye' and those, 'Whose general condition is known to affect the ocular apparatus'.

In 1934 a School magazine, 'The Bone', was founded. The students began to establish a library. In 1935, a Students' Union was formed embracing the magazine and study circle. There were outings to Hayling Island in 1937 and 1938.

Despite the criticisms of the School by the Select Committee in 1935, the students enjoyed their Christmas Party that year. There was a fancy dress parade judged by the Dean and Dr Wood. 'The most amusing event of the evening was the performance of short sketches by some of the students depicting incidents at the BSO and including impersonations of School officials and members of faculty.'[11]

The Journal of Osteopathy for September-October 1936 carried congratulations to John F. Kemp, winner of the Dorothy Wood Gold Medal. It claimed, 'Mr Kemp has winning ways, a wonderful weight (13 stone) a wandering wallop with his right. Maybe No. 3 is the reason for my writing these nice things about him.'[12]

In 1934, in addition to its official gown, hood and cap, the School adopted its colours and its crest, with the dictum: *Pro Natura Veroque,* later changed to *Pro Natura et Veritate*

In 1936 the Registrar told Shilton Webster-Jones, later to become Principal of the School, that his application for the post of Superintendent was unsuccessful, because the School was establishing a new policy regarding this appointment. However, he was offered the newly-created post of Assistant Registrar for a period of one year with a salary of approximately £125-£150 per annum. This was renewed. He was also expected, within reason, to fill the breach when members of the staff were unavoidably absent and, in addition, to give one or two lectures regularly per week. In 1939 he was appointed Registrar with Middleton as Deputy Registrar and Director of Clinics.

A Committee of Investigation, appointed by the Council of Education, dismissed Elsie W. Wareing, (the first graduate of the School and Littlejohn's assistant). She objected to this contending that it was illegal. However, the Board of Governing Directors confirmed the Committee's action. The Board also considered trying to recover the gratuity paid to her on termination of her employment, in view of her subsequent objections.

In 1938, probably as a result of gaining accreditation with the GCRO, BOA members Jocelyn Proby, R. Hope Robertson and O. B. Deiter joined the Faculty. In 1939 the Council of Education consisted of the Dean, Hall, Tanguy, Canning, Webster-Jones and James Littlejohn (Registrar). Proby and Middleton later joined.

In 1939, Dr Deiter conducted a regular weekly course of lectures on technique. A Faculty room was designated. There was a possibility of the Sheffield Clinic affiliating with the School, but a lack of finance hampered progress.

A representative of the European Chiropractors' Union (Mr Bradbury) wrote to the School suggesting co-operation in trying to prevent the various 'Nature Cure Bodies' from granting Diplomas.

In June 1939 the Council of Education were concerned that the teaching of anatomy at Chelsea Polytechnic was far from satisfactory and the school might teach this themselves. However, by October, following the outbreak of war, Chelsea Polytechnic had closed, so other arrangements had to be made. (See below).

The BSO had its Ladies' Osteopathic League for, 'The furtherance of the cause of Osteopathy in Great Britain by means of social activities, by raising funds and generally to aid the work of the British School of Osteopathy'. It was equivalent to the Ladies' Association of the BOA.

The Journal of Osteopathy reported a bazaar held by the Ladies Committee in the Livingstone Hall, Westminster, on 9 February 1935, which ended with H. P. Herbert's play, 'Two gentlemen of Soho', performed by the BSO Students' Dramatic Society.[13]

Before the outbreak of War: A Student Summer Outing in 1939

Just prior to the outbreak of war the students at the BSO had a Summer outing. The description is in stark contrast to what was to happen that Autumn. They:

'Met at Buckingham Gate at 10.30am and were transported by car owners among them to Badger Hall, the delightful country home of Dr Littlejohn. At least one party, we are sorry to report, got lost on the way, but arrived in time for the picnic lunch and the liquid refreshment which Dr and Mrs Littlejohn had so kindly provided. There was no lack of amusements and the afternoon—except for the time given to a delicious strawberry tea—was spent in playing darts, tennis, croquet, table tennis and rounders, while, for the less energetic, there was quiet strolls through the many acres of unspoilt country which forms the estate of Badger Hall. One event of the day was a cricket match—Staff v. Students. This proved to be great fun—the students winning the match by some five runs—probably gained when the Staff were incapacitated by mirth at the brilliance (sic) of the students' batting. After a most enjoyable supper, carpets were taken up and then on with the dance to the strains of the radio—back to London-tea!-bed! A glorious day—many thanks to Dr and Mrs Littlejohn.'[14]

The Edinburgh College of Naturopathy, Osteopathy and Chiropractic

A Prospectus for the College for the session 1935-1936 indicates its Principal was Norman Harris, a Diplomate of the American School of Naturopathy and Chiropractic, Triple Diplomate in Naturopathy, Osteopathy and Chiropractic UAOCN, Member of the American Naturopathic Association, Member of the World League of Naturopathy, Member of the National Association of Naturo-Therapeutic Physicians and Surgeons, and President of the United Association of Osteopaths, Chiropractors and Naturopaths of Great Britain and Ireland. The Secretary's Office was: 42 Moray Place, Edinburgh 3.

The Edinburgh College and its related professional body, the United Association of Osteopaths, Chiropractors and Naturopaths of Great Britain, considered that it was essential that a Natural Healer should include all three therapies in his or her practice. It rejected those individuals or Schools that claimed any manual manipulative method to be a complete system of healing in itself. Osteopathy and Chiropractic were considered complements of Naturopathy.

They claimed that the whole conception of natural healing was opposed at every point to the teachings and practice of orthodox medicine. Therefore it followed that the teaching of Naturopathy and its complements, Osteopathy and Chiropractic, should present revolutionary differences, but most (then) so-called schools of natural healing did not do so, for their curricula were modelled after those of the medical schools, such that, 'They are but cheap plagiarisms'.

The College was critical of many drugless methods in that they were considered positively harmful and many more were without value. 'The 'drugless' practitioner through false, conventional teaching, has inherited too many medical fallacies, and cares for his patients too much in accord with these fallacies. He treats disease by name; he treats disease symptomatically; he treats 'disease'. By employing merely local treatment he leaves the essential systematic derangement and its causes neglected, untouched, and even unsought. Symptoms only receive attention and these symptoms will certainly cease when their antecedents are corrected — they will not cease before.'

The Prospectus considered that the chief concern of practically all of the schools of Naturopathy, Osteopathy and Chiropractic was to be able to present timetables comparable with the schools of medicine, because they yearned to be indistinguishable as possible from them. It considered that, 'All these courses are conventional curricula, aping and perpetuating all the vicious nonsense that conventional teaching imposes, including, of course, the long barren vacations without which it would be so difficult to spread out 3 or 4 weary academic years....It is surprising to discover that so many teachers of these subjects are hide-bound by every convention of false orthodoxy they purport to condemn.'

The Edinburgh College ruthlessly discarded accepted conventions of teaching 'medicine', 'Because such teaching means the perpetuating of bad methods; unscientific, disproved premises; unnecessary time-wasting subjects; untenable false dogma; illogical confused thinking; and finally a puzzled graduate, outwardly word-perfect for examination purposes, but inwardly frustrated, unconvinced and without the true self-confidence and faith which only the acquirement of irrefutable knowledge can give.'

The curriculum of the Edinburgh College was arranged to cover 'exhaustively' the whole field of Naturopathy, Osteopathy and Chiropractic, including all ancillary subjects, in one year.

Prospective students were required to be between the ages of 16 and 65 and to satisfy the Principal that their general education was of a standard necessary to enable them to complete the course. The total fees for enrolment (one guinea), tuition (60 guineas), examination (two guineas) and the diploma (one guinea) were payable in advance. Examinations were written, oral and practical and those successful were awarded the Triple Diplomate in Naturopathy, Osteopathy and Chiropractic (ND, DO, DC) and admitted as Practitioner Members of the United Association of Osteopaths, Chiropractors and Naturopaths of Great Britain and Ireland.

The British Institute of Naturopathy and Osteopathy (BINO)

The British Institute of Naturopathy and Osteopathy wrote to the BOA in February 1935, with the intention of establishing a college of Osteopathy at Matlock Bath, Derbyshire. It became operative in 1938 and lasted until 1947.[15] A Prospectus of unknown date indicates that the Principal was S. W. Daley-Yates ND DO PhB (abbreviations as stated), Council Member of the British Association of Naturopaths, Registered Member of the British Federation of Natural Therapeutics, Member of the Institute of Botano-Therapy and Fellow of the International Faculty of Sciences. six collaborating Faculty were listed, including G. Daley-Yates.

The British College of Osteopathy

A. S. Harding at the BSO received a letter from this College dated 28 May 1937 indicating it was located at Masson House, Matlock Bath, the same address as BINO (see above) with clinics also at 29 Lampton Road, Hounslow, 13 Goodmayes Road, Goodmayes and 84 Barrington Drive, Glasgow. Its Principal also was S. W. Daley-Yates, but with qualifications now listed as DSc DO (Lond) PhD. In the Prospectus for 1937-1938, they are listed as DSc DO (Lond) ND. The course was of four years, each of nine months and led to a Diploma in Osteopathy.

The Training of Nature Cure Practitioners

The Nature Cure Association of Great Britain and Ireland (NCA) was located at 10 Pembroke Gardens London W8. Its Executive Council consisted of: B. St John Doherty, Stanley Lief, Harry Clements, Milton Powell and Leslie Korth.

In the mid 1930s a group of naturopaths approached the BSO with a view to a closer working relationship with it, possibly to provide a course, but the BSO rejected the proposal. The group therefore decided to form their own teaching institution with a 'holistic' view,[16] but there is also evidence that a similar approach was made again in 1948 (See Chapter 9).

In 1936, the London School for Natural Therapeutics closed down to make way for a college run by the NCA. An appeal was launched by Stanley Lief for funds to do so. This was the predecessor of what was to become the British College of Naturopathy, though without a building students were initially nomadic and visited practitioners.[16]

In an article Lief said, 'The establishment of the college will mean the realisation of a dream that has existed with me for years For years I have been aware that the future of the Nature Cure Movement in this country would ultimately depend on whether we have a really dignified, adequately equipped, and a properly staffed training centre'.

In March, 1938 the NCA and College and Clinic was founded at Wyndham House, Wyndham Place, Bryanston Square, London W1, on a 20 year lease. It was opened by George Mitcheson MP. It was closed in 1939 as fire bombs set the roof alight. The repository in which its furniture was stored also later burned down.[15]

In a letter to A. S. Harding at the BSO, dated 16 October 1936, reference was made to the four year course of training required to qualify as an osteopath and naturopath, the first two years to be undertaken at medical college and the following two years at a training college, which the NCA proposed to have ready for students probably by the following September. In a booklet entitled, 'Training of Nature Cure Practitioners', reference was made to the teaching of Osteopathy and manipulative therapy and osteopathic diagnosis in the third and fourth years. A minimum of 700 individual treatments was an essential condition for admission to the final examination.

British Osteopathic Hospitals

The BSO planned to have residential wards at 16 Buckingham Gate in 1930. (See Chapter 2). A hospital fund was in existence in 1932. In 1933 reference was made to plans for two wards: The J. Martin Littlejohn Ward and the Sir Herbert Barker Ward.[17] *The Journal of Osteopathy* for October-December 1935 also referred to an intended British Osteopathic Hospital and the slow gathering of funds for 'indoor cases'. A residential osteopathic sanitorium existed at Stone Cross, Hall Green, West Bromwich, supervised by Arthur Millwood.[17]

The British Osteopathic Mental Hospital Limited

A proposal for such a hospital was outlined in a 14 page booklet, bound but undated, written by R. Hope Robertson MB, ChB (Edin), DO (USA), a Kirksville trained osteopath practising in Leeds. It is presumed to have been written before World War II, though no earlier than 1938.

The booklet began, 'The Company is being formed for the purpose of establishing an Osteopathic Institution in the precincts of London for the treatment and care of patients of either sex suffering from mental and nervous diseases....'

The nature of Osteopathy was then discussed. 'Osteopathy covers all fields of the art of healing, as does Orthodox Medicine. All diseases of the mind and body come within its scope....There is no disease and no disturbed condition of the mind or body that Osteopathy cannot influence.'

The value of an osteopathic hospital was then introduced. It claimed, 'It is beyond question that by osteopathic treatment in a properly equipped Institution at least 65% of all these patients (with schizophrenia) and also a large percentage of patients suffering from other mental diseases could be completely cured and restored to their former health.'

Reference was made to the American Osteopathic Mental Institutions that, 'Are and have been for many years, the most flourishing Institutions of the kind in the world. The most important is the Still-Hildreth Osteopathic Sanatorium, Macon, Missouri, established in 1914....'

Schizophrenia was then discussed and some basic statistics on recovery. 'The average rate of recovery, based on the results of our state institutions, varies from 3% to 7%. The statistics show that in checking over 1,000 cases, which have been in the Still-Hildreth Sanatorium during the past 19 years, the rate of recovery was 33%....In early cases, patients that were ill six months, or less, the recovery rate was 68%.'

Hope Robertson claimed that during his eight years of osteopathic practice in Leeds, he had, 'Proved by experience and practice that he can cure at least 62% of thoroughly representative cases of dementia praecox (schizophrenia) of two years standing and 90% of cases taken in their early stages'.

It was considered that, 'The fundamental principle of osteopathic treatment is the correcting of physical causes, which, through their adverse influence on the autonomic nervous system, bring about disturbed circulation, the underlying factor of this disease....Most mental diseases are the result of a starved or toxic brain the function of which cannot be normal. Treatment is primarily adjustment of structure to restore normal function.'

Dietetics and hydrotherapy, such as hot packs, prolonged baths and colonic irrigation were considered powerful adjuncts to treatment. In addition, regularity and routine, recreation in wholesome sports and games, pleasant surroundings and friendly care were believed important, together with occupational therapy for chronic cases.

On 1st January 1938, 131,952 persons were under care in county and borough mental hospitals. Only 8,500 were discharged during 1937. It was estimated that over 40% of the inmates of mental institutions were schizophrenics. The total expenditure by Local Authorities in England and Wales on mental hospitals and patients therein during 1935-36 was £9,737,047.

Hope Robertson was aware that, 'The medical profession and Ministry of Health appear to take the view that Osteopathy is an experiment and still in its infancy'. He went on to state: 'This is proved to be fallacious by the fact that it has, as already stated, flourished in America for many years....In 1931 there were over 8,000 osteopathic practitioners. We now have over 500 gentlemen of proved ability practising the profession in Great Britain, including about ten fully qualified members of the medical profession.'

It was estimated that the capital necessary to rent and equip the proposed Hospital and to commence and establish its working would be approximately £20,000, that would include: one matron, 15 nurses, ten maids, three cooks, three scullery maids and two gardeners. Dr Robertson's fee was to be agreed. Patients would be charged ten guineas per week. It was estimated the hospital would provide for 40 patients on a profit-making basis.

'The Institution proposed to be established would provide for each patient being placed under the care of a physician who specialises in Psychiatry. The grounds of such an Institution would be extensive with facilities for walking, tennis, croquet and other games. Ample physical equipment, both indoor and outdoor, inductive to a good environment would be furnished, and for indoor recreation a library and music room would be available in addition to amusements in the form of reading, dancing, cards, chess, billiards, moving pictures and music.'

'A well balanced, wholesome diet is essential in all cases, and in selected cases special diets are beneficial. The milk and most of the fruit and vegetables, it is anticipated, would be supplied from the garden and farm of the Hospital.'

The booklet concluded that, 'The Hospital will be near London and thus afford students from the Schools of Osteopathy every opportunity of attending lectures and clinical demonstrations. Furthermore, it will undoubtedly be of substantial help to all practising medical men and osteopaths in as much as they will have at their command facilities for the treatment and care of those mental cases where hospitalisation is absolutely necessary.'

Lionel Atherton and Triunism

A lecture given by Lionel Atherton DO MI Inst BTH (London) was reported in the *Brighton Standard* of 7 March 1936, on 'Triunism — athreeway form of healing based on Osteopathy, Psychotherapy and Medical Botany'. It was founded upon the application of Eastern knowledge of medicine to Western clinical practice. He claimed he had an orthodox medical training (his qualifications do not indicate this) and he was a rich man as, 'He was in receipt some time since of a fortune from a grateful patient'. He claimed to be founder of the first British osteopathic hospital, with which was incorporated the Atherton Triune Healing Home, situated near Dorking. Prospective patients could make appointments by arrangement with the Secretary at the Hotel Metropole.

The British Institute of Osteopathic Research (BIOR)

During the proceedings of the Select Committee, Sir Arthur Robinson in presenting a Memorandum on behalf of the Minister of Health, commented:

'That the proper action at present is to set on foot an organised and careful scientific enquiry into the principles and practice of Osteopathy by a body suitable for the purpose.'

The osteopathic profession responded to this. The BIOR was formed with the main object of promoting such careful and scientific enquiry and research into this new art of healing, 'Advancing the prestige of Osteopathy and conducting actual research. The work...will collate existing knowledge of osteopathic results, and add new materials gathered from the field of practice, confirmed by laboratory and other diagnostic methods.'

Discussions regarding its formation began in November 1934. It was registered on 7 October 1935, though *The Journal of Osteopathy* October-December 1935 claims it was founded in November 1934, prior to the meeting of the Select Committee of the House of Lords.[18], 'It expressed our wishes and our determination to make Research the great work of the future...before the question was mooted at the hearing.' Darlison (the Hon Sec.) did the spadework for the scheme. Members were from the BOA, OAGB and GCRO, i.e. it was non-sectarian and non-political.

The 1935 July issue of *The British Osteopathic Journal* claimed that the Institute, 'Has now definitely commenced activity. The principal work for a time will be the collecting of case histories from practitioners, for which purpose a special case history sheet will be supplied by the

Institute. By this means much valuable information regarding the symptoms, the peculiar conduct and the effects on the body of the various diseases will be secured. From time to time it is proposed to issue bulletins containing the conclusions drawn from a study of this data, which will be available to practitioners.'

'Experimental research work will only be possible when the Institute is in possession of funds for the purchase of necessary apparatus, and also, for the securing of services of a research physiologist. Donations to the Institute are therefore urgently needed and should be sent to the Hon. Secretary, The British Institute of Osteopathic Research, 16 Buckingham Gate, London SW1.'

In the Annual report of the BIOR in December 1936, Darlison indicated that there had been encouraging results and referred to a magnanimous donation from the Osteopathic Trusts Fund, enabling the Institute to be incorporated and to proceed entirely free of debt. Further material was also to be provided by the BSO, through the improved organisation of the clinics.

Case history sheets were produced by a Case History Sheets Committee for use by the profession. The Data and Collation Committee concentrated upon the compilation of data on cases of asthma, hay fever, sciatica and low-back conditions generally.

A research library was set up, which was in contact with the A.T. Still Research Institute.

Bulletin No 1 of the BIOR (19pp), dedicated to osteopathic practitioners, was issued in 1938. It was mainly an appeal to the profession for assistance in the work by reporting cases and an indication of the lines along which the research would progress.

An appeal was made by T. E. Hall ('We need statistics') and he requested X-ray negatives of the lumbar-sacral region be sent to 50 Great Cumberland Place, London W1, 'To warrant further research into the type of articulating facets that make up the lumbar-sacral joint. The direction and relation of spinal compensation following mechanical disturbance in the pelvis and/or lower extremities would appear to be almost entirely determined by the type of facet present in this area. Outstanding features, or brief notes accompanying the radiograph would be welcomed by the Investigating Committee.'

An account of seven patients followed, though with no conformity of headings. A collation was made of current cases in 1939. 77 were listed. On a separate sheet (date unknown, but possibly as above) a further 24 cases were listed.

It lists the Members of Council as:

Dr J. Martin Littlejohn (President)
Dr W. Kelman MacDonald (Vice-President)
T. Edward Hall DO
R. W. Puttick DO (Los Angeles Cal)
T. Mitchell-Fox DO
Edwin Miller DO (Phil Pa)
R. H. Banbury DO
Dr D. Wood-Hall
J. J. Darlison MA (Cantab) DO
Jocelyn Proby MA (Oxon) DO (Kirksville)
Dr J. Littlejohn Hon Treasurer
J. Canning DO Hon Secretary

In May 1939, Lester B. Emerson was elected onto the Council, a chief representative in the UK of the Health Spot Shoe Co, of New Cavendish Street, London W1. H. C. Middleton was also elected at that time.

The Working Committee consisted of five members. 28 Members were listed in total.

The Scottish Osteopathic Research Institute (SORI)

The SORI was Inaugurated at the Annual convention of the BOA in October 1935.[19] In its Memorandum of the Constitution, it claimed that its purpose was, 'To conduct Clinical and Laboratory Osteopathic Research'.

Under 'Method' it stated, 'The work will take the form of a scientific investigation into Osteopathy for the benefit of humanity and alleviation of suffering. The work will be done in the Laboratories of Edinburgh University, and will be under the direction of W. Kelman MacDonald, M.D. (Edin.), D.O. (Kirksville, USA) and carried out by fully qualified research workers appointed by the Council of Management of the Institute.

'Dr Kelman MacDonald will on the completion of this constitution, hand over to the Council of Management a sum of £900 or more, which has been collected by him and his friends from patients who have benefited from osteopathic treatment. This sum, with any additional sums that may be received, will form the nucleus of the fund required to carry out the purposes of the Institute and to pay the necessary outlays incurred therewith.'

'The Institute will be under the direction of a Council of management of not less than 3 and not more than 12 persons, who will have responsibility for the conduct of the Institute and the finances thereof, and generally everything connected with the Institute other than actual research work.'

The President of the Institute was The Most Honourable The Marquis of Linlithgow, Viceroy of India. The first Council of Management consisted of Sir Robert Gordon Gilmour, of Craigmillar as Chairman and Mackenzie Fortune Esq. as Honorary Secretary and Treasurer. Members, who each held office for one year were: Sir John Buchanan-Jardine, William Leng, Rutherford Fortune Esq. and J. Taylor Grant.'

The work was carried out under the guidance of an Osteopathic Advisory Committee, appointed by the British Osteopathic Association:

Kelman Macdonald MD, DO
George Macdonald MB, ChB, DO
R. W. R. Watson MB, ChB, DO
R. Hope Robertson MB, ChB, DO
T. S. Torrance MB, ChB, DO
L. W. Betournay DO
J. J. Dunning DO

The British Osteopathic Review for November 1935 carried an advertisement for an experienced, whole-time physiological research worker for three years in the first instance with a salary of £500. Facilities for the work were to be provided in the medical school of the University of Edinburgh. It claimed that the work would be under the Scientific Advisory Committee appointed by the Medical Faculty of the University of Edinburgh and the Osteopathic Advisory Committee.[20] The work was expected to occupy at least seven years. Applications were to be sent to Dr Kelman MacDonald, 40 Drumsheugh Gardens, Edinburgh.

In February 1936, *The British Osteopathic Review* carried an apologia: 'The Faculty of Medicine [of Edinburgh University] have not appointed an Advisory Committee to control such research work, and so far no such arrangements have been made with the individual Head of any Department to have research work carried out within the University Laboratories...It appears that the main stumbling block is that the subject of osteopathic research is a very difficult problem and would require for its satisfactory handling the whole time services of a complete team of workers each being a specialist in his own line of research work.'[21] In May 1936, Dr Kenneth Mackenzie, an experimental physiologist, started the research.

'In the First Report of the Institute of 1937, reference was made to the Select Committee of the House of Lords. During the hearing of the evidence it had become clear that there was a lack of scientific evidence in support of the contentions of the osteopathic witnesses. Though much valuable work had been done by Louisa Burns in the United States of America, the value of the work was lessened by the fact that it was not done in a laboratory of recognised scientific standing. It is of paramount importance, therefore, to realise that the work of The Scottish Osteopathic Research Institute is carried out in a laboratory of international repute.'

In the Report of the House of Lords, the Committee paid, 'A tribute to the ability and sincerity, of Dr Kelman MacDonald, the representative of the British Osteopathic Association....Dr Kelman MacDonald acts as the Director of the Scottish Osteopathic Research Institute.'

The report of the SORI claimed: 'In particular it is the osteopathic spinal bony lesion which is the subject of this research. It was decided that some organ should be used as a biological test of the influence of the osteopathic causative factor.'

'The white rat was chosen as a large number of cases with identical injuries must be studied. It was considered sufficiently physiologically akin to the human species; easy and inexpensive to maintain; anatomically well known; rapid in gestation and large enough for the accurate performance of experiments. The ovary of the rat was selected for biological tests as it lends itself to accurate observations of function.'

Work was conducted to test the validity of the statement, 'That lesions of definite regions of the spinal column cause changes in the organs associated with these regions by way of the sympathetic nervous system'. The ovary is sympathetically innervated via the 2nd and 3rd lumbar segments. It was assessed whether lumbar lesions cause infertility.

A 'considerable number' of rats were lesioned by hand and mechanically and single and multiple traumatisations of different vertebral segments tried more or less at random. 'The hand (especially that of a trained osteopath) is a very flexible instrument capable of appreciating slight protuberances, such as the spinous processes of the rat, even when covered by a layer of skin, capable of applying finely graduated pressure and appreciating slight movements of the joints to which pressure is applied.'

A complex machine was devised which went through four stages of evolution, with an electro-magnetic hammer. 'With a weight of 4 Kgs (about 9 pounds) on the weight pan and 500 blows from the hammer, which weighs 25 gms and delivers 8 blows per second, there is produced a definite lesion in the spine of the rat, which can be recorded by X-ray photography. The total work done amounted to 2.4 Joules.'

The results gave definite evidence that sterility would result in certain cases, and that the exact region of the spine in which crucial results could be expected was the third lumbar segment. Of the six lumbar segments of the rat, lesions in the upper or lower pair of vertebrae had no effect. This was followed up by the examination of the tissues of the animals by sectioning, staining and photomicroscopy.

The X-ray photography posed difficulties due to the flexibility of the spine, the size of the object and the lack of co-operation of the rats in keeping still (!) and in the interpretation of the X-rays. Drs Mackenzie and MacDonald gave independent written reports of their findings together with two independent experts who were unaware of the details of the experiment.

In 1937 the BOA minutes recorded that an Osteopathic Research Institute, presumably the SORI was affiliated to the BOA, employing a full time scientist and two laboratory assistants and a part time histologist. A lesioning machine used was to be exhibited at the AOA conference.

It was considered that these experiments raised some interesting problems. How is the sterility brought about? Why is sterility not absolute — for in every case some lesioned animals remained fertile? Can sterility be removed by corrective treatment? However, the research methodology had major limitations.

The Lumbar Club

The Lumbar Club was formed by a small group of British osteopaths, 'In an effort to provide facilities for research in practical osteopathic technique and body mechanics.'[22] Its task was, 'To maintain a high standard of "ten-fingered" craftsmanship among osteopaths'.

It claimed, 'The osteopathic practitioner may be justly proud of his skill as a psychoanalyst, a dietician, or a laryngologist; he may be a master of bedside mannerisms, but as an osteopath, unless he is possessed of a highly developed manipulative technique, he remains a mere 'engine wiper'.

The first meeting of the six foundation members took place on 18 January 1937. The club met once a month. Papers were read followed by discussion and demonstration.

One of the rules of the club forbade the discussion of political matters relating to Osteopathy. It awarded annually a silver badge and one year's membership to the student of the BSO who did the best practical work during his or her final year.

The Officers of the club in 1937-38 were T. E. Hall, R. K. Hardy and James Canning. A 'Day Book', contains the accounts of the 'Lumbar Club' for 1938 and 1939 and the membership list: H. C. Middleton, A. T. (John ?)Leary, T. E. Hall, J. M. Littlejohn Jr, S. Webster Jones, J. Bishop, J. Canning, R. K. Hardy, W. Gilmour and H. Trill.

There are records of savings certificates held by the club in March-July, 1942.

A similar club existed in America: The Atlas Club.

Osteopathy in Germany and the Osteopathic Olympic Committee

In 1936 Dr W. J. Douglas visited the Winter Sports at Garmisch-Partenkirchen where he demonstrated osteopathic technique at the invitation of the Sports' doctors. Douglas had been in practice in Paris for three years previous to this and was the sole osteopath working there. He was Vice-President of the AOA in 1935.

Volkische Beobachter, the official newspaper of the National-Socialist Party founded by Hitler, in 14 February 1936 asked the question, 'What is Osteopathy?' Douglas so impressed the doctors that he and a team were invited to the International Conference of Medical Advisers for Athletics in Germany in Berlin held under the auspices of the Reich government.[23] One of its Honorary Presidents was Reichsminister Dr W. Frick. It was claimed to be the first time Osteopathy was officially introduced to Germany and demonstrations were given relating to athletic injuries, as a preliminary to the XI Olympiad.

The first session of this conference was held in Berlin from 27-31 July 1936 at the Kroll-Oper. 35 countries were represented and five languages were spoken. Over 500 practitioners were registered and more than 75 papers read. Dr G. Wagner, Reichartztefuhrer and President of the Conference stressed the fact that all doctors should realise healthy people require as good doctoring as sick people. He said he was anxious that all visitors should feel entirely at home in Berlin and that when the time came for them to return to their native lands they would leave the Reich City with the fixed impression that the people of the German nation had but one thought and one aim, and that was International Peace. 'Dr Wagner expressed himself most sincerely and his words were received with prolonged and delighted applause.'

The contributions of the British osteopaths who participated were:

E. T. Pheils: Discussed Principles of Osteopathy followed by a demonstration of manipulation of cervical vertebrae;

W. Kelman MacDonald: Discussed the causes and treatment of low backache, illustrated by moving pictures and lantern slides;

C. L. Johnson: Demonstrated methods of bandaging and strapping sports injuries;

J. J. Dunning: Provided moving pictures of the Rice-Webster technique of diagnosing and treating vertebral lesions;

O. B. Deiter: Gave a paper on tennis elbow, followed by a demonstration of osteopathic manipulative methods of treatment.

During the Olympic games one or more members of the committee attended the Olympic Village each day and treated competitors. American osteopaths were led by Dr H. E. Litton of Kirksville.

On 1 August three German newspapers made reference to Osteopathy.[24] According to the *Berliner Tageblatt* an Olympic Osteopathic Committee of American and English osteopaths visited the sports therapy institute at Eichkamp, at which, 'Through medical manipulative therapy and orthopaedic measures it was proved that sports lesions can be healed'.[25]

The *Frankfurter Zeitung* wrote:

'The doubts which might have existed regarding their methods which generally necessitate rather severe manipulation will have disappeared almost entirely following the demonstration by an extensive film by Dr Kelman MacDonald of Edinburgh, Scotland. Though at the first moment, in spite of its entire absence of pain, one cannot help getting the impression of it being rather a gruesome cure, the practical success of this re-adjustment method was aptly proved by numerous X-ray pictures of the spinal column before and after the treatment. His explanations and his film were received with great interest. Much special interest was given in this connection to the manner of treatment of the tennis elbow by Dr Deiter— symptoms of this kind in the elbow not being entirely due to playing tennis—by which through simple manipulating massage healing was forced. It is a good method although to many it will appear extraordinary, the more so in most cases one must give careful treatment to sensitive joints.'[24]

Morganpost wrote:

'The participants of the Congress had come to hear and learn what their American colleagues had to tell them about the method of Osteopathy which is rather unknown in Germany. Osteopathy aims to keep health in an ill body which is still not ill, and help to move those forces which operate against illness. The osteopaths try to show by their method that every illness gives simultaneously some kind of change in the spine. As therefore a changed bone structure is the origin or goes simultaneously with every illness, the treatment must specialise on the bones and joints. If you correct the spine of the chest area you can help asthma and heart trouble and stomach and bowel diseases. It is said that ill nerves can soon get better by helping the circulation in the spinal cord. Also it is said that many diseases of the ears, eyes, nose and throat can be helped through osteopathic treatment because in these cases the muscles of the spine reflect and draw together so that when they are loosened by osteopathic manipulation the complaints very speedily disappear.'

35 members of the AOA arrived in London on 23 August to spend the final week of their tour there, having visited Holland, Germany, Austria and France.

Litton was widely quoted in British newspapers that poor, cheaply fed children enjoy better health than rich children. According to him, children of rich parents in the US are under-nourished, under weight and have a tendency towards curvature of the spine. Edward Hall wrote a comment in the *Journal of Osteopathy*: 'What a pity that Dr. Litton couldn't find the time during his stay in London to take advantage of the invitations he accepted for himself and his party to visit the British School of Osteopathy, look it over, and partake of luncheon with its staff. After all, it's only 50 yards from Buckingham Palace at 16 Buckingham Gate, SW1.'[26]

Journals

The *Journal of Osteopathy* was first produced by the BSO in 1929. By 1939, there was a problem of the cost of production. Hall considered this was due to faulty organisation and threatened to resign from the editorial staff, but was persuaded to continue by the Council of Education. In October, the Council of Education decided to issue it in a reduced form, as a war emergency issue.

In December 1933, a Committee was elected by the BOA in order to publish *The Osteopathic Review*. It was edited by Dr O. B. Deiter and issued quarterly, price one shilling. Members received two copies free. Several issues carried on the front cover a photograph of the Walton Heath Osteopathic Hydro at Kingswood Court, Tadworth, Surrey. The Principal was Sydney A. Cullum DO.

By 1935, it was decided that while it was still to be the Journal of the BOA, it was to be published independently. Deiter took it over but the BOA still wanted editorial control. Later it was considered that Deiter had gone back on an agreement by refusing to allow the BOA Council to have anything to do with the journal. Deiter appointed a new Editorial Committee and resigned from the BOA. However, by 1937, it was decided that the journal was again to be published by the Association.

The British Osteopathic Journal was started in January 1934 as a quarterly journal by the IAO, 'To stimulate inquiry and dispel prejudice'. The volume for July 1935 had an article: 'British Osteopathy. The School and its Founder, by J. J. Darlison MA (Cantab.), DO'.

In volume 11 (July 1936) the editorial address is given as 546 Eccleshall Road, Sheffield 11. In its 12 pages, there is an editorial from a grateful patient, with the editorial comment, 'Another human document showing how Osteopathy has helped a man from the darkness of despair to the sunshine of confidence and good health'.

Other articles were on: Feet, hips and spine; The British Institute of Osteopathic Research; An Osteopathic Fundamental; The Journal and its Readers; Good health (by Herbert Milne) and Hydrotherapy (by R Neville Coleby).

The National Society of Osteopaths had its own journal, '*The Osteopath*'. Volumes 1 and two appeared in December, 1937.

Osteopathic Books

During the 1930s a number of osteopathic books were published in Britain. In 1931 Ethel Mellor wrote, *Manipulation as a Curative Factor*, published by Methuen, price ten shillings and sixpence.

Captain Gerald Lowry (one of the first graduates of the BSO) wrote, *From Mons to 1933*, which carried a foreword from the Rt. Hon Lord Ampthill, who claimed, 'I myself am a firm believer in Osteopathy. Captain Lowry cured me of painful sciatica', and Field Marshal Viscount Allenby. Lowry went on to write *Helping Hands* (1935) and *The Feet in Relation to Health*. (Date unknown).

In 1933, L. C. Floyd McKeon wrote, *A Healing Crisis*, published by Michell Health Products, Weston Super Mare, price five shillings, followed by *Osteopathic Polemics* in 1938, published by C. W. Daniel Company Ltd.

In the 1930s George MacDonald and W. Hargrave-Wilson published *The Osteopathic Lesion* (Heinemann) and Kelman MacDonald, *The Scientific Basis of Osteopathy*, based on the seven Bulletins of the A.T. Still Research Institute and articles from the Journal of the AOA.

J. J. Darlison's *The New Art of Healing, Osteopathy* (1935) was obtainable through W. H. Smith and Son Ltd, price one shilling. In his Foreword of 1 November 1935, Littlejohn explained how Darlison spent three years studying traditional medical healing, but developed hearing disability due to active service as an artillery officer in the Great War. 5000 copies were sold by January 1936.

In 1937, J. M. Dent and Sons Ltd published *What is Osteopathy*, written by Charles Hill, Deputy Medical Secretary of the BMA and the 'Radio Doctor', and H. A. Clegg, Deputy Editor of the BMJ. The book carried a foreword by H. G. Wells:

> 'It is in the nature of man to be rebellious against his medical director. Man is born recalcitrant, protesting, and many of us even at the moment of birth require slapping. The doctor is not alone in his unpopularity. The hatred of teachers is almost as widespread, and of priests even more so. It would be easy to take sides in the matter if the doctor proved always right. Unhappily he is often wrong....I do not like baiting medical men. My friend G. B. Shaw does. He fails to control those natural resentments that I keep so beautifully in hand....This book tells the story of Osteopathy calmly, but with a twinkle of amusement that sometimes gives place to a twinkle of indignation. Plainly Osteopathy, considered as a system of medicine or as anything more than the manipulative side of surgery, is impudent balderdash. Mr friend Sir Herbert Barker, now practically reconciled to the medical profession, explains on every possible occasion that he is *not* an osteopath.'

The Foreword, however, did not reflect what followed, namely a rabid condemnation of Osteopathy, as revealed in the proceedings of the Select Committee of the House of Lords. In their conclusion the authors wrote:

> 'We claim to have shown that the theory of Osteopathy is based not only upon insufficient evidence but upon insufficient

knowledge of what must be the basic sciences of any system of healing which claims to be scientific. Andrew Taylor Still for whom belief was stronger than reason, preached his doctrines with religious fervour. For him statements need not be supported by logical argument, because Osteopathy was God's Law. Upon our profound disagreement with the theoretical basis of Osteopathy is based our opposition to its recognition by the State in the form of Statutory Registration.

To the osteopath in search of state registration we would say: Get your name on to the medical register; learn all about disease and health in the medical schools and pass the necessary examinations; then specialize in the osteopathic technique if you wish to. If it is found that osteopathic manipulation has something which medical manipulation has not, then this something else will have to be included in the therapeutic equipment of the practitioner of Medicine.'

Sydney Horler wrote of the book, 'Throughout the 212 pages of this book the joint authors have done their very best to hold the healing art of Osteopathy up to the most virulent ridicule, and in fairness, I must say that many of the things they "expose" would have put me off going to any osteopath for life, if I had not proved beyond any possible doubt that Osteopathy can do things which ordinary Medicine is utterly unable to accomplish'.

In the media

The Proceedings of the Royal Society of Medicine Section on Physical Medicine in November 1932 contained the address of the President, Sir Robert Stanton Woods, who referred to Osteopathy and supported the view that the medical profession should be the body to decide what is truth. He was against Schools of Osteopathy doing this as they would be one-sided.[27]

Dr Ethel Mellor wrote in *The Spectator* on 9 August 1935:

'Why will medical men of high standing...continue to repeat that osteopaths trace all disease to...pressure on nerves and arteries of misplaced and maladjusted bones...of the vertebral column? This, despite its refutal by men of high standing in their own profession, as by osteopaths themselves, and witnesses before the recent Select Committee of the House of Lords. I do not say that the pressure does or does not exist, but that a belief in such pressure is no part of the osteopathic teaching....Moreover, the implication of scorn... like a boomerang, rebounds on the medical profession, for the possibility of such pressure and its relationship to disease is to be found in serious medical writings of a 100 years ago with basis in medical writings of the previous century. The whole of our medical knowledge (has been) accumulated step by step throughout the centuries, by the patient experiments and by the observations of workers all over the civilized world.

Only through unity can the benefits of healing be made available to all men; hence every citizen has an interest in the conduct and outcome of the 'scientific' enquiry tentatively suggested by the representative of the Ministry of Health in evidence before the Select Committee. Unity and not two schools of healing will the better serve our public good.'[28]

In 1938 the Medical Defence Union wrote to Ethel Mellor DSc DO asking her to refrain from using the title 'Doctor'. She attempted to sue the MDU for libel, stating that she was a Doctor of Science of Sorbonne University and Doctor of Osteopathy in the US. Lord Hewart said there was no evidence of defamation and the case failed.[29]

In 1936 Sir Morton Smart, the manipulative surgeon, was declared by some press literature to be the King's official, personal osteopath.[30] At the Select Committee at the House of Lords (1935) he had given evidence against the recognition of Osteopathy. (See Chapter 5).

On 11 September, 1936 the *Daily Express* mentioned that Austin Munks, winner of the Senior Manx Grand Prix Motor Cycle race, owed his success to a Ramsey osteopath on the Isle of Man. Munks could not previously grip properly with his left hand.

In *The Telegraph and Morning Post* on 2 October, 1937, H. L. Eason, Principal of the University of London, referred to, 'The idle and the ignorant rich frequented the osteopath, the chiropractor and other miracle mongers'. Floyd McKeon of Blackpool responded on 6 October. *The Sunday Pictorial*, the following day made reference to the value of osteopathic treatment to restore health, of people over 50 in a home for destitute men, the Embankment Fellowship Centre, Belvedere Road, South-East London.[31]

J. J. Darlison and Edwin Miller on behalf of the BSO discussed Osteopathy at Trinity College, Cambridge Medical Society. The meeting was reported in the *Cambridge Daily News*.[32]

On 24 March 1936[33] *The East Anglian Daily Times* mentioned

Osteopathy in Ipswich and again on 31 January 1939 it reported that Osteopathy was making great strides forward there. The *Sheffield Star* on 7 February 1939 noted that a group of osteopaths were to form a clinic in Sheffield to be opened in March. The *Sunday Pictorial* on 29 January 1939 reported a case of a boy unable to walk or stand. Three hospitals had given him up. Following osteopathic treatment he could sit up, move his hands and arms, speak a little bit, 'And most wonderful of all, take those few steps which show that shortly he will be able to walk.'[34] *The Times* on 9 February 1939 discussed the GCRO and in the *Sunday Express* on 12 February, Viscount Caslerosse praised treatment by osteopaths.[34] *The Evening Standard* on 20 April claimed that patients do go to see osteopaths.[35]

References

1. *The Journal of Osteopathy*. (1931). October, III(1):3.
2. Darlison, J. J. (1935). <u>The New Art of Healing, Osteopathy</u>, p. 23. (London: W. H. Smith & Sons).
3. Puttick, R.W. (1956). <u>Osteopathy</u>, p. 46. (London: Faber & Faber).
4. *The British Osteopathic Review*. (1936). Osteopathic Association clinic. Successful annual bazaar. February, 3(1): 106.
5. *The British Osteopathic Review*. (1936). Osteopathic Association clinic. May, 3(2): 121.
6. *The Journal of Osteopathy*. (1935). October-December, VI(5 & 6).
7. *The Osteopath*. (1937). December, 1(2): 15.
8. *The Osteopath*. (1937). Osteopathic research. December, 1(2): 6-9.
9. Report from the Select Committee of the House of Lords appointed to consider the Registration and Regulation of Osteopaths Bill [H.L.] together with the proceedings of the committee and minutes of evidence. (1935). 3058-3107, pp. 210-212; 3174-4111, pp. 216-259. (London: HMSO).
10. Darlison, J. J. (1935). Free treatment for the poor. *The British Osteopathic Journal*, July: 5-6.
11. *The Journal of Osteopathy*. (1936). BSO students' party. January-February, VII(1): 8.
12. *The Journal of Osteopathy*. (1936). Congratulations. September-October, VII(5): 8.
13. *The Journal of Osteopathy*. (1935). February-April, VI(1 & 2).
14. *The Journal of Osteopathy*. (1939). The students' union. July-September, X(3): 5.
15. Chambers, M. M. (1995). The British Naturopathic Association. The first fifty years. (British Naturopathic Association).
16. Dr Ian Drysdale, Principal of the British College of Osteopathic Medicine. Personal communication
17. *The Journal of Osteopathy*. (1932-1933). December-January, IV(2):3.
18. *The Journal of Osteopathy*. (1935). The British Institute of Osteopathic Research. October-December, VI(5-6): 1.
19. Deiter, O. B. (1935). Notes by the Editor. *The British Osteopathic Review*, November, 2(4): 68.

20. *British Osteopathic Review.* (1935). November, 2(4): 86.

21. *British Osteopathic Review.* (1936). February, 3(1): 103.

22. Middleton, H. C. (1937). The lumbar club. *The Journal of Osteopathy*, July-September, VIII(3): 9.

23. *The British Osteopathic Review.* (1936). Osteopathy in Germany. May, 3(2): 121.

24. *The British Osteopathic Review.* (1936). Notes by the editor. September, 3(3): 144-145.

25. *The Journal of Osteopathy.* (1936). Osteopathy at the Olympic Games. September-October, VII(5): 2.

26. Hall, T. E. (1936). Comment. *The Journal of Osteopathy*, September-October, VII(5): 7.

27. *The Journal of Osteopathy.* (1932-1933). IV(2).

28. Darlison, J. J. (1935). <u>The New Art of Healing, Osteopathy,</u> pp. 15-16. (London: W. H. Smith & Sons).

29. Editorial. (1938). *The Journal of Osteopathy*, IX(2): 3.

30. *The Journal of Osteopathy.* (1936). September-October, VII(5): 1.

31. *The Journal of Osteopathy* (1937). October-December. VIII(4):3-4.

32. *The Journal of Osteopathy.* (1936). Osteopathy at Cambridge. January-February, VII(1): 2.

33. *The Journal of Osteopathy.* (1936). March-April, VII(2).

34. *The Journal of Osteopathy.* (1939). Editorial. January-March, X(1): 4-5.

35. *The Journal of Osteopathy.* (1939). April-June, X(2):5.

Chapter 9

The 1940s — War and After

The Impact of War on Osteopathy

Osteopathy, like all professions, was seriously affected in the first half of the 1940s by the Second World War. Physical and other stresses, both in war service and on the home front, resulted in many people needing osteopathic treatment, but as many osteopaths and osteopathic students were called up for service, there were far too few osteopaths to provide this.

The BOA asked the profession for volunteers to work in its clinics. Osteopaths not called for service were asked to assist those who were, by managing their patient lists in return for half of the fees. There were osteopaths who needed to rent rooms, as their consulting rooms had to be given up for wartime use.

In 1939 Floyd McKeon approached the Minister of Health seeking to make Osteopathy available to those engaged in war. The Minister replied that he was, 'Only concerned with the arrangements for civilian casualties....The decision as to the appropriate ancillary treatment for particular casualties must rest with the physician or surgeon in charge of the case.'[1]

In 1940 Kelman MacDonald contacted the Minister of Pensions for a permit to treat war injuries at the BOA clinic, but was refused. In September 1939, the BOA and GCRO offered their services to the war effort and in November, the BOA offered its services to the Canadian Forces. Dr Callum of the BOA said it seemed a pity that young graduates could not make use of their qualification instead of just being put in the firing line. In April 1944, American-trained osteopath Stephen Ward, who eventually managed to get himself transferred to the Royal Army Medical Corps, though unable to practise in it, wrote to ministers regarding BOA members becoming part of the Corps and establishing osteopathic clinics in command centres. The matter was referred to the

War Office. Ward was to make a name for himself in another capacity in the 1960s. (See Chapter 12).

The BSO also made representations to the Ministry of Health, the War Office, the Admiralty and Home Office asking for recognition of osteopaths in National Service and pointing out how osteopaths would be of use. The replies were mostly negative. Questions were also asked in Parliament.

In July 1940 Lord Elibank, Streeter and Webster-Jones had an interview with Malcolm Macdonald, the Minister of Health. It became apparent that the difficulty of osteopaths being employed as such in National Service could be overcome if the term 'Osteopathy' was dropped and a status adopted equivalent to that of masseurs, teachers of medical gymnastics, or Swedish drill.

Hope Robertson saw the Director General of Medical Services of the RAF in 1941 suggesting that the air force might make use of osteopaths' services and also assist the BSO by attracting students to the profession. The Registrar of the BSO forwarded to the Air Ministry information they requested.

In 1944, Philip Jackson reported to the BOA that the 'Vice Dean of the BSO, Dr Edward Hall, was doing much osteopathic work for the paratroops', but the proposed transfer of an osteopath, Mr Kemp, that year, to the 6th parachute division, was refused as Brigadier General Rowley Bristow claimed the available orthopaedic service was adequate.

The BOA also requested the release of practising osteopaths and students from war service. In 1940, at a GCRO meeting, it was agreed to send deputations to the Ministry of Health and Ministry of Labour asking for osteopaths to be placed on the list of reserved occupations. The former was not supportive, but Ernest Bevin, the Minister of Labour and National Service said he would do what he could. He paid an unofficial visit to the BSO and enquired about the use of Osteopathy in industrial fatigue. The BSO's Registrar requested the Ministry of Labour to postpone students' military service, at least until their examinations, but the Ministry claimed it only acted on advice from the Ministry of Health, which was not supportive. As a result, the School was deprived of both current and prospective students, which had a devastating effect on it financially.

In 1943, the BSO compiled a list of men in the forces for whom it might be possible to secure release, and graduates not in the forces for whom it might be possible to secure deferment. Keith Blagrave was so released from munitions work and appointed Clinic Director at £6 per week. In December of that year the BOA again considered the means of getting men released from the forces to work in its clinic. 26 members of the GCRO served in the war of whom four were killed.

This lack of official support for Osteopathy contrasted with Royal patronage: Queen Elizabeth, (later the Queen Mother), who suffered from a stiff neck on a visit to Birmingham, was treated by a local osteopath, Elmer Pheils. Brian Inglis (1964) commented: 'From that time on, any attempt to harass Osteopathy by coming down on a doctor who recommended it in place of orthopaedic treatment might have given more trouble than it was worth.'[2]

Many children were evacuated from London during the war. As close links still existed between the BOA and AOA, the BOA in 1940 arranged evacuation of children to the US, and placement with patients.

The Vice-Dean of the BSO proposed that the School be used as an Emergency Casualty (First Aid) Centre staffed by voluntary personnel. In 1940, plans were submitted to the Medical Officer of Health for Westminster, who visited the School. The Local Authority, however, was obliged to provide equipment and bear additional expenses. O. B. Deiter had a sympathetic hearing from the Ministry of Health on the matter, but when the Dean wrote to the Minister. The latter replied that they could not make use of the clinic as several casualty stations were already redundant and the building was not sufficiently strengthened to be even an unofficial First Aid post.

The BOA-BSO Conflict

1940 saw a flare up of the old animosity between the BOA and BSO. In the Province of Ontario the BSO had been on the list of approved schools for teaching Osteopathy, but late in 1935, following machinations by the BOA, it was deleted from the list. As the School itself had not been notified, it asked Ontario to confirm if this was so and if it was, whether it could be reinstated. Proby spent a year in Canada during which time he investigated the matter and requested a reconsideration of the status of the School, as it was by then on the GCRO Register. He was sent copies of letters from Kelman MacDonald, Frederic Davis and C. L. Johnson (President of the BOA) received by Ontario, which, 'Contained statements not in accordance with the facts'. Johnson had advised against recognition and had made derogatory statements regarding the School and Register. The School decided to report the matter to the GCRO. Proby wrote to the BOA, 'I would be greatly obliged if you would let me know whether or not the BOA recognises the

BSO and if you would consider that this School should again be placed on the list of approved Schools in Canada, particularly in the Province of Ontario.' This placed the BOA in an embarrassing situation. Pheils suggested that the BOA should make a plain statement, that the BSO and its graduates were recognised by the GCRO, but not by the BOA and that it, 'Could not give them any advice as to whether or not the BSO should again be placed on the list of approved schools in Canada'.

In 1942, Proby sent a letter to the President of the BOA asking him to try to change the attitude of the BOA and its members to the School. He wrote, 'It is impossible to build up a satisfactory teaching institution unless the whole of the profession is behind it.' Jackson commented at a committee meeting of the BOA that he thought that perhaps Proby's complaint was justified. Barber agreed that the only hope for the BSO was for the BOA to, 'Get behind it and make a good school of it'. Lean said, 'The great difficulty was that they say one thing and do another. We had had that trouble since the very beginning. It seems impossible to find out exactly what their standards of education really are.' The BOA President met with Proby to discuss the matter, but the outcome is unknown.

A BOA College and Hospital

Even as early as 1940, Osteopathic Trusts, which were financing the BOA clinic, desired a closer co-operation with the BOA to form an osteopathic college and hospital. The BOA launched an appeal in 1944 to clear the clinic of the Docker debt, to open more clinics, and for an osteopathic college and hospital. This was particularly necessary as it was uncertain if the Home Office would allow further osteopaths from America into the UK after the war.

The GCRO and Registration

In 1942 Lord Elibank resigned as President of the GCRO and the Rt. Hon Lord Strabolgi, who wished to introduce another Osteopaths Bill, replaced him. Streeter, the Chairman of the Register, also resigned and in 1943 Frederic Davis replaced him. The Earl of Mansfield was President from 1945-1947, followed by the Hon B. L. Bathurst QC, when a paid assistant was appointed to reorganise the administration.[3] In 1945 W. Kelman MacDonald was Registrar. During the war it was impossible to operate an agreed constitution effectively and the Register was unable to achieve smooth running until 1947, at which time the Articles of Association were modified under Bathurst's guidance. There were two major amendments, adopted on 18 March 1950:

a) To have one grade of membership only;

b) To set a time limit for (1 January 1951), for admission of applicants who were not graduates of recognised schools, but in active osteopathic practice for not less than five years. They would be required to appear before an examining board, in order to become Associate Members, following which membership would only be permitted to graduates of approved institutions. (Article 11). This was announced in a wide range of newspapers and magazines ranging from *The Times* to *The Vegetarian News*.

131 applications were received from such unregistered practitioners, but only 60 returned the application forms of whom 48 were invited for examination. The Examining Board consisted of a medical doctor, a US osteopathic graduate and two members of the BSO Faculty. There was a viva voce examination and practical examination. 45 appeared and 15 were elected to membership.

The National Society of Osteopaths applied to enter the Register in 1943. Members were required to take the Register's examination.

The Beveridge Report

There was concern in 1942 by both osteopaths and patients regarding the Beveridge Report on Social Insurance and Allied Services. Patients would cease to be able to choose their medical treatment and unregistered practitioners would not be able to practise under Common Law.[4] Osteopathy would be restricted to being undertaken only under the control of a registered medical practitioner.

The GCRO formed a Parliamentary Committee: the BOA represented by True and Cooper; the Register by Webster-Jones and Davis and the OAGB by Mitchell-Fox and Hall, to consider what approach should be made to the Minister of Health. While there was little hope for recognition of osteopaths, they proposed that the Bill dealing with the State Medical Service include a clause enabling osteopathic treatment without medical supervision. Before the White Paper of 1944, Lord Strabolgi, Lord Teviot, Sir Henry Baddeley and others made a deputation to the Minister of Health, Henry Willink.

A questionnaire was sent out to members of the OAGB regarding the Beveridge Report. A general meeting of all osteopaths was planned for 11 November 1944 at the Mayfair Hotel, with Lord Strabolgi as Chairman, but the BOA considered this date too early and wanted to draw up a statement of aims and a statement for the Minister of Health, to be sent initially to the OAGB.

In November 1944, the meeting of the Parliamentary Committee of the GCRO was suspended as Davis, the Chairman and representatives of the BOA resigned (for reasons unknown). The BSO representatives on the GCRO pressed for a general meeting of the Register at the earliest possible date.

A letter was sent from the Board of the BSO to the President of the BOA (Jean Johnson) urging a joint meeting regarding the Beveridge Report. Even by 1945, no acknowledgement or reply of any kind was received. The OAGB and NSO were disgruntled that the Joint Committee to approach the Minister of Health had collapsed.

In November 1944 Christmas Humphreys, at a BOA Council meeting stated that he had, 'The lowest possible view of anything coming from the Minister'. He warned that, 'Every form of unorthodox healing is going to be stamped out'.

Christmas Humphreys repeated this warning at a further BOA meeting in April 1945, drawing parallels with the Herbalists Bill of 1941 which was, 'Rushed through the House of Commons at the height of the War, protests all round; rushed through the House of Lords in such a way that the Lord Chancellor himself apologised afterwards for having been made a fool of in pushing this thing through with a powerful combine behind it representing the chemists; a sop thrown to them about taxation'. It nearly happened to osteopaths with the Medical Appliances Bill of 1936....'You jolly nearly got stamped out then.'

He referred to the Tavistock Clinic as, 'The finest organisation of its kind in the psychological world' (he was on the Committee) that was completely left out of the White Paper. 'If that is how they are treating their own men, some of them famous doctors, how are they going to treat completely unorthodox things. What a hope! Don't let us have any false friendships here. This is war.'

He warned: 'There is a need for ears and eyes in Parliament and to discover from doctors the policies of the Ministry of Health. One has to watch the GMC. It is ten years behind the general body of practitioners and the Permanent Ministry of Health officials — they are just as bad — hopelessly out of date.'

He considered that, the Ministry of Health will attempt to stamp out Osteopathy. It was, 'Attempting to grasp more and more control for the government, including over the doctors....The whole policy of the medical profession as a whole, as I see it at the moment, is to grasp the maximum amount of control over all forms of healing and to say that that which does not accept their curriculum does not exist and shall be stamped out....People may not claim or attempt to heal such and such diseases....You want to be very careful before you put your head into that lion's jaws.'

He recommended having a Standing Committee of Osteopathic Associations and to completely empower them to act on behalf of everybody in defence of osteopathy—'a collective watch dog....'Watch, watch, watch; have your ears in the House of Commons; have your spies among the doctors; know exactly what is in the wind everywhere.'[5]

MacDonald said that without the BSO the progress in Osteopathy would not have been nearly as good as it is. He likened it to what the Labour Party had done to the Conservatives.

In 1945 a resolution was passed that the BOA invite all osteopathic bodies to form a 'Standing Joint Defence Committee' to defend the practice of Osteopathy, with particular reference to possible legislation. The BOA considered the representatives might be: Davis and one other from the Register; Hall and Canning from the BSO. The OAGB was considered really to be the BSO and was substituted for it. The NSO would have only one representative, Rutherford,—'their standards are low, but their enthusiasm is high'.

The GCRO were of the opinion in 1946 that the Committee should be reformed and consist of two members from the BOA, OAGB, Society of Osteopaths and GCRO Council. The BOA, however, did not wish to join as they did not consider it appropriate to approach the Minister of Health at that time.

The British Health Freedom Society

In 1943, the British Health Freedom Society (BHFS) was formed of some 2,000-3,000 lay people and non-medical practitioners, by Stanley Lief, John Wood and J. J. Darlison, with Webster-Jones as an adviser, to protect the interest of patients of unorthodox practitioners in the light of the Beveridge Report. There were some 50 branches. The aim was to establish the right of any member of the public to go to any practitioner (whether recognised by the medical profession or otherwise) for treatment, without penalties or loss of benefit under the proposed National Health scheme and under the Industrial Injuries Bill. The BHFS advertised in *Health for All* and the BSO displayed BHFS literature in its clinic. Osteopaths encouraged support from patients.

The School was approached to send a representative to a meeting, arranged by the BHFS, of MPs and 'unorthodox practitioners' held in the House of Commons in November 1945. Miss Beresford and the BSO Registrar attended as observers on behalf of the OAGB. A further meeting was held in December between Mr House MP and practitioners' representatives. T. Edward Hall and C. R. Morton (Secretary to the BSO Board) attended only in a watching brief, as it was felt the School should not be concerned with this matter.

In 1947, a Joint Committee of Practitioners' Associations was formed to negotiate with Aneurin Bevan, the new Minister of Health, for inclusion under the National Health Act. It became the General Council of Natural Therapeutics and the following year, the Incorporated Society of Registered Naturopaths, at which point the OAGB withdrew.

The BSO in the War Years

War broke out in 1939 just three weeks before the start of the new term. Chelsea Polytechnic closed due to the war and so basic science teaching was undertaken by the faculty, with unexpected advantages, e.g. reduced travel time for students and the course being more relevant to their needs.

Due to the financial state of the School, for reasons discussed, graduates were asked to support it financially, to recommend patients for X-ray and to recommend prospective students. No expenditure other than was absolutely necessary for the routine work of the school was to be incurred without reference to the Board.

Clinic income was considerably reduced. It was hoped this trend would be reversed, so it was decided to continue with the then present staff for three months. The hours of attendance of students at the school were revised to enable the building to close earlier.

In *The Journal of Osteopathy* for 1939 Webster-Jones wrote an article on 'The School in Wartime'. 'Attendance of patients at the clinic fell alarmingly. The children's clinic was particularly affected by evacuation. Patients presented with symptoms consequential to the war: street falls in the black outs, back strain due to filling sand bags and "warden's feet". Those previously engaged in sedentary work now found themselves engaged in manual tasks for which they were unaccustomed.'[6]

On 15 November 1939 at 7.30pm the BBC made the first osteopathic announcement over the National wavelength: 'The Clinic of the British School of Osteopathy, 16, Buckingham Gate, London SW1, has not been evacuated and is open for the treatment of patients from 9am to 6.30pm. I will repeat the address....'

In July 1939, Dr T. Mitchell-Fox wrote on behalf of the School to Lord Hailey offering to train refugee students as osteopaths. Applications were made to the Home Office for permits for five refugee students. Three were admitted, but certain 'difficulties' later arose with the Home Office.

The Council of the Jewish Emergency Medical and Dental Association opposed refugee doctors being trained by the School, or being helped to set up as osteopaths. The Chairman of the Board of the BSO wrote answering their criticisms and setting out the position of the School and of Osteopathy. Professor Samson Wright requested further details of the training given at the school.

Among the new students in 1939 was an E. Deutsch, aged 19. He was recommended by the War Registers Internationale. He was described in the BSO minutes as, 'Austrian refugee. Jew-unorthodox'. He was admitted to the course, 'Provided that permit, hospitality etc. were satisfactorily arranged'.

Dr Bak, a refugee doctor with a Viennese medical qualification, taught physiology, histology, physiological chemistry, laboratory diagnosis and pathology. She also provided a laboratory service in urinalysis and blood analysis for the profession. No further refugee students were admitted, because, 'With one or two exceptions the arrangements had broken down'. The BSO wrote to the Czech Committee regarding a Miss Kraus. The Student Loan Fund provided fees for two refugee students, A. Peczenik and P. Marcovic, but Marcovic was called up for service with the Czech legion. All efforts to secure exemption failed. E. M. Tiger, a Viennese refugee and law graduate, with a specialist interest in forensic medicine and experience in anatomy and physiology, was sponsored and accepted onto the course with two years' credit. He applied to the Student Loan Fund for assistance, but was interned.

In 1940, Robert Adams, described in the Council of Education minutes as a 'Jamaican Negro' applied for the course. There were no new students in 1942. In 1943 the Board of Governing Directors decided that no further students were to be enrolled until after the war, unless the Council of Education requested the Board to reconsider this. However, a Dr Abrahams was enrolled for the medical practitioners' course that year. Hall indicated the difficulty in providing a full syllabus for one student. It was suggested Abrahams visit individually those Faculty who were not available on the School premises. In 1944 there were 44 applications for enrolment, but only two paid enrolment fees.

Even in 1940, there were problem students. A Miss H. caused considerable trouble by her behaviour in class and was a disturbing influence on other students, and her fee cheque had been returned twice by the bank. Another student was suspended for financial reasons.

Requests were made to reduce the rent of Buckingham Gate, but these were refused. By the end of 1940 the School was in a serious financial position. In 1941, the landlords were pressing for the rent. Littlejohn paid them £200 and offered to forego interest on his loan until further notice. Eventually the rent was reduced to £150 pa. The

BSO applied to Osteopathic Trusts for financial help. Treatment of injuries caused by air raids was publicised in an attempt to maintain the clinic's numbers and income. Rooms were let. A donation of £800 was received. In 1941, a Bulletin covering the activities of the School was published. It was sent to regular readers of *The Journal of Osteopathy*, which it replaced, appealing for funds.

An attempt was made in 1940 to get newspapers to accept photographs dealing with the work of the School. The clinic was advertised in six local papers (though with no response) and a circular sent to about 111 large stores, factories, restaurants and to foot clinics, which were also visited. Lapsed patients were notified that the clinic was still open. A panel of speakers was identified for clubs and societies. At that time an Osteopathic Advice and Information Bureau existed at 31 Lyndhurst Avenue, London SW16.

In 1932-1933 Littlejohn had received donations from members of the profession and others for the foundation of an osteopathic hospital. Proby wrote to him in 1940 regarding the position of the fund and requesting an advancement, but Littlejohn refused, claiming that the fund was registered and could not be legally used for another purpose. However, in 1942, a loan of £200 was made to the School out of the fund.

In 1940, members of the Board agreed to contact personally all those who could be of financial assistance, with full details of the seriousness of the situation should the School fail to continue its activities. They decided on a further appeal to the profession and to consider ceasing activities of the School and liquidation of the Company. The School also explored introducing Deeds of Covenant for seven years to raise finances.

Even by 1944, the response of the Appeal was small. In that year it raised £167 and eight shilings, collecting boxes £86 five shillings and tenpence, and the first instalments on deeds of covenants £81. There were some enquiries following publicity in the *Daily Sketch*. A patient offered 'a juvenile dancing display' to aid clinic funds. There was an Appeal to graduates to accept patients only able to pay a small fee and to donate such sums to the school.

The School also suffered some war damage, particularly to the entrance of the building and a claim for compensation was later made. The damage was not as severe as that received by the naturopathic college at Wyndham Place. In 1944 the BSO decided that new premises were needed.

In addition the BSO was faced with other crises. In 1940, due to ill-health, Littlejohn ceased active involvement in the School and did not attend meetings. He wrote to Webster-Jones indicating that he had been in hospital for two weeks and had X-rays to find out the real cause of the trouble. He was suffering general weakness. Middleton and Webster-Jones took over his teaching.

To make matters worse, in January 1940, Edward Hall wrote to the Dean, criticising the School and resigning from the Board and other offices. Mitchell-Fox attempted to ascertain if his decision was irrevocable, as it was felt at that time that changes in the Board were undesirable. At a Board meeting in March, Hall explained his resignation was the cumulative result of a series of small incidents over a long period. His resignation was accepted with regret. However, in December, the future of the School looked so bleak that a letter was sent requesting him, 'To give the Directors the benefit of his knowledge to the School and his special organising ability, at this difficult period'.

In 1941, Dr Hope Robertson visited Hall to discuss how he (Hall) could assist the School. The Board invited him to meet them to express his personal views for the future of the School. Hall suggested ways of raising funds, one of which was to place collecting boxes in waiting rooms of practices. By 1942, the collection boxes had been delivered to Hall, but there was a problem distributing them. County Societies of Osteopaths, particularly the Northern Counties, were approached. Boxes and letters were sent out, but only nine replies received. An Appeal letter to osteopaths was also written by Proby and 3,000 copies printed.

Following Hall's resignation, Jocelyn Proby was appointed Deputy Dean of the BSO, but he had a two days a week post with the Huntingdon Agricultural Committee. An application was sent to the Minister of Labour to secure his release to spend more time at the School. In 1943, however, he moved to Ireland and Philip Jackson replaced him on the Board. Proby resigned in March 1944, 'Due to the exceptional circumstances of the war'.

After Proby's departure, in 1943, Hall was re-appointed Vice-Dean for the duration of the war, at £300 pa and re-elected as a Governing Director. He declined to accept the sum, but accepted payment of expenses up to a maximum of that figure. There was strong opposition to the appointment. Proby, who was instrumental in Hall's return, received letters from the Dean, Deiter, Terry Short and Mitchell-Fox and a telegram from Hope Robertson indicating their concern. Webster-Jones and Middleton resigned as a consequence of the re-appointment. Their resignations were accepted by the Board with regret. It recognised that much of the work they had undertaken and accomplished had been, 'For motives entirely divorced from financial and purely for the good of the school and clinic'. They were interviewed in the hope that they would continue teaching. The roles of Registrar and Director of Clinic were kept in abeyance.

In March, 1943, Webster-Jones wrote to the Board of Directors that he had been an official of the School for seven years and his resignation, 'Arises from no personal animosity to Mr Hall, but solely because, from past experience, I feel I could not work with him again'. He initially agreed to continue to lecture as a member of the Honorary Faculty, but then, as neither he nor Mr Middleton had been consulted over the appointment of Hall, he withdrew this offer:

> 'I do suggest that there is, gentlemen, such a thing as courtesy and consideration to old servants, who have worked hard thro' extremely difficult times with very little help to keep the School and clinic going. They took over the teaching of anatomy and physiology when Chelsea Polytechnic closed down which entailed long hours of study and preparation in their spare time mostly during air raids. They built up the clinic again after the Blitz when patients fell to a very small number and, with the exception of three days when the building was severely damaged by blast, they maintained an uninterrupted service throughout, with no breaks for holidays. I shall continue to help the School in any way open to me, for it is very near to my heart.'

The Secretary to the Board and Jocelyn Proby both replied. Proby regretted Webster-Jones's decision and indicated that he could not understand the reasons for it and stressed the importance of members of the profession working together if it was to progress.

Canning also wrote to Webster-Jones on 11 March concerning his and Middleton's resignations:

> 'Dear Webber
> There is one point I wish to make quite clear because you may have a false idea about it. It is this. Proby quite independently arrived at the decision to bring Hall into the School again.... I had a hope that both of you might be big enough to let Principles rise above personalities especially as you know from inside the pettiness, jealousies and indifference which

have obstructed our professional development. Your refusal to work with Hall is a personal disappointment to me. I fail completely to understand the antipathy for one whose qualities seem to me essential to the progress of both School and profession at present. I can only make a comparison with Churchill, who for so many years was rejected and damned by lesser minds. Yet now he is the vital leader of the day. Hall has Churchillian qualities. He likewise has the same faults and these I know well. In my opinion he has a rare combination of fine qualities which are to be found nowhere else amongst our bare 300 practitioners. No where can I see a sign of leadership yet Hall has the quality in a high degree. He had vision and a forward looking mind, great energy and organising ability and can achieve so many things which are impossible to others.

He is a fine osteopath and a natural teacher and possess the capacity of the Old Dean for (?) devotion and neglect of his own interests in favour of Osteopathy. In addition his ready generosity and instant response to any appeal for help is phenomenal. The only name which occurred to anyone about the School who needed help was Hall's. I doubt if help was ever refused....As always the only real enemies of Osteopathy are osteopaths. It is a depressing reflection. I hope that you may take second thoughts on the matter.'

In his response of 14 March, Webster-Jones indicated that he knew the proposal came entirely from Proby:

'We quite sincerely believe that the Board's decision is a grave mistake, not from the least personal animosity to Hall. I have never disagreed that Hall is a fine osteopath and generous and I owe him a personal debt of gratitude as a teacher of technique. But I would suggest that his present position in regard to the School and the profession rather disproves what you say of his capacities as a leader &c. I am very surprised at the Board's decision, which I fail to understand....My decision so long as Hall's appointment stands, is irrevocable.'

His letter to Arthur Millwood provides some background to these events and his intent to stand against James Canning for election as Graduate Representative on the Board.

'Canning is the retiring Graduates' Representative, and so far as I know, is willing to stand again. I have been asked to accept nomination, and I have agreed to do so. In ordinary circumstances, I do not know whether I should have stood against Canning, but after what has just happened, I feel I should definitely do so, as I do not consider Canning has represented the opinion of the majority of graduates.

You will remember that Hall walked out on us at the BSO in 1940, resigning after a most unpleasant row with the Board and after sweeping general criticism of everything and everybody. Shortly afterwards, the Dean had to give up on account of failing health, which meant that the rest of us, Middleton and myself for the most part, had to take over the Dean's and Hall's lectures, most of which we had to prepare during the Blitz.

Since then we have kept the School going and built up the clinic again to a really flourishing concern. Now, without asking our views on the matter, or giving us the least hint of it, the Board has brought Hall back again as Vice-Dean with an allowance of £300 for expenses. This is all a result of Proby's influence as Acting Dean.

Proby, who has been Acting Dean since Xmas, has now decided to return to Ireland, which he can do being an Irish citizen, until after the war. Having done so, he will not be able to come over to England except on a special permit. He thinks the BSO needs a leader (which nobody denies), and that Hall is the right person for the job. After all that has happened this is quite incomprehensible to us. I gather that the Board has taken into consideration the possibility of our resigning, but apparently were of the opinion that the exchange would be worth it....I understand that Terry-Short vigorously opposed the proposal as did Dr Littlejohn, but neither were at the Board meeting concerned....I gather that Hall did not seek to return, nor was he very keen to do so, but that Proby wanted him to.'

Littlejohn wrote to Webster-Jones on 26 March:

'I am going to ask you to withdraw your resignation and will you for me please ask Mr Middleton to do the same. My sons agree with me. You have both been such workers in the school and clinic....I am still the Dean of the School and no one can do anything against my wishes....I would like to see you and Middleton some evening here if you could arrange it. We must all try and keep together so as to maintain the School....'

They were interviewed by the Dean in April. Following a Board meeting, Canning wrote:

'I feel strongly that I should have been more insistent that our recent School problems should be handled more from the sympathetic than the official standpoint. I regret this and blame myself for it, because the others do not see the inside workings of the School as I do.'

(He was in the School much more than other members of the Board).

Proby wrote: 'With regard to your resignation, the Directors feel that they have no alternative but to accept it with very great regret.'

Saul wrote to Webster-Jones on 13 April expressing the concerns of the Northern Society of Osteopaths and that, 'They had placed it in my hands to try and find some means of getting you to return to the BSO'. Webster-Jones replied thanking him for his concern, but the appeal to reconsider his actions should be directed at the Board. 'If we agree to withdraw our resignations we shall once again expend our efforts in bolstering up an inefficient and inexperienced administration while the School gradually goes to pieces before our eyes.'

In May, Saul indicated that he had written to Proby regarding the matter. Webster-Jones replied again expressing his disappointment in the Directors with whom an informal meeting was held. He had hoped that he would be approached officially to return to the School and expressions of regret made privately would be made official. They were not forthcoming. Webster-Jones and Middleton did agree to continue lecturing in an honorary capacity and by July Webster-Jones was elected Graduate Representative on the Board in place of Canning. Middleton also became a Board member.

Webster-Jones corresponded with solicitors (Blakeney & Co.) regarding Hall. They wrote to him in March 1943:

'Referring to your call on me, I think it first of all advisable to point out to you that the Law of Slander is complicated. What I have to warn you against is, that a personal attack on

Hall must be limited to his conduct within the 4 walls of the
Clinic and School, otherwise he might be able to attack you,
by suggesting you were malicious in your statements because,
as a result of his appointment, you and your Colleague have
reverted to a lower status. You must studiously avoid any
reference to drink and schizophrenia.

I would suggest that you emphasise the following-

1. The shortage of lecturers at the time when Mr Hall refused
to extend the number of his lectures, whilst Mr Middleton
and you stepped into the breach and gave additional lectures.

2. The history of the Board's disagreement with Hall.

3. Your opposing advice with regard to administration and the
finance of the clinic, by which, in spite of criticism, you have
enabled the same to continue.

4. The present problem, is to carry on during the War with
reduced staff and reduced income, but you and Mr Middleton,
cannot work with him.

5. Whatever his abilities, lack of harmony between you would,
in turn, damage the well-being of the School and clinic. You
could say that personalities would be bound to arise over
methods of procedure, therefore, in fairness to him and the
Board, it would be better, the Board having made their choice,
for Mr Hall to have a clear field of action.

6. You are only too pleased to remain a member of the faculty
and to continue with your lectures.

7. It seems strange that the Board should have reversed their
policy which led to Mr Hall's original resignation, and the
officials remaining loyally by them during the intervening two
years should now be ignored, in spite of the fact that they have
kept the ship afloat.

No doubt you and Mr Middleton would like to come and have a
chat with me and criticise my suggestions, at the same time offering
yours. I have probably missed out quite a lot.'

Further correspondence took place in April, June and July, but in
view of later events, it would seem that Webster-Jones and Middleton
did remain at the School

All this was against the backcloth of War. As an example, in
October 1943 an air raid warning sounded and Webster-Jones had to
leave the Council of Education meeting of the BSO to report for fire
watch duty.

The afternoons were shortened because of blackouts and there were fewer Faculty because of call up. The teaching of pathology, medical and surgical diagnosis and bacteriology particularly suffered. Stoddard had hospital duties; Deiter and Edgar Martin Littlejohn were engaged in active service (in which the latter died in 1944). By 1941, due to a shortage of teaching staff, the hours of certain subjects no longer complied with those agreed with the GCRO, though every effort was made to see that standards were kept up. The GCRO was informed. Kelman MacDonald, representing the GCRO, was satisfied that the School was doing its best to maintain standards. In 1944, there was discussion with Lord Hankey on post-war training and a revised curriculum. Higher educational standards were planned for the School and promotional literature was compiled.

Four diplomas were issued in 1941, three in 1942 and four in 1943. One diplomate in 1943 was Charles Graham Lief, the son of Stanley Lief (the founder of what was later to become the British College of Osteopathic Medicine). He reported for military service later that year and was killed in action in March 1945. In 1944, Peczenik (who had taken a break in his study) and Dr Abrahams were the only two diplomates. In 1942, Dr Dorothy Wood, the wife of Edward Hall, did not consider it desirable to present her gold medal and a certificate was granted in lieu. It went to Bruggemeyer. She later severed her connection with the School, having made 'certain general criticisms' of the administration.

There was a drive to increase the use of the BSO's X-ray equipment by London osteopaths. In 1941, it had to be moved to a safer site, but as the risk was considered to be as great in the basement of the building, no action was taken. The radiographer became ill and it proved impossible to obtain the regular services of a replacement, which resulted in loss of revenue. Middleton and Miss Higham obtained instruction in its use from the Medical Supplies Association. In 1943, Proby wrote to the President of the BOA drawing attention to the X-ray facilities for use by practitioners and suggested some assistance in teaching from members of the Association.

Initially, the clinic was open from 10.00am to 7.30pm in the Summer months. In 1940, it was decided to open at 9am and also in the lunch hour and not to close in August, as had been the custom. Staff took holidays in turn. By the end of 1940 patient numbers were almost up to pre-war standards with 250 patients a week, of which 16-18 were new cases and the income was £28. By 1942 over 300 patients a week were treated. An income of £48 per week was recorded in 1943, but then fell due to the shortage of operators. Personal approaches were made to the profession to assist. Employees of Southern Railway were referred.

There were only two clinic assistants, who did three sessions each, and four students. The students worked two morning sessions each and also one evening session after lectures. The balance of 18 clinic sessions was covered by paid operators at ten shillings and sixpence per session. A ten shilling allowance was made for operators who travelled long distances. It was considered undesirable for clinic operators to have private patients. Permission initially given to Middleton and Webster-Jones was withdrawn, but this ruling was relaxed in 1942 by the Board as a temporary emergency measure and the 'microscope room' was used by them for private patients. Of the seven shillings and sixpence patients were charged, two shillings went to the clinic fund and sixpence for the upkeep of the room. In 1942, a decision was made that stockings need not be worn by lady operators on clinic duty, but slacks were not allowed.

In 1942, a gynaecological clinic was held by Miss Bishop, in a separate part of the building from the general clinic, with only fourth year students present, though not for the gynaecological examination.

From 1943, the number of 'foot cases' increased as a result of the Central College of Chiropody meeting at the school on Sunday afternoons. Keith Blagrave attended the meetings, 'To protect the property and interests of the school'.

Edwin Miller proposed to reopen the Ear Nose and Throat (ENT) clinic on two afternoons a week. There were complaints from students that his teaching was inadequate and that he really did not want students present. He also sought support from the School for his claim for exemption from National Service, although he had only just rejoined the School. He was also not a member of the GCRO, which recommended he should take a course at the School, the fee for which was 25 guineas. As he could not pay, it was reduced to £20. Miller expected financial remuneration for working in the ENT clinic. It was later considered that there was no immediate need to re-open it as it was not a bona fide teaching clinic. By 1949 Canning and Middleton saw appropriate ENT cases.

A special course for medical practitioners. was advertised in *Medical World*, but Canning felt that it should not be pushed too much as many graduates may not join the profession afterwards. Dr J. P. Henderson was the first to complete it. Dr Gibson also enrolled and later taught minor surgery.

Due to a national demand for paper salvage, in 1943 records prior to 1936 were scrapped to save space and to help the war effort. The history of osteopathy in Britain would be the richer if this had not occurred.

Due to the paper shortage, supplies of the prospectus ran low. A leaflet was produced to replace it and 500 copies printed, but in 1944 350 copies of the 1938-39 prospectus were found and the preface rewritten.

An unqualified bone setter, M. V. Langley, claiming to have been 'Blake's assistant', applied to work in the clinic in 1942, in order to obtain material for a book on Osteopathy. He was advised that he would hardly be a suitable person to collect material for this purpose and that he was unacceptable to the School in any capacity other than as a student.

In 1944, the BSO wrote to Lord Hankey regarding grant-aided education, but he recommended delay in proposing Osteopathy for inclusion in the list of professions that were part of the scheme.

The Osteopathic Educational Foundation

Kelman MacDonald addressed a meeting of the Register in 1945 regarding a pamphlet he produced entitled, 'A Memorandum on Osteopathic Education'. He visualised a second School/College, to be run by the BOA and suggested the Register should promote a financial campaign supporting Schools, including the BSO, research and the general advancement of Osteopathy in Great Britain. He considered that, there were not nearly enough properly qualified osteopaths to meet the rapidly rising public demand for osteopathic treatment. The BSO representatives supported the scheme and the Council adopted it with MacDonald as organiser. It was launched in Manchester in January 1945. Further meetings took place in London.

Hall wrote to MacDonald and the Northern graduates requesting that the appeal be directed to patients and not osteopaths, as the BSO already had an Appeal to graduates and the two would clash. In March, osteopaths of London and the South met MacDonald. The Osteopathic Educational Foundation (OEF) of the GCRO Ltd was formed. As the BSO was initially the sole beneficiary it wanted a representative on the Committee. Hall was proposed.

The OEF was located at 12 Clarges Street, Piccadilly, London W1. Its main purpose was to establish or aid in establishing and maintaining one or more schools or colleges for the purpose of training and educating osteopaths, but also, 'To establish or aid in establishing and maintaining schools, classes or other means of instruction for nurses, masseurs and persons engaged in or assisting nursing and treating the sick, injured or infirmed', and to borrow or raise money for the purposes of the Foundation and to invest the moneys not immediately required for its purposes.[7]

By 1946, 45 out of 144 registered osteopaths had contributed to the

OEF, which had received nearly £3,500. An early payment was £600 to the BSO, including £300 to cover war damage. With the death of Kelman MacDonald in October 1946, the activities of the Foundation were temporarily interrupted, until the appointment of A. W. Ellis as Appeal Secretary in July 1947. A large scale appeal was then conducted.

One of its first activities was to publish of *The Osteopathy Quarterly*. In addition, a new series of Osteopathic Information Bulletins was issued: No.1: Osteopathic treatment in acute diseases; No. 2: Posture and Body Function; No. 3 (1949): Osteopathy and medicines. The second Bulletin contained an Appeal to re-house the BSO as the lease on 16 Buckingham Gate had nearly expired.

Development of Naturopathy

In 1945 the Nature Cure Association (NCA) and British Association of Naturopaths (BAN) merged to form the British Naturopathic Association (BNA). The original intention was that both associations should wind up and form a new one, but for historical reasons members of the BAN joined the NCA, the title of which was then changed to the BNA. Stanley Lief was the first President and re-elected the following year. A General Naturopathic Council was formed in 1946 to deal with parliamentary issues consisting of seven members of the profession, four being members of the BNA: Stanley Lief, Percival Scarr, William Bone and Milton Powell.[4]

In 1948 the BSO received a letter from Percival Scarr, the Secretary of the BNA, to explore the possibility of co-operation in the training of osteopaths and naturopaths. The proposal was for the first two years of the course to consist basic sciences, common to all therapies, followed by a further two years taught by tutors from each therapy.[4] The Vice-Dean, Middleton and Proby had an informal meeting with the College Committee of the BNA to discuss initial training at the BSO, but there was no progress.

A BNA London Group was formed in 1946 that provided postgraduate lectures and demonstrations. There were plans to re-form the college and a college fund was set up.[4]

At an Extraordinary Meeting of the BNA held in Edinburgh in October 1948, discussion took place regarding starting a college to replace that of the NCA destroyed in the war. Whether this was the cause or the consequence of the failure to proceed with a joint course with the BSO is unknown. There was an appeal for funds. The British College of Naturopathy part-time course began on 5 January 1949 with Stanley Lief as Dean. Clifford Quick taught physics and chemistry;

Brian Youngs, biology; Stanley Lief, philosophy of nature cure and dietetics and Arthur Jenner, the general administrator, taught anatomy, physiology, and physiotherapy. There was no clinic at first. It began in a room made available by a BNA member, Vincent Evans. It then moved to the rooms of the Dean, Stanley Lief, in Park Lane, until 1951.

In 1949 Hector Frazer, whose wife had been treated by Lief, bought a house in Holland Park Avenue to lease to the college for 21 years at a modest rent, but permission was not granted for change of use to a clinic or college.[4]

The British Institute of Naturopathy and Osteopathy, founded in 1938 by S. W. Daley-Yates, closed in 1947 as the correspondence course was considered inadequate. From 1944 graduates became members of the Natural Therapeutic Association (NTA). Council members of the NTA went on to form the Guild of Naturopathy and Osteopathy (GNO) in 1949, with Daley-Yates as first President. They planned to establish a 4 year course. The BNA considered that the qualification of some of the NTA members precluded them from BNA membership.[4,8,9]

The Natural Therapeutic and Osteopathic Society and Register (NTOS) was formed in 1948. Under its auspices, Horace Jarvis founded The Croydon School of Osteopathy and became its Principal. It provided nine hours training a week for three years.

The BSO after the War

In 1945, the average weekly clinic income was just over £36, increasing the following year to over £44 with an average income per patient of two shillings and fourpence and three shillings and tenpence, respectively. In 1947, the situation stabilised and the average weekly income was £45-£49 with the income per patient the same. Weekly income rose to as high as £61 in 1948 and was £64 in 1949, but the income per patient did not. In 1946, students were required to attend a minimum of six hours a week in clinic, replacing the previous requirement of third and fourth year students to treat 700 patients in total.

The balance and interest on the loan for the purchase of the X-ray equipment was paid. After several changes of radiographer, Mr Meyern took over as radiologist, having been trained by the Medical Supplies Association, until a new radiographer was appointed, who was 'very capable, though not actually qualified'. A brochure advertising the X-ray department was produced in 1946.

The children's clinic was reopened in 1946, headed by Constance Smith. Muriel Dunning (nee Higham) joined her in 1948 and they ran it together until 1949, when Constance Smith resigned. At that time 4th year students also contributed to it.

A clinic was established at 388 City Road by several members of the clinic staff, who applied for its affiliation to the School. Objections were raised as they acted without consultation or co-operation of the school's officials. In 1949, attempts were made to start an evening clinic. Canning and Middleton volunteered to assist.

The Publicity Committee met regularly and appointed a public relations officer from April 1945, but he was not re-appointed in 1946.

In April 1945 the purchase of the lease of 1 Collingham Gardens, South Kensington was discussed, but did not proceed as the Dean did not approve, as he had previously advanced a large sum to the school and also there was no suitable clinic accommodation close by. It was decided to remain at Buckingham Gate for at least a year. It was considered how best to use the premises. The value of the lease at Buckingham Gate was revised by the Dean's solicitors. Repairs and redecorating were planned following war damage.

The post of Registrar had not been filled for some time. Webster-Jones was appointed for three and a half days a week.

The National Services Act delayed the release of prospective students from National Service and hence opening of the school was postponed. In 1945, three students enrolled, including two medical students. Several applications from prospective students were received. A question was asked in the House of Commons regarding the refusal of grants to ex-servicemen to train as osteopaths. Early in 1946 there was still no fixed date for opening the School, though former graduates were coming out of the forces and reporting to it. A 'refresher course' was arranged for three students. Later that year 18 students had enrolled, though some had not as yet been released from the forces. A formal re-opening took place on 16 September (a day before the course started) with the Ladies' Osteopathic League providing refreshments. Graduates, faculty and friends attended.

The Registrar still had difficulty in placing first year students in external, pre-medical courses, all of which were full. It was impossible to continue the pre-war arrangement with Chelsea Polytechnic, the first year course having been suspended. The possibility of courses at the London County Council (Norwood Technical Institute or Northern Polytechnic) and the University Tutorial College was suggested.

In 1946, the BSO sought approval from the GCRO for modifications of the regulations for first year training for selected ex-service personnel for two years. Prospective students were Flight Lieutenant B. J. Beech and D. N. Goodall. The latter graduated from New Jersey College in 1928, was 50 years' old and had 17 years in practice as an osteopath. He joined the course with three years' credit. He had previously been associated with the National Society of Osteopaths. Stanley John Wernham applied to complete the course and was credited with three years on the basis of work previously undertaken at the School. He was to attend clinic on Tuesday morning and two hours on the Wednesday and to make up his full complement of clinic at Xmas and Easter.

The Curriculum Committee of the BSO met with MacDonald from the GCRO. There was an urgent need to standardise nomenclature and terminology. A new prospectus was produced.

The London College of Osteopathy (LCO)

In July 1945 George MacDonald presented a report from the Education Committee to the BOA Council:

'As there is much demand made on medical students' time...it was agreed that there was no possibility of interpolating an osteopathic course during the student's undergraduate career. Accordingly it was decided that a school to teach Osteopathy as a post-graduate course to individuals who were already on the medical register was what would be required.'

A full-time course of one year was recommended, of nine months, (1, 080 hours) of instruction: 36 hours on principles, 144 hours on practice, 216 hours of technique, 144 hours of demonstrations in clinics and 540 hours on actually giving treatments. If there were two treatments per hour each student would give 1,080 treatments, three patients an hour 1,620 and four patients an hour 2,160 treatments.

There would also be a course of two or three hours a day, six days a week, including Saturday mornings, over a period of two academic years (72 weeks), i.e. approximately the same number of hours. The object of the second course was to attract young medical graduates, who were perhaps doing hospital appointments, or some other special work in London, but who were also anxious to become qualified in Osteopathy, but to limit this to six students at most. 'It is the young fellows we want mostly, who want to become specialists.'

The object of the School was to teach osteopathic principles and practice as taught in the recognised American colleges. Great care would be taken only to accept students who were anxious to become practising osteopaths, and to avoid, as much as possible, giving a smattering of osteopathic technique which an individual could apply as an adjunct in general medical practice.

It was decided that there should be a Principal, an Honorary Dean, a full-time salaried osteopath as Sub-Dean, a lecturer on the Principles and Practice of Osteopathy, who would be in charge of the clinic and the general attendance at the School, and a number of honorary teaching osteopaths who would teach technique and would supervise the actual treatment of cases by the students. It was considered ideal to have an honorary osteopath for every two students, but there would be no disadvantage in having a larger number of honorary osteopaths than this. As many people as possible were to be attracted to the School to give the students a varied training.

With regard to a full-time osteopath, it was agreed that they should probably be paid £1,000 a year, free of Income Tax, to 'get the right man', who would almost certainly have to be imported from America, so that they could be assured of having the right principles and practice as taught in America. It was considered he would also have to have experience of running a clinic. It was agreed that a confidential letter should be sent by the Committee to the Deans of the various colleges in America asking if they would look out for such a person. Cooper intimated that he might possibly be going to America later in the year, and it was agreed that he should interview some of the possible candidates at that time.

The intent was to start the school in October 1946, even if they only had a few students. 'It would be better to have a few good students than a large number of inferior ones.'

It was agreed that the Committee should draft out a clear-cut scheme to present to the BOA for discussion. Osteopathic Trusts would engage a secretary to work out the details of the School. The Committee was unanimously of the opinion that there would be no difficulty in getting enough money for this scheme. It was hoped that once the scheme was started, no matter in how small a way, it would eventually grow so that they could have their own radiological department, their own biochemical department, 'And so on—in fact all the possible investigations that were required in ordinary practice even to the possibility of having some beds for in-patients'.

Pheils was concerned that Osteopathy was not dragged in the mud and become simply an adjunct to the general practice of medicine. It would be necessary to get students to sign a declaration of what they intended to do. Jackson considered that the scheme would draw a dividing line between the osteopath with a medical degree and the one who had not. Pheils considered it would be similar to what happened with psychotherapy. MacDonald considered it might not be a bad thing to have two types of osteopath. Jackson thought it might open the door to legislation for the medically-trained osteopath, leaving the other one outside. The Chairman considered that, 'It will definitely increase the standards and then the man from the BSO would have to be a better trained man'.

Sutcliffe Lean claimed it would be a case of history repeating itself. Some years ago, the Littlejohn group went to the Board of Trade and said: 'There are enough osteopaths English trained in this country to handle all the people who want treatment; therefore forbid American osteopaths to come in'. They got that through. George MacDonald indicated that this was very different from what Dr Jackson was visualising; that was a Home Office Aliens decision. Bullus said that he would like to see Osteopathy instilled in them before they were fully trained in medical schools. MacDonald said that there was no time at medical schools. There could be open lectures on a Saturday morning once a month. 'If we could even get these lads interested in their 4th or 5th year...it would be a good thing.'

Pheils stated, ' I think your force in Parliament will be much greater if you have an institution like this, coupled with others. If you go up just on the credentials of the BSO to get anything, you are up against a stone wall...and it is easier for us to make that sort of institution creditable than to be mixed up with something into which you can shoot holes from every angle.'

Philcox referred to a scheme in 1937 to have a college and hospital and everything. 'Is something like that on a smaller scale absolutely impossible, i.e. to have an osteopathic medical school?' He was critical of four years' medical training followed by nine months' osteopathy. 'A great deal will depend on the people who are teaching. That is the reason we want to get the best man we can from America.'

The Council accepted George MacDonald's proposal. A building was considered in 1945, but it had not been inspected. Osteopathic Trusts had over £8,000 at that time from the Davenport Estate and refunded from the Inland Revenue. If they went ahead with a School they would need to use the BOA clinic, but there were tenants there. They had paid £2,900 to keep the clinic afloat. The BOA was also getting closer to settling with the Docker estate. They considered it would pay to take over the clinic. The cost would be £9,000. There was concern regarding ownership of the clinic. It was intended to be the BOA clinic, but the name was changed to the Osteopathic Association Clinic on account of entry into directories etc.

In 1946 there were still links between the BOA and AOA, the former sending representatives to the AOA Annual Convention. A letter was received from the Board of Trustees of the AOA regarding the LCO, that, 'They concur in desire of the BOA to elevate their standards of education, and in that concurrence recommend to them that they follow the standards of education as set up by the Bureau of Professional Education and Colleges of the AOA'. In reply, the President of the BOA pointed out the number of hours devoted to osteopathic medicine at the LCO was 1,260 against 1,060 recommended by the AOA and requested the figure be passed to the Bureau.

Osteopathic Trusts agreed to purchase the remainder of the lease of Docker House at Dorset Square for £9,000. Major Lockwood (the organising secretary) said that these decisions would mean that the Trust would spend all its money and an Appeal for funds for the college and clinic would have to be launched. Pheils felt that, 'Osteopathic Trusts had never spent money more wisely....When we have sufficient graduates we could have our own institution from beginning to end. It was a very wise step which would enable Osteopathy to face the world and all its criticisms—something that would be an everlasting credit to Osteopathy.'

A 'Faculty of Osteopaths' was proposed consisting of all members of the BOA practising osteopathy in the UK, with a manifesto that, 'They believe that while the osteopathic factor in disease must in future be fully recognised and its usefulness taught in all medical schools, Osteopathy should be practised by specialists, who should not only be masters of the principles and technique of Osteopathy, but should also have a general knowledge of the Science of Medicine. As it is impossible at the moment for such knowledge adequately to be obtained in this country, other than in medical schools recognised by the GMC, the Faculty of Osteopaths hopes to produce in the future osteopathic specialists drawn from the graduates of such schools.'

In 1946 the LCO came into being offering a postgraduate course in osteopathic medicine for registered medical practitioners. It planned to operate for one to two years before applying for official recognition by the Register.

A Symposium on the Future of Osteopathic Education was held at the Waldorf Hotel, Aldwych, London in June 1946. The special topic for discussion was, 'Should Osteopathy be taught as a postgraduate medical speciality, or as a four to five year course at an osteopathic school?' It was chaired by Clem Middleton, who, 'Regretted the absence of many BOA members in this stimulating discussion'.

George MacDonald supported the case for teaching Osteopathy as part of the orthodox medical course. 'As a medical specialist, the osteopath would be able to play an important part in the new health schemes.' The original objective of Kirksville College was that Osteopathy should be part of Medicine. Altering and improving the practice of Medicine'. He considered that the high degree of skills in medical diagnosis could only be obtained in a medical school and separate schools of Osteopathy would mean unnecessary duplication.

R. F. Miller replied, contrasting the methods, purpose and curricula of orthodox medicine and osteopathic training. He considered orthodox teaching covered too wide a field and lacked a philosophy. Osteopathy, however, had an active philosophy. He feared that on amalgamation, Osteopathy would be bogged down in the large medical curriculum; the concept would be lost.

Edward Hall contended that the osteopathic student, 'Must soak himself in his osteopathic environment. He must be taught to think Osteopathy and Osteopathic Theory first, last and always'.

Webster-Jones argued, 'Orthodox medicine tends to regard ill health as a disease of a particular part of the body....Osteopathy regards the patient as an individual and tries to discover within the body the cause of his loss of health and, by removing it, thus release the patient's own vital forces of recovery. The AOA compromise with orthodoxy has led to a progressive deterioration of osteopathic principles.'

The Chairman concluded, 'In the present incomplete state of medical knowledge, there was need for a variety of schools, each searching for truth, but as science progressed the true nature of disease would perhaps become more apparent and the approach to treatment narrowed down. Then it may be possible to see more clearly how Medicine should be taught, but until then, systems such as Osteopathy may best serve humanity as independent studies.'

At the BSO, the Public Relations Officer felt that some attempts should be made to reconcile the differences apparently existing between it and BOA. Discussion took place between Webster-Jones and George MacDonald regarding this, but the outcome is unknown.

The BOA and OAGB

It became apparent that further influx of American-trained osteopaths into the UK was unlikely, partly because of the dollar-sterling exchange rate and partly because it looked as if the NHS would exclude private practice outside of it.[10] Immigration of US citizens was also restricted (See above).

There was concern regarding the maintenance of standards of practice. Sutcliffe Lean at a BOA Council meeting said, 'That the Register upholds osteopathic standards is not true. I have been powerless to prevent putting at least 12 people on the Register who have not been through an osteopathic college'.

The Presidents of the OAGB in the1940s were:

1944	Webster-Jones
1945	Willis Haycock
1947	Patrick Saul
1948	James Canning
1949	H. Clem. Middleton

1946

The National Health Act was passed in 1946, and came into operation in July 1948.

Following a BHFS meeting in December, a questionnaire was sent to all practitioners regarding their training. George House MP visited the BSO and clinic, but the BSO would not associate itself with the Joint Practitioners' Association of the BHFS.

The BSO had invested £300 in the PO Savings Bank. Littlejohn had waived interest due to him for a considerable period and Proby considered the priority should be to pay him back. Major James Littlejohn discussed this with his father. £500 was eventually paid to Littlejohn and £100 per quarter. By 1947, the School had over £2, 000 banked, but repairs were necessary to the building due to war damage and dry rot.

In 1946, the remuneration of faculty was one guinea per lecture, though some faculty forewent all or part of their fees.

In view of the publicity in the press of the Inaugural Dinner and opening of the London College of Osteopathy in September, the BSO decided to organise a similar function.

The School submitted details of a postgraduate course for Membership Examination to the Register.

On 5 October 1946, Stephen Ward joined the BSO Board, by invitation of Jocelyn Proby, to replace Philip Jackson (See Chapter 12).

1947

Dunning sent a letter asking the BOA to apply on his behalf for a special service medal for his work during the war in treating General Eisenhower and other high ranking American army officers. The BOA decided this would not be fair to other BOA members.

A letter was received by the BOA from Dr James Cyriax who was writing a book on Osteopathy and wanted to visit the college and clinic. It was felt that he was not the right person to write about the college.

J. Guymer Burton wrote *Osteopathy Explained* which went through several editions. By the 4ᵗʰ edition it had sold 7,500 copies. The 5ᵗʰ edition was published shortly after his death in 1968.

At the BSO, Hall resigned as Vice Dean and as representative on the OEF. John Martin Littlejohn wrote to Webster-Jones in April 1947, in handwriting difficult to read, that he had been laid up a few weeks. 'My best wishes as always to the BSO for its success and good will. My personal greetings for your appointment as Vice Dean, after all the years you have been associated with the BSO....I trust you will make a great success and keep things going as I have tried to over so many years....My kindest regards to you and your dear wife and family, ever faithfully yours...'

Littlejohn died on the 8 December 1947. (See Chapter 3). There was an intake of eight students in both 1947 and 1948 with 24 students in total at the School.

Middleton introduced discussion of the teaching of cranial technique.

Neville Coleby, who had been killed on active service, had bequeathed £500 to the OAGB. A Trust was set up, 'For the furtherance of the Science of Osteopathy'. It was proposed that it be used to establish a number of bursaries and/or scholarships for BSO students. Two students in 1948 had their fees covered for three years, on condition that they assisted part-time at the school for one year after qualification.

In 1947 a Postgraduate Committee was formed. The first postgraduate course was in May 1948. All graduates and qualified osteopaths were invited. The fee was ten guineas. Five Pounds and five shillings was paid per lecture, but many lecturers refunded their fees. The first course made £205 ten shillings and eightpence for the School. It was decided to make this an annual event.

'Sammy' Ball and Stephen Ward were External Examiners at the BSO that year. Stanley J. Wernham passed and was given a Diploma.

A revision course to gain MRO membership was provided at the BSO at a cost of ten guineas. The National Society of Osteopaths expressed thanks for this.

1948

In February 1948, the BOA considered inviting graduates of the BSO to lectures. It was agreed not to do so officially, but if members of the BOA wanted to invite individuals from the School they were at liberty to do so.

A multidisciplinary meeting of some12 people (mostly osteopaths, but also herbalists and naturopaths) took place in the Oakhurst Residential Resort, Hastings, through the initiative of Ken Basham, an osteopath and naturopath and author of several books. (*Feminine Ailments* was published in 1952). He also organised seminars and study weekends. From this meeting a study group was formed that in 1960 became the Fellowship of Osteopaths. This was the beginnings of what was to become the College of Osteopaths.[11]

In early 1948, following Littlejohn's death, the BSO received letters of sympathy from Kirksville and Chicago. Kirksville published an obituary in '*Stilleto*', the college magazine. At a meeting of the Register it was decided to open a fund for the purpose of establishing a twofold memorial to Littlejohn — a visible memorial and a scholarship.

After Littlejohn's death, Herbert Milne of Blackpool was suggested as a third Trustee, but the Trust Deed could not be located. The other Trustee, Dewar, was thought to have a copy, but he had moved, his new address was unknown and he was absent from the country on government business.

A Committee of Hall, Canning, Webster-Jones and Webb discussed the appointment of a new Dean at the BSO. The title of the position was changed to that of 'Principal' and Webster-Jones was appointed on 22 May 1948.

The lease needed renewal. £5,000 had to be raised for this. A Building Appeal Committee was set up. Appeal meetings were held at Liskeard, London and Manchester. It was felt that the OEF should handle the Appeal.

Due to the gold shortage, it was still impossible to award the Dorothy Wood Gold Medal. A certificate and monetary prize (£5) for the purchase of books was awarded to Murray Silverstone.

The British Osteopathic League

The preliminary organisation was described in *The Osteopathic Quarterly* in 1948. It stated that:

'The excellent response to the appeal for volunteer helpers (made in the July issue of *The Osteopathic Quarterly*) makes it plain that there is a need for a carefully planned organisation. It has been decided to form a British Osteopathic League, a 100% *lay* organisation of supporters of, and believers in, Osteopathy—in one overworked but expressive word, Osteopathy "fans".[12] The purpose of the League is to organise public enthusiasm for Osteopathy in this country and properly to concert the efforts of all who desire its advancement. The Osteopathic Educational Foundation is the sponsor of the British Osteopathic League; but after the League is set up it will run itself. It will be an independent body but will donate to the Osteopathic Educational Foundation whatever profits accrue from its activities.'

There was a Central Committee and Regional Committees. The first progress report was published in the following edition.[13]

The objectives of the British Osteopathic League were:

(a) The widest possible enlightenment of the public concerning the osteopathic system;

(b) Development of the professional status of Osteopathy in Great Britain;

(c) Maintenance of the full liberty of the individual to obtain osteopathic treatment without restriction;

(d) The promotion and organisation of social functions of all kinds designed to raise funds for and behalf of the Osteopathic Educational Foundation;

(e) The country-wide distribution of the Directory of Members of the Register of Osteopaths and other reading matter which emanates from an authoritative source;

(f) The development of the largest possible league of supporters of Osteopathy.

One supporter organised two whist drives, as a result of which the sum of 12 guineas was paid into the funds of the OEF. Derek Oldham (a well-known singer), and Miss Iveson, a pianist, offered to give a recital in aid of the osteopathic fund.[7]

A preliminary conference took place on in March 1949 and meetings in April and June. About 100 persons were present on the latter occasion.[14] A successful bazaar was held in September, opened by Helen Cherry, 'The young stage and screen actress'.[15]

The Osteopathic Quarterly

Following the first issue in January 1948, it was published quarterly sent to subscribers, but also available through newsagents. The first

Editorial was written by T. E. H. (T Edward Hall?), who also contributed two of the five articles.[16]

It claimed, 'The broad purposes of this new publication are that it shall be a voice for professional Osteopathy and that it shall form a link between the qualified practitioner and the lay public, of whom so large a section sympathises with the principles and objects of the profession. Until now, there has been no satisfactory medium for keeping them informed about the achievements and scope of Osteopathy and the deficiency has deprived them of many possibilities to indulge a proselytising zeal, which is one of the most precious assets of this growing profession.'

The first volume contained articles on: John Martin Littlejohn: An appreciation by T.E.H.; A Consideration of Asthma by Willis Haycock; Heredity and the Spine by R. F. Miller; Jaundiced Views on Osteopathy by H. Milne and The Acute Shoulder by T. Edward Hall. There were also notes on the OEF and the BSO. Advertisements were carried for 'Ultratherm Short Wave Therapy', 'Camp Sacro-iliac Supports' and 'Bristow Faradic Coils for all general treatments'.

Further articles in Volume 1 (1948) included several by A. W. Ellis: Osteopathy and the public; The first osteopath: Notes on the autobiography of A. T. Still and Second day of term at the British School of Osteopathy. Other articles were on: Constipation (J. W. Terry-Short); On footwear for infants (A. Williams); The relation of micro-organisms to disease (Jocelyn Proby); The importance of posture (H. C. Middleton); Heredity and predisposition (T. Mitchell-Fox); I accuse the doctors (Sydney Horler); Exercises in relaxation (Willis Haycock); What osteopathy does for tonsillitis and catarrh ('The Practitioner') and One way of qualifying (Bertram T. Fraser)—a criticism of someone who claimed to be an osteopath, naturopath and chiropractor, having obtained his qualifications by correspondence course.

It publicised that it was preparing a National Appeal for funds to secure the lease of 16 Buckingham Gate.[6] Further advertisements appeared for 'Remedial Herbs' and 'Little Toddlers Infants Flexible Footwear'.

In a letter to the Editor, an E. Pierpoint wrote:

'May I be allowed a few lines of your valuable space to make what I feel is a justifiable complaint. It was in the first place a rude shock to discover that under the threat of dire penalties I was to be compelled to pay National Insurance. It was an even ruder shock to discover that having paid the contribution demanded, I had lost more of my freedom in the sense that my own action placed an embargo on free choice of treatment. The point is, medical treatment in the past failed to alleviate my troubles and without bias towards either side or resentment towards orthodoxy's failure, I have in recent years, been treated by osteopaths on numerous occasions with complete success for a variety of ailments. It is only natural that I wish to continue, as indeed I shall, but my resentment is justified when I realise that payment of a compulsory levy does not entitle me to obtain help towards the sort of treatment of which from experience I have need, and for which, it seems, I must now pay twice.'[17]

The Editor referred the writer to a petition to contract out of the National Insurance Scheme. A form of declaration was available from KRP publications Ltd.

1949

The closure of the GCRO for direct entry (Article 11) was announced.

In 1949, there were only three students at the LCO, but there were 15 enquiries from doctors. At a BOA Council meeting Pheils and Jackson (the President of the BOA) expressed concern that the dwindling number of American-trained osteopaths would have serious implications for the future of Osteopathy in Britain. There was also concern by Jackson of the antagonism between the BOA and the Council of the Register, but Pheils said he could not see where that came from.

After being cured by an osteopath, when all the doctors and specialists he consulted about his condition had done him no good, Sydney Horler wrote an article in the *Sunday Dispatch* on 19 September 1948.

'I ACCUSE THE DOCTORS

says *SYDNEY HORLER*
famous Crime Writer
WHO PUTS HIS CASE AGAINST A BLIND SPOT IN MEDICINE'

It engendered a huge response of letters, over 1,000 in two days. He then wrote a book, published the following year entitled, 'I accuse the Doctors. Being a candid commentary on the hostility shown

by the Leaders of the Medical Profession towards the healing art of
Osteopathy; and how the public suffers in consequence'. He claimed:
'I have no doubt that this book...will meet with fierce opposition from
the Medical Profession, and all those who believe in orthodox healing.
They will pour contempt upon it. But they cannot destroy the evidence.
The truth will stand any scrutiny.'

The foreword explained that the book was written out of gratitude
for being cured when he was quickly becoming a permanent cripple,
and from an overwhelming desire to place the knowledge he had gained,
'Before all my fellow sufferers (the name of whom must be legion) in
order that they may benefit in the same way as I did. I intend in this
book to tell the truth about Osteopathy as it was revealed to me, and
also the truth about the fierce hatred and violent prejudice which the
leaders of the Medical Profession show towards Osteopathy.'

In February 1949 *Picture Post* carried an article on 'Osteopathy
at Work' sub-titled, 'A rival or ally for the doctor?' Written by Fyfe
Robertson,[18] it began:

'For 70 years, Osteopathy—a system of healing without
surgery or drugs—has steadily gained ground. Though it lacks
an established scientific basis, it can claim remarkable results.
Today many doctors regard osteopaths as rivals or as quacks.
One day they may welcome them as allies. Most people know
very little about Osteopathy, and that little is usually wrong.'

It ended:

'It is reasonable to hope that one day Osteopathy will be given
its due place in a general system of healing which will include
the best of every system. The sick are not interested in the
vested rivalries of different schools; they are interested only
in being made well.'

In November 1949, George Bernard Shaw sent a hand-written
postcard in response to an appeal by the OEF. His response is somewhat
surprising given that he was a friend of Elmer Pheils:

'I cannot connect my name with any of the 1,000 opathies in
the world. After an extensive trial of Osteo I am convinced
that though it can correct traumatic lesions permanently its
correction of reflexes is only momentary and useless.'

In June 1949 there was a service in Commemoration of the Science and Art of Healing at the Cathedral Church of Christ, Canterbury, to open the Canterbury Festival. All present were in some way associated with the country's medical profession, except those of the GCRO, the BSO and two Associations. A. W. Ellis, in *The Osteopathic Quarterly*, wrote:

'They walked in plain clothes, for as yet the osteopathic profession in this country has no raiment or insignia for occasions like this. It cannot be denied in any quarter that the public regard for the non-medical, properly trained osteopath is today high indeed and that there is a growing awareness of the work that is being done by the General Council, voluntary body though it is, to enhance the professional status of the qualified practitioner. Individual members of the medical profession are now coming to appreciate this and the association of the two schools of thought, slight though it may have been, should not fail to lessen the bitterness which in the past has separated them. *There is no time when in their very hands is the issue for good.*' [19]

At the BSO, the landlords (Christ's Hospital) agreed a 21 year lease as from September 1948.

Over £5,000 was collected for the Guarantee Fund (mostly from the OEF). There was a problem of depositing more than £500 in the Post Office, a situation described as 'Gilbertian'. The matter was drawn to the attention of the Chancellor. £5,000 was paid into a joint account with Christ's Hospital.

Repairs and decoration of 16 Buckingham Gate began in the Summer vacation, but they were still disruptive in December. A licence was needed from the Ministry in order to do the work and war damage needed to be agreed with the War Damages Commission. New display boards were created for the front of the building. On 8 December Lady Hankey unveiled a memorial portrait of Littlejohn by R. G. Lewis. It was considered a striking likeness. Lewis had only a black and white photograph to work from. On the day, Lord Hankey distributed diplomas, prizes, and the Gold Medal certificate and an honorary diploma to Jocelyn Proby. Ellis, the Appeal Secretary of the OEF, was thanked for raising over £5,000 for the Guarantee Fund. Over 100 people were present and admired the redecoration of the building.

Sub-tenants were asked to vacate the property and the top flat was acquired for student use.

The training of visually impaired students was re-considered and rejected.

There were still conflicts among BSO Faculty. Hall wrote a letter to Webster-Jones, dated 13 October 1949:

'My Dear Webster-Jones
I feel I must protest in some measure about last night's meeting of the Technique faculty. I think it was to say the least, a most inopportune moment for Mr Currie to be invited to attend the meeting. Admirable graduate and student as he is, he is not a member of the Technique faculty.
I protest also against Mr Middleton's denial that he ever received a condensed copy of the Physiological Movements from me, especially in view of the fact that two minutes later he stated that in any case he did not agree with them. These two statements are decidedly contradictory.
I should like to ask when and how was I displaced as Chairman and Head of the Technique Section of the faculty? As far as I am concerned this is a minor matter but the casualness of its occurrence speaks volumes.
As it is impossible for Mr Middleton to be wrong, I have no doubt he will be very grateful to take over my teaching on Wednesday afternoons from two to 3.'

Webster-Jones replied the next day:

'My Dear Hall
Thank you for your letter. I think Wednesday's meeting of the Technique Faculty was a most unsatisfactory one clearly demonstrating the need for a full and frank discussion of the teaching of technique in the School. Your sweeping criticisms of the teaching of the physiological movements require justification; and they are most distasteful to your colleagues who are responsible for teaching the students...
The best way to settle the question at issue will be for each of us to receive a copy of your notes before the next meeting, so that we may be able to discuss the points involved with full knowledge.
I am not sure that you had been displaced as Chairman and

Head of the Technique Faculty. If you had wished to take the Chair at the meeting, then why did you not do so? I was the last to enter the room on Wednesday, to find that the Chair had, apparently, been left for me to take. I, therefore, took it without thinking, as I am used to doing at School Committees. I greatly resent your implication that there was anything intentional towards yourself on my part, and that "the casualness of the occurrence spoke volumes."

Actually as it turned out I think you were more free to speak your mind outside the Chair. Perhaps you would like to invite another member of the Faculty to preside at the next meeting; Dr Stoddard for instance, who is not actually teaching technique.

May I suggest to you, in all sincerity, that you have not, during the past two years, really led or directed the technique teaching at the School. How can we hope to stabilise our methods and settle points of difference if you resign your only hour of teaching just because of a disagreement at a meeting with a more junior member of the Faculty. Neither Mr Middleton nor any one of us is infallible; nor does any of us desire to lecture in your place. Apart from the value of your contribution to the teaching, we all have more than enough to do already.

We simply must thrash out this impersonally in the interests of the School, and its technique teaching. The matter is urgent, as there is danger that the students may be confused by contradictory teaching. Our methods have so far produced very good osteopaths, and they will continue to do so if we all work together....'

Profile: S. Grierson ('Greg') Currie

In 1991, S. Grierson Currie began to frequent the students' bar of the BSO. Although not always welcome, given his frequent intoxication and his over-fondness for female students, he would reminisce on the past. He sent a hand-written letter (3.12.91), describing his time as a student at the BSO (graduating in 1949) and then a typed letter describing how he became an osteopath.

'The Students' Union was defined. I re-started it, as its 1st Hon Sec—I forget who was Chairman (Could it have been John Wernham?). I did just meet our Dean—J. Martin Littlejohn—before he died. The Vice-Dean T. E. Hall held the

BSO together. Jimmy Littlejohn (younger son of J.M.L.) tried to teach me the Principles of Osteopathy. His elder brother— J. M. Littlejohn FRCS*—taught me the anatomy of the skull. Joyce Bishop and Keith Blagrave and Clem Middleton and Webber and others taught me a bit BUT the only true teacher I had was John Ghyll Dixon at 140 Harley Street. One of the early (? founder) members of the GCRO with the Drs MacDonald etc. I learnt more about my craft from him than from anyone else.

I was not one of the pioneers of osteopathy in England—I was in the second stream. Still pioneering—still striving— for what? Respectability, recognition—or what ? No. I think I personally was concerned with learning more about this marvellous art form because I am a firm believer in the Healing Art and it was when Science was introduced that I believe Medicine went wrong.

When I started the BSO Faculty were: Dean: J. M. Littlejohn, Vice-Dean: T. E. Hall, S. Webster-Jones, J. H. Clem Middleton, J. Canning, Joyce Bishop, Keith Blagrave, Hardy, Jimmy Littlejohn, J. M. Littlejohn FRCS*, Alan Stoddard, Ledermann, E. L. Meyer, Miller (dietetics),

X-Ray—Daisy Browne went from BSO to Dorset Square— followed by Jane Kelly (Decd). Office—Secretary Joan O'Keefe, former parliamentary sec to MP for Horsham. Mother of Deelan O'Keefe FRCS who lectured in pathology. Both went to Kenya—Deelan became an orthopaedic surgeon there. Clinic receptionist and almoner Winifred Horsey— became Wyn Currie (His wife)'.

* It was actually James Littlejohn, who was the FRCS as an ENT surgeon.
From the typed letter:

'As an enthusiastic rock-climber, I was climbing on Dow Crags, Coniston, Lake District, on Easter Monday 1936. We were doing a climb described as "supersevere" only to be attempted in dry weather wearing rubber shoes. It was dry, the sun shone warmly over a beautiful winter scene, and melting snow ran freely down all the gullies. So we climbed the notorious Hopkinson's crack on the middle buttress on Dow Crags in nailed boots.three of us. Winston Farrar, Head

Librarian, Leeds Central Library, and poetry in motion to watch when he climbed—was leading. I seconded and Phil (a Buddhist) and a beginner was 3rd. I will not waste time about that exhilarating climb, except that we made it. We were so late, that the others of our party had left to return to the Mines House Youth Hostel, for the much needed evening meal.

In order to get back before all the grub was eaten, the three of us were taking every short cut we knew. This is why we glissaded down 300 feet of steep snow slope. My own descent was unusual, I did it face down, headfirst, out of control, at the speed of an express train. Which to cut out any more to do, is how I became an osteopath. When the doctors and surgeons had frightened me to death with warnings of an ankylosing spondylitis if I continued to abuse my body (I was a gymnast) my new girl friend who was a masseuse at Champneys told me about Osteopathy. I went to see Jack Stables in Bradford. He was the No 1 graduate of the Looker College...As a physiotherapist myself, when I got off Jack Stables plinth after the first visit, I said, "What is this you've got that I know nothing about". John Stables encouraged me to go to the BSO and find out. He was too old to join the newly-formed Register being about 80 when I knew him in 1936.

I got the job of physiotherapist in charge of the newly-opened medical and swimming baths in Epsom in February 1939, just so that I could sign up to study Osteopathy. Then of course, the war, and I spent 6 years in the navy in Naval Hospitals, Plymouth and Mombassa, as a physiotherapist, but believing in Osteopathy and reading about it.

When I was demobbed in January 1946, I couldn't wait to sign up. With my background and experience, I could have taken the two year course, and I'm glad I didn't but elected to do three years (?) and go over anatomy and physiology again. The grind was good for my war-addled brain, and the depth at which we covered these two essential subjects was much more thorough than for physiotherapy.

The BSO had been closed for most of the duration of the war, and was reopened in September 1946. For the month before it reopened I spent several days each week helping out wherever I could. All the treatment tables, library books, and surgical instruments were piled up in the cellar. So I tackled the task of moving the tables upstairs to wherever they were needed.

I must have cut a strange figure to clinic patients, climbing up those steep stairs with a plinth on my back, but it was the easiest way to move them. Then I set up the library and fitted out Minor Surgery. By this time it was time to become a student once again, and put the war behind me.

I was not in the first wave of osteopathic pioneers, of course, but I can claim to be on the tail of the second wave. We were still rugged outlaws from the world of respectable medicine. I just met the Dean, J. Martin Littlejohn before he died, but was never taught by him.'

References

1. McKeon L. C. Floyd (1939). Osteopathy and war casualties. *The Journal of Osteopathy*, October-December, X(4): 6-7.
2. Inglis, B. (1964). Brian Inglis gives a personal view of the manipulators. *The Sunday Times*,1 March: 34.
3. Daniels, B. A. (1997). A Brief History of the GCRO. Annual Report for 1997 and News Bulletin. No. 35, GCR 6/97, pp. 41-50. (Reading: The General Council and Register of Osteopaths).
4. Chambers, M. M. (1995). The British Naturopathic Association. The first fifty years. (British Naturopathic Association).
5. Minutes of the meeting of the Council of the British Osteopathic Association held on Friday April 13th 1945.
6. Webster-Jones, S. (1939). The school in wartime. *The Journal of Osteopathy*. October-December, X(4): 8-10.
7. *The Osteopathic Quarterly.* (1948). The Osteopathic Educational Foundation. Six months' progress. 1(1): 29.
8. Power, R. (1984). A Natural profession? Issues in the professionalisation of British Nature Cure, 1930-1950. Dissertation submitted as course requirement of the CNAA MSc in Sociology, Polytechnic of the South Bank.
9. Spenceley, W. Historical flow chart. In Power, R. (1984). A Natural profession? Issues in the professionalisation of British Nature Cure, 1930-1950. Dissertation submitted as course requirement of the CNAA MSc in Sociology, Polytechnic of the South Bank.
10. Dutton, C. (1991). Obituary: Dr Sammy Ball. *The Times, 3 December* 1991.
11. Hugh Hellon Harris. Personal communication.
12. *The Osteopathic Quarterly.* (1948). The British Osteopathic League Preliminary organisation.1(4): 116-118.
13. *The Osteopathic Quarterly.* (1949). The British Osteopathic League. First progress report. 2(1): 25-27.
14. *The Osteopathic Quarterly.* (1949). The British Osteopathic League. Celebrating the inauguration. 2(3): 85-86.

15. *The Osteopathic Quarterly.* (1949). The British Osteopathic League. A successful bazaar. 2(4): 115-117.

16. Editorial. (1948). *The Osteopathic Quarterly*, 1(1): 1.

17. *The Osteopathic Quarterly.* (1948). 1(3): 90.

18. Robertson, F. (1949) Osteopathy at work. *Picture Post,* 26 February, 42 (9): 10—14.

19. Ellis, A.W. (1949). The Canterbury festival. Commemoration of the Science and Art of healing. *The Osteopathic Quarterly*, 2(3): 63-68.

Chapter 10

The 1950s — Shrugging off the Cobwebs

The 1950s was a period of development for the profession, shaped by a new generation of osteopaths, trained post-war.

In 1950 15 osteopaths joined the GCRO under Article 11, which closed the following year. It was a 'grandfather clause' enabling registration of those osteopaths who had not been taught at a recognised college. The closing of Article 11 marked the end of an era.

In 1950, yet again, registered medical practitioners were instructed not to co-operate with unregistered health care practitioners, including osteopaths. Those osteopaths working with doctors, could only work as auxiliaries, which many refused to do, for example at the Nature Cure Clinic founded in 1928 in London, osteopaths and naturopaths had worked alongside doctors to provide treatment for the poor.[1]

In the early 1950s, Enton Hall, an Osteopathic Resort and Health Farm near Godalming, Surrey, was at its prime. Its Principal was R. Atkinson Reddell DO MRO.

The 3rd Annual Convention of the Societe des Recherches-Osteopathiques was held in London in 1958, opened by the Mayor of Kensington. The programme included a presentation by Stewart B. Humphry on osteopathic diagnosis and by Albert W. Priest on osteopathic gynaecology. Albert Rumfitt and Webster-Jones gave accounts of Osteopathy at the BCN and BSO, respectively. An exhibition of radiographs was lent by the 'Radiological Department' of the BSO. There were French lecturers and a technique film and dinner and dance until 2am.

The 'Boneshakers' Club' met regularly in the 1950s to discuss osteopathic technique. In June 1959, it presented a silver plate to T. Edward Hall on the occasion of his marriage, on which were inscribed the signatures of its members: Ralph B. Goldie, David Wainwright, Eddie Gilhoolie, J. Barclay Baird, James Hopkiss, Rex Shaw, J. Guymer Burton and Maitland Buchanan.

Presidents of the OAGB in the 1950s were:

1950	Harold Mather	1955	Jocelyn Proby
1951	Harold Banbury	1956	J. Guymer Burton
1952	Keith Blagrave	1957	Conrad J. Barber
1953	Muriel Dunning	1958	James Hipkiss
1954	Alan Stoddard	1959	Donald Turner

At the GCRO, the Hon B. L. Bathurst (Viscount Bledisloe) was President until 1959, S. S. Ball was Chairman, Shilton Webster-Jones was Vice-Chairman, R. F. Miller was the Registrar and A. W. Ellis was Secretary to the Registrar, later replaced by R. A. Oakshott.

Outside Interest

James Cyriax wrote a letter to the BSO regarding the second edition of his book, '*Osteopathy and Manipulation*' and asked for authoritative statements on the principles and practice of Osteopathy. A sub-committee consulted a solicitor. The School replied, 'As stated in our previous correspondence with you, the theory referred to by you, viz. that all diseases come from the spine, <u>never</u> has been held or taught by the British School of Osteopathy. No further communication should be made in writing and no verbal statement made at any interview unless a solicitor is present and a verbatim report made by a stenographer'.

Dr Myron Beal from the USA visited the School in 1950, having been asked by the Secretary of the AOA to provide his personal views on it. He suggested that full details of the syllabus should be sent by Webster-Jones to the AOA. It was decided that while full facilities would be given by the BSO to Beal, no official approach would be made by the School to the AOA, unless requested by the GCRO.

Naturopathy and Osteopathy

In 1951 the BNA decided to create a Register of 'qualified' practitioners, but this was opposed by more than 20 members, most of whom were BSO graduates and registered with the GCRO. They resigned from the BNA.[1] In 1951 and 1952, the proposal to include the term 'Osteopathic' in the title of the Association was rejected.

The BNA, however, decided to grant Diplomas in Osteopathy, 'To be at least as high a standard as other existing osteopathic institutions', as well as Diplomas in Naturopathy. Those who qualified would be able to use the title, 'Registered Osteopath (BNA)'. Not surprisingly, the GCRO objected to this and in 1954 threatened to take legal action. Three representatives from the BNA met three from the GCRO. The BNA agreed not to use the designation, though BNA members who were Registered osteopaths could use the term, 'Registered Naturopath and Osteopath'. As from 1953, membership of the BNA was only open to graduates of the BCN, the first of whom emerged that year. In 1959 the GCRO met with the Executive Council of the BNA with a view to co-operation. Such discussions were to continue for a further three decades.[1]

In 1951, the BCN course consisted of weekend and evening lectures, 12 hours a week. Attendance from 18.00 to 21.30 was required during weekdays and a Saturday morning clinic. There were seven lecturers. There were 28 students at the college in 1953. The first graduation ceremony took place that year at Cairns Hydro Hotel in Harrogate.[4]

In 1953, postgraduate weekend courses in Osteopathy and Naturopathy were offered, including an advanced course on Osteopathy and one on Physical Therapy and Neuro-muscular Technique provided by Stanley Lief.[1] In 1956 a 4-year course was proposed. The college was registered as a Company in March, 1956. By the following year it had 40 students. It was hoped that being filmed by *Pathe Pictorial News* would raise its profile.[1]

In 1951 the Vice-Dean of the College, Arthur Jennings, managed to obtain rooms in Craven Terrace, Lancaster Gate, London W2.[1] In 1953, Hector Frazer found a building at 6 Netherhall Gardens, Hampstead, North London for which he paid £10,000, together with a further £5,000 for repairs and alterations. The original house was designed in 1882/3 for the artist Thomas Davidson. The design expresses the architect's, 'Individual interpretation of the Queen Anne style'. (British College of Naturopathy and Osteopathy Prospectus, undated).

The official opening of the building, named 'Frazer House', took place on two October 1954. Stanley Lief launched the College Foundation Trust in an attempt to raise a further £50,000. The following year Hector Frazer moved out of his flat in the house to create more space for the College and an X-ray machine was purchased. In 1959, Frazer arranged for the transfer of the freehold of the property to the BNA as a gift and to double any sum of money raised, up to £25,000.

Other Schools and Colleges

In September 1951, 'The Maidstone Osteopathic Clinic' began in the consulting rooms of S. John Wernham.[2] Its objects were to provide persons of limited means with free osteopathic treatment (though they were encouraged to make a voluntary contribution) and to be a teaching clinic by providing new graduates from the BSO with the opportunity to gain experience under the supervision of a senior member of the profession.'

The clinic depended on private subscriptions and donations from patients. It was opened formally at 30 Tonbridge Road on 11 August 1953, when the old X-ray unit of the BSO was sold to John Wernham for £50, 'In view of the great assistance Mr Wernham at Maidstone had given, in various ways, to the school and the OEF'.

In 1955, the GCRO accredited the LCO, which became the London College of Osteopathic Medicine (LCOM), but the student intake was small.

Osteopathic Publications and Publicity

The Osteopathic Quarterly was at its peak in the early 1950s. The series had a 'Portrait .Gallery' of well-known osteopaths and supporters: Harold Mather, R. F. Miller, Viscount Elibank, A.W. Ellis (drawn by Laurie Taylor), R. Harold Banbury, Murray R. Laing, J. K. Blagrave, Muriel Dunning, Herbert Milne, Sammy Ball and Lord Hankey. Leslie Korth wrote an article on 'Hypnotism and its use in Osteopathy' and 'Health from Sea-water' and Arthur Millwood on 'How do you Chew?' 'Simon Simplex', the pseudonym of Clem Middleton, wrote a series of articles on Osteopathy, 'The Day in the Life of a Spine' and how osteopathic treatment is given, illustrated by Laurie Taylor. Five of the articles with their illustrations were bound into a 31 page booklet published by the Osteopathic Publishing Co Ltd, 20 Buckingham Street, London WC2, entitled, 'A day in the life of a Spine and other Diversions', price one shilling and sixpence.

In 1956 Volume 9 of The Osteopathic Quarterly appeared as only two issues. By volume 10 (1957) it was incorporated in a magazine entitled 'Osteopathy' and in 1958 in 'Your Health' which continued publication until 1960. In the OAGB September Newsletter of 1959, the editor referred to the Osteopathic Publishing Co Ltd working on a scheme with Messrs W H Smith & Sons to establish 'Your Health' on bookstalls, but it would incur a substantial expense in promotional advertising. The presentation and contents of the magazine were to be kept in a popular form to be attractive to the general public. A circulation of at least 15,000 to 20,000 was aimed for so that it could then, 'Be used to publicise the osteopathic approach to the maintenance of good health, and the treatment of those illnesses which react particularly well to Osteopathy'. This never transpired. A new series of The Osteopathic Quarterly was introduced in 1967, published at 30 Tonbridge Road, Maidstone.

Proceedings of the Osteopathic Association of Great Britain No. 1 appeared in 1956, No. 2 in 1958 and the Journal of the Osteopathic Association of Great Britain Vol. 1 No. 1 in 1959.

In 1953, a Dr Ledermann wrote a book on *'Natural Therapy'* and in 1955, the second edition of Jocelyn Proby's *'Essay on Osteopathy. Its Principles, Application and Scope'*, of 44 pages was published by the Osteopathic Institute of Applied Technique, to which profits went and also to the OEF. In 1956, Faber and Faber published R. W. Puttick's *'Osteopathy'*. On 10 October 1951, a reader of the *Daily Mirror* requested in the 'Live Letters' column, a cure for sciatica. She was recommended to write to the GCRO at 12 Clarges Street, London, W1, for the name of an osteopath. 847 letters were received at that address.

In 1951, Stanley Matthews, 'The Wizard of Football', had his injured foot treated by an osteopath and the boxer, Randolph Turpin, told the *Daily Express*, 'The reason I'd done my hand, according to the osteopath who looked after me then, was that I was punching two stone above my weight'.[3]

Research and Scholarship

In 1952, Freda Sharpe at the BSO devoted one year, half time, to reviewing Littlejohn's notes on osteopathic practice, with special reference to technique and also acute diseases, but her work was criticised as, 'More a resume of the notes and less in the nature of comment'. Hall agreed to supply more material, including the Dean's own notes. Middleton also gave her advice and guidance.

In 1957, there were concerns regarding the publication of Littlejohn's lectures in the first edition of *The Maidstone Yearbook* as sources, dates, comment and annotation were omitted. The Council of Education of the BSO were uncertain they had convinced John Wernham of the unsuitability of publishing the lectures without these. A letter was considered requesting that before publication of further extracts, advice be sought, but it was not sent. Further discussion was deferred until the next issue was to be published. The outcome of this is unknown.

In 1958, James Canning raised the question of what action could be taken to preserve and utilise Littlejohn's 50 years' experience evident through his lecture notes. As much as possible of the material was to be accumulated. A Committee was appointed to do this consisting of Canning, Hall, Webster-Jones and P. R. Stanley.

In October 1955, J. Guymer Burton (Vice-President of the OAGB) produced a summary of replies to the OAGB questionnaires returned on professional fees, circulated the previous September. 'The object of the enquiry was to enable the Association to give factual information to the Principal of the BSO in response to his request for guidance in replying to enquiries from recent graduates regarding the usual professional fees charged by members of the Association.'

Replies were received from 54 members of the Association: 17 in Central London, 4 in London suburbs, 13 in provincial cities, 10 in rural towns and 10 in industrial towns. All stated they accept patients at a lower fee in cases of need. 26 believed new graduates should charge a full fee; 30 were against this. 38 allowed half an hour per treatment; some recent graduates three-quarters of an hour. A few treated 3-4 patients an hour.

The BSO: Student Recruitment

At the BSO in 1950, the building had been put in a good state of repair. 32 students attended the School in October. The increase in students in 1951 required changes in the school routine, timetable and clinic attendance. Problems, however, later arose in recruiting students. Student numbers in 1954-55 were: eight, seven and six in the second, third and fourth years and in 1957, the respective numbers were six, three and three.

Arthur Millwood suggested advertising for students in larger provincial newspapers and certain health journals. Advertisements were inserted in six principal newspapers, but no students were obtained. Further advertisements were placed in the *Evening Standard, Daily Mail and Daily Express*. In 1954, practically no students were recruited through members of the profession. Students differed from those entering in previous years, being generally younger and with little or no knowledge of Osteopathy or experience of it, and with financial difficulties. A brochure and pamphlet were produced to attract students onto the course. The concern regarding student recruitment was brought to the attention of the OAGB and a scholarship sought from the OEF.

The absence of student enrolment in February 1955 caused the Principal great anxiety. Suitable publicity was needed. Members of the OAGB were asked to promote the course. Large numbers of prospectuses were sent to the Ministry of Labour. A special brochure was published, '*Osteopathy as a Career*'. East Suffolk Education Committee made a grant to a student, the first such award to study Osteopathy.

The BSO: Curriculum Developments

In accordance with a decision by the Council of Education of the BSO in 1950, a series of Faculty meetings was held to discuss the curriculum. This was a major turning point for the School, involving a shift from Littlejohn ('classical') Osteopathy to a more rational approach.

The change in part was motivated by a need to make Osteopathy more acceptable to orthodox medicine, but also through a desire to make it more understandable by students. These changes were not welcomed by all Faculty. In 1951, the Board considered the Council of Education should devote more time to developing the curriculum and proposed delegating to the Clinic Committee and the Executive Committee more of the School administration. In 1952, the Council of Education met regularly to discuss the curriculum.

It was agreed that in the second year practical anatomy should consist of introductory osteopathic work, such as handling of joints, simple movements and soft tissue work.

In 'Practice', the osteopathic concept was to be stressed. Among particular disorders to be considered were to be pneumonia, prostatic conditions, uterine misplacements, blood diseases and diabetes, with diagnosis and orthodox treatment outlined, together with the osteopathic approach. The curriculum in the early 1950s was:

First year: Chemistry, physics, biology.

Second Year	*Third Year*
Anatomy (and embryology)	Principles and diagnosis
Practical anatomy	Practice (3rds and 4th)
Physiology (and histology)	Pathology (with 4th)
Applied anatomy (Pt 1 Somatic)	
Introduction to Osteopathy	Orthopaedics and Neurology
	Applied Anatomy of the foot
	Technique
Dietetics	
Tutorial clinic	
Principles of technique	
Fourth year	
Practice	Specialities
Applied anatomy II	Surgical diagnosis
Technique	Medical (Clinical) Diagnosis
Tutorial clinic	ENT
Pathology	Paediatrics and skin
Comparative therapeutics	The eye in general practice
Clinical demonstration	Psychology
Minor surgery	Gynaecology

In 1954, it was agreed that a practical test in technique was to supplement the written examination in this subject.

The Council of Education again reviewed the curriculum in 1955, starting with Practice taught by Webster-Jones, Middleton, E. M. Page, A. Stoddard and Dr Ledermann. The osteopathic approach was to be emphasised, based on Littlejohn's lecture notes and personal experience.

In 1957 Sunday technique sessions were held by Edward Hall, with the assistance of demonstrators, in the large lecture hall. Some clinic cases of special interest were presented.

'Principles', taught by Webster-Jones since the 1940s, was revised and devoted mainly to the nature of health and disease, the history of medicine in relation to the inception and development of Osteopathy, linking the newer concepts of medicine with osteopathic teaching. It included discussion of the osteopathic lesion—definitions, pathology, local and remote effects.

In 1958, Webster-Jones suggested that there was a need to establish a department in the School for the teaching of Basic Sciences as there was a serious loss of students by sending them for tuition elsewhere. In 1959, Audrey Smith prepared a tentative syllabus. Dr Pentney proposed that the first and second years should be integrated and the School should move away from having an 'academic' first and second year. 'This would help the students overcome the dullness of swotting an academic subject for a set examination and make him think for himself. He would then when entering his clinical years be better equipped in general for investigation and treatment of patients.' However, this view was rejected as it would have presented administrative and technical difficulties and lecturers experienced in clinical work would be needed.

Commencing October 1959, a course in comparative anatomy and physiology was delivered, during which physical and organic chemistry and the appropriate physics were incorporated, for example the function of respiration was traced through plants, the lower forms of life, fish, birds, quadrupeds and humans. During this section the physics of movements and behaviour of gases etc. were emphasised and the physico-chemical processes of osmosis interpolated. This improved student numbers as they undertook the basic science course in the first year, or joined the second year with appropriate A levels.

In 1958, Heads of Technique and Practice were proposed, though Stoddard and Pentney thought this premature in view of the size of the student intake. Eventually, two appointments were made: Stoddard for Practice and Edward Hall for Technique. Hall was soon replaced by Clem Middleton. Osteopathic Diagnosis was revised and taught by Audrey Smith, and Colin Dove updated and took over the teaching of Principles, relieving Webster-Jones of both of these subjects.

The BSO: The Clinic

In 1951, for a trial period, the clinic opened from 6-7pm, but students were unco-operative and claimed it interfered with their evening studies and they often left early without permission. There was also little demand for treatment at that time of day. The clinic then closed at 6pm, but opened at lunchtimes instead. It opened on Saturday mornings too (and lectures also took place then), but this ceased in 1958 due to staffing difficulties.

Graduates were encouraged to continue to work in the School's clinic for at least a further year, without teaching duties. They were appointed at ten shillings and sixpence a session. ten clinic assistants worked 20 sessions. They were graduates of at least one years' standing. In 1952, clinic assistants were given the status of tutor operators and their pay increased to one guinea a session. This was the beginning of tutor-directed teaching in the clinic. Until then, students treated patients without necessarily being supervised by a qualified member of staff. If patients were few, a co-operative member of staff might provide a demonstration.

In 1950, the clinic was run by Senior and Junior Clinic Superintendents paid £300 p.a. and £250 p.a., respectively. The Senior Superintendent was present three mornings and two afternoons and alternate Saturdays mornings and was responsible to the Council of Education for the general running and management of the clinic, kept case records and advised and assisting the Junior Superintendent, who was required to do two mornings and three afternoons and alternate Saturdays. All graduates of the school were eligible to apply and the posts were advertised in the *Osteopathic Quarterly* and on the school notice boards.

The number of new patients rose from 20 a week to 50, though with some fluctuation. 16 patients an hour were treated in the clinic and sometimes there was congestion. Over 600 patients were treated a week at one point in 1955. There was, however, a lack of new patients in the children's clinic.

The number of students in the clinic increased from 11 to 14. In 1957 there were 38.5-48 clinic sessions a week, with 18 senior clinic assistants. Patient numbers were 1388-2252 per month, of which 145-294 were new compared to 1502-2109 and 161-338, respectively for 1956.

The 1951 influenza epidemic affected the numbers of operators and patients. New patients had to wait two to three weeks for an appointment.

The number of hours of clinic duty of students was increased to a minimum of 900 for the third and fourth years. In 1951, All third and fourth year students attended two morning or afternoon sessions and one evening per week. They also worked two weeks in the long vacation and two days in each short vacation.

Students working in the children's clinic only attended the general clinic one evening a week. In the early 1950s, every student spent one term of their last year in the children's clinic. In addition students were encouraged to assist during vacations. A practical technique class with lectures on treatment of children was provided one hour a week in the fourth year. Children's Christmas parties were popular and successful. Over 70 children attended the Christmas party in 1951, despite the premises being inadequate for such a number.

A sports injuries special clinic was proposed in the Clinic Superintendent's Report of 1955. It was run by Greg Currie for a trial period before being discontinued.

In 1951, there were plans for a for an extension of the clinic. Webster-Jones and James Littlejohn approached Miller and Ellis of the OEF for funds. It gave £750. Permission for the extension was initially refused by the Ministry, but the School reapplied, as there was a change of government. In 1952, Marples of the Ministry of Health, a patient of Webster-Jones, gave his full support to the licence. Christ's Hospital, the lease-holders, also initially refused permission. In 1953, an architect submitted plans for the extension. It consisted of an Almoner's Office, Staff Office, three cubicles, a waiting room and separate cloakrooms for male and female staff. It was completed in December 1953.

In 1953, a Mr Robertson spent two days a week in the clinic on a sponsored research project working on sciatic neuritis. After eight months he became ill and was unable to continue. Anthony Marsh took over until 1954, although the treatment routines used by Robertson were retained. In 1954, clinic staff were encouraged to carry out and publish original clinical research.

The Littlejohn Lecture

The first Annual Meeting of Faculty took place on 6 December 1951. That year it was decided that a Dr J Martin Littlejohn lecture was to be given annually to faculty on subjects of interest and importance to Osteopathy. The Board donated ten guineas, 'Or such larger sum as the Board may approve'. It initially took place at the Annual Faculty Meeting, preceded by a report by the Principal on the work of the School over the previous year, proposals for the forthcoming year and the distribution of Diplomas. The first lecture was given in 1952 by T.

E. Hall on Littlejohn's contribution to Osteopathy. James Littlejohn said afterwards, 'Surely the word "Lecture" is a misnomer. What we heard tonight was an oration in the truest meaning of the word'. It was followed by a dinner for Faculty and their guests. 34 people attended.

The 1953 lecture was given by Jocelyn Proby on, 'The Place of Osteopathy in Modern Therapeutics'. The Faculty meeting was not held immediately preceding the Memorial Lecture as in the previous year, as there was a small attendance and non-Faculty guests were present. In 1954, John Martin Littlejohn Jr agreed to give the 3rd memorial lecture on some aspect of his father's work, but then asked for this to be deferred until 1955, so Webster-Jones gave it on, 'Osteopathy as Revealed by the Writings of A. T. Still'. In 1953, a patient of Hall's provided a board to commemorate the lectures.

These lectures continued annually, with the exception of 1958. In 1955, John M. Littlejohn Jr was again asked to give the lecture, but refused. Willis Haycock delivered it instead on, 'The Expanding Concept of Osteopathy', at the OAGB Convention, held at the Mayfair Hotel. Copies were sent to American colleges. The next lecture was given by James Canning on, 'Osteopathy—a Basic Therapy'. Canning and Webster-Jones considered that the lecture did not lend itself to publication, but the Board disagreed. The 1957 lecture was given by Middleton on, 'Osteopathy in Visceral Diseases.' Apparently wide differences of opinion were aired. At the 1959 lecture held at the Charing Cross Hotel (rather than the Mayfair Hotel as in previous years), Muriel Dunning spoke on, 'Osteopathy and the Development of the Vertebral Column'.

The BSO: Other Developments

From an income of £866 and expenditure of £840 in 1950 there was a steady trend over the next few years of expenditure overtaking income. In 1950, a letter was sent to the profession from Ellis of the OEF and Webster-Jones, putting the case for support of the School. A target was set by Ellis of £1,500. There was a request from students for more school furniture. Tables and chairs were purchased.

In 1952, the students' library had fallen into a bad state. It was discussed whether it was the responsibility of the School or the Students' Union. It was agreed that it was the former, but a librarian was appointed by the students at an honorarium of £5 per year.

There was a proposal for the amalgamation of the BSO and LCO and of the Osteopathic Trusts and the OEF. A meeting occurred led by the Hon B. L. Bathurst and Christmas Humphreys. Following correspondence it was decided not to proceed.

Stoddard proposed that a textbook on osteopathic technique as taught at the School be prepared. A Subcommittee was appointed— Stoddard himself, Middleton and Hardy. All members of the technique teaching staff were asked to participate. Several meetings took place and progress was made in 1953.

In May 1952, Dr and Mrs Fryette of Beverley Hills, California were the guests of honour at a dinner at the Mayfair Hotel, organised by T. E. Hall, 'An old personal friend of Dr Fryette'. Fryette had studied under Littlejohn in Chicago and developed osteopathic techniques. About 30 well-known British osteopaths attended, including Dr Murray-Laing on behalf of the BOA. Fryette also lectured to the students at the BSO on, 'The total lesion'. He was given an honorary appointment to the Faculty of the BSO and an Honorary Diploma.

The Fryettes re-visited the School again in June 1955 while on holiday in Europe. He met technique faculty and presented a copy of his textbook to every graduate present. They were the principal guests at the Faculty Dinner, to which all 'medical' members of the faculty were invited.

Webster-Jones was re-appointed as Principal for a further three years in 1951 and again in 1954, but then Edward Hall suggested a committee be appointed to define the office of Principal and the duties involved.

In 1951, Dr James Littlejohn resigned due to other commitments. This was a break in the family tradition of association with the School. Hall wrote to Webster-Jones in 1956 that he had decided to withdraw from the BSO. Given his later involvement with the School, it would seem it was from teaching rather than the Board. In 1959, Canning, who had been a Director for many years, resigned, having been ill since 1957.

There was a need for another School official. In 1953 Audrey Smith offered to work in the School and help in the clinical and teaching work. She became 'Registrar' mainly for the purpose of compiling and maintaining clinic records and statistics. From 1952 to 1954, 1,700 cases were analysed from the clinic discharge book.

In 1953, in view of its nearness to the palace, the building was washed down and re-decorated for the Coronation.

In 1953, the Board approved the award of Fellowships for selected individuals.

In 1955, final payment of the loan (without any interest) from Littlejohn to purchase the building was made to his son, Dr James Littlejohn.

In 1956, students objected to an increase in examination fees by the Board, which sought legal advice. The increase was to be applied only to referred and new students.

W. C. Bruggemeyer asked the Principal to review the situation regarding admitting other visually impaired people on to the course. This was considered impractical as the special teaching required could not be provided.

Dr Edgar Culley, who graduated from Kirksville in 1900, was one of the first osteopaths to work in Australia. He developed a Trust Fund to assist students in Osteopathy. Fryette sent the Fund a BSO prospectus and a commendation. Consequentially, at least £500 was to be sent to the School each year for a trial period of three years as the, 'Edgar W. Culley Students Fund for meritorious applicants who need financial help'.

In 1957, following the death of Mr Ellis and the litigation in which the GCRO was evidently engaged, both the GCRO and the publishing company were in 'low financial water.' The GCRO was housed in Buckingham Gate and the Registrar, R. F. Miller, requested a reduction of 50% in the rent. Concern was expressed in 1958 regarding accommodation of the Register in the BSO building and that, 'Impartiality and independence could be compromised in certain circumstances'.

Proby's Paper

Some ten years after the re-opening of the School, (April 1957) Jocelyn Proby produced a paper on the state of the BSO. It is of interest in that it provides an insight into the challenges it experienced at that time. He considered that the termination of the Principal's present term of office (which did not take place) might provide an opportunity to make some changes. He was concerned that they were not getting enough students of the right type. Most of the students were female and he considered an attempt should be made to attract men to the School, by modifying the entrance requirements and possibly also the nature of the course.

Proby considered that they had pushed up the standards to a point which made student recruiting harder than it ought to be. He then proposed running the course on a part-time basis, at least in the first year or two, though it might have meant lengthening the course. He then discussed the organisation of the School. There were long periods during the week when there was really no one with seniority or real authority in the building. He considered either the Principal should be there for a much greater proportion of the week, or perhaps better, he should have a deputy. He felt that that the medical influence in the School had become rather too strong and a determined effort must be made to bring the students more in contact with more of the senior and experienced members of the profession.

He suggested that the Board of Directors should be strengthened with new blood and to increase the permanent salaried staff of the school to two, i.e. a Principal and Vice Principal, or alternatively to have a more highly paid Principal who would be there for a larger proportion of the time.

He recommended that a small committee should be appointed to decide what changes in organisation were necessary and what personnel required in different capacities. This was undertaken. Webster-Jones as Principal devoted two and a half days a week to the School and Audrey Smith became his personal assistant, covering part of the remainder of the week.

References

1. Chambers, M. M. (1995). The British Naturopathic Association. The first 50 years. (British Naturopathic Association).
2. H.G.D. (1955). The story of the Maidstone Osteopathic Clinic. *The Osteopathic Quarterly*, 8(2): 25-28.
3. Editorial. (1951). Sportsmen and Osteopathy. *The Osteopathic Quarterly*, 4(3): 88.
4. Dr Ian Drysdale, Principal of the British College of Osteopathic Medicine. Personal communication.

Chapter 11

The 1960s

Professional matters

In 1964 the GCRO had a debt of over £117, such that the Secretary voluntarily proposed a cut in his own salary.[1] A Public Relations Officer was appointed, initially part-time, then full-time. In 1965 an 'Osteopathic Information Service' was formed, establishing for the Press, TV and radio as 'a single authoritative source of information'.

Statutory recognition was again under consideration. In 1960 a spokesperson for the Minster of Health indicated that in order to win over the doctors the profession must first demonstrate that it could regulate itself. The 1965 GCRO report noted:

'Popular journals are already tending to crusade in favour of Osteopathy and to attack the medical profession for its alleged refusal to acknowledge the benefits of osteopathic treatment. They could both stimulate public demand for Osteopathy to be brought into the National Health Service and embroil our profession in an unwanted controversy with the doctors.'

A Status Planning and Publicity Committee in 1965 decided to, 'Abandon recognition as a target, In fact to wash it right out of our philosophy',·as independence might have been lost and osteopaths made subordinate to doctors' and Osteopathy might become a 'Profession Supplementary to Medicine', as was so for physiotherapists, and the opportunity to diagnose lost.

The Kidderminster Corporation Bill, presented to Parliament in January 1969, threatened the right to practise of various health professionals within its precincts. Osteopathy was not included, but the GCRO saw the Bill as a threat, established a political pressure organisation,' and requested the Ministry of Health to withdraw the offending clause. The London Borough of Redbridge attempted to enforce a classification of an osteopath's practice as, 'An establishment for massage and other similar treatment', which created great offence.

An amalgamation between the GCRO and OAGB had been considered for over a year before a meeting took place in November, 1966. The argument for separate bodies was that the GCRO represented the public and therefore another organisation (the OAGB) was needed to represent the profession. A similar debate was to be repeated in 1992. However, in 1967 differences between the two organisations may have had deeper roots in that many who were active in the OAGB were those who had failed to be elected onto the GCRO Council.[2] On the same day, in the morning the AGM of the GCRO resolved that a joint working party be set up to produce an Amalgamation Plan and in the afternoon the AGM of the OAGB resolved to produce a Demarcation Plan. Some osteopaths left one meeting to vote at the other. In 1967, there was a postal referendum, completed on 1 June. Demarcation received 56.4% of the votes.[1]

In the 1960s both the Guild of Naturopathy and Osteopathy and the GCRO agreed not to use the term 'Registered Osteopath'. Members of the GCRO used the term, 'Member of the Register of Osteopaths' and designated themselves MRO.[1] Members of the BNA continued to use the term 'Registered Naturopath and Osteopath'.

In April 1968, the GCRO brought a case against the Register of Osteotherapists and Association of Naturopaths, whose members used the post-nominal letters 'MRO'. In the High Court, Mr Justice Pennycuick granted the GCRO a perpetual injunction and awarded costs. The GCRO, however, were aware that further legal actions could result in, 'A searching scrutiny of the conduct of its affairs'.[1]

In the 1960s Air Chief Marshal Sir William Elliot was President of the GCRO, with Viscount Bledisloe as Vice-President. 'Sammy' Ball was Chairman in 1960 and Philip Jackson from 1961 to 1967 when R. F. Miller succeeded him.

In 1964 there were 215 members of the Register and by 1969 251, but the numbers of new members barely exceeded the losses. 54 members were threatened with 14 days' notice of termination of membership unless they paid their subscriptions.[1]

Presidents of the OAGB in the 1960s were:

1960	E. W. Twinberrow	1965	Donald F. Norfolk
1961	S. Grierson-Currie	1966	Reginald W. Carpanini
1962	Stanley Holditch	1967	Leonard C. Nugent
1963	Arthur J. Smith	1968	Lutchman M. Naidoo

1964   Audrey E. Smith

After 1968, Presidents were in office for three years.

In 1969 the OAGB had a dinner in the House of Commons hosted by The Rt. Hon Sir Peter Rawlinson QC, MP.

In November 1968, Herbert Milne wrote a memorandum to the OAGB entitled: 'Osteopathy—What is its Future?' He expressed concerns regarding Osteopathy at that time:

'As I sit back and reflect on my many years in the practice of Osteopathy, the development of the BSO, the Association and the Register, I am filled with deep concern for the future of our profession in Britain. From the early days, 40 years or so ago, to today, I see a contrast that startles me. The pioneer spirit that then obtained, linked with a keenness to know in all matters pertaining to theory and practice...was linked with a faith that was the result of the success seen in practice, and the fuller realisation of the broad base of Osteopathy as it was and could be made to serve ailing individuals.

The profession exhibits a keenness that I am sorry to say, is not apparent to anything like the degree it was then....As the growth in knowledge and fitness went on, the image that inspired it was the concept of Osteopathy as a system and not just a technique....

Compare this to the picture today in which the public image is so widely held, that Osteopathy is something useful for painful joint disorders and, possibly, bronchial asthma and another oddment or two within the body. Shades of Still! To my mind this public image is at least partly accountable for the small number of students at the School, and can one wonder at it when a prominent official of the BSO gave his interpretation of Osteopathy on television that, "We find in osteopathic practice that a great many of the aches and pains, disorders and stiffness and the weaknesses that are common today are the result of minor mechanical disorders in the body...the main fact being that the diagnosis of these disorders is really the basis of Osteopathy". If it is—God save us! In no part of the statement was there any reference to spinal lesions (minor or otherwise) being capable through the influence of nervous connections, of affecting visceral function. This sort of thing is to deny by default the very basis of Osteopathy.

But this television presentation is topped by an open denial,

proudly stated in a letter to *The Lancet* some time ago, in which
a prominent member of the Register "explained" to its readers
that:—"No responsible osteopath would any longer associate
the vertebral lesion with visceral disturbance"....Anyway, if it
is true, it signs the death warrant of Osteopathy....In the light
of this, is it not time that a careful re-appraisal of our position
should be made and an authentic statement, prepared for
public information, so that a true image may be formed, which
would give to the profession a full concept of the amplitude of
practice which is essential to both confidence and dignity....
To carry out this aim, I would suggest that a committee be
formed representing the School, the Association and the
Register, to strive to work out the pattern of a basic theory
which will meet the demands of the Select Committee of the
Lords.'

Milne then went on to, 'Offer a contribution which may be of value
in assisting the committee (if it is formed) to arrive at a conclusion on
the matter'.

He then explained a neurological connection between the
musculoskeletal system and the viscera, though his argument is difficult
to reconcile with the science of 1968, let alone with that of today. He
claimed that the sensory mechanism in the peripheral nerve consists
of three systems: deep sensibility (pressure and movements of parts);
protopathic sensibility (capable of responding to painful cutaneous
stimuli. This is the great reflex system) and epicritic sensibility (by
which we gain the powers of cutaneous realisation). 'If it is correct as
we have striven to show that in the evolution of disease, whatever the
initial influence may be, the passage from physiology to pathology is
always associated with the neural changes in the spinal cord and its
appendages due to, now, the capacity of the irritant to produce the
spinal lesion.'

On 1 March 1964, the *Sunday Times* carried an article on, 'The
manipulators, a personal view' by Brian Inglis.

With the death of James Canning in 1961, Lord Hankey in 1963 and
Lord Semphill in 1966, the profession lost three loyal supporters.

Profile: James Canning

James Canning, born in 1885, initially trained as an architect and
surveyor in his father's office and designed buildings in Manchester and
later banks in Africa. Having contracted malaria, he returned to the UK

and decided on Osteopathy as career. He joined the BSO in 1925 and graduated as student number 16 in 1929, a contemporary of T. Edward Hall. He then joined the Faculty and made important contributions to curriculum developments. He served on the Council of Education and Board of Directors, where he was known for his honesty and integrity. He was a proponent of 'Littlejohn' Osteopathy and was also a competent artist. In 1937 he married Joyce Bishop. Edward Hall was the best man at the wedding. In the Book of Remembrance at Aldershot crematorium, under the crest of the BSO, is inscribed, 'James Canning, Osteopath. Loved and honoured for his skill and dedication as a healer, and for his integrity as a man'.

The BSO: Recruitment

In 1963 the London County Council approved grants to suitable students for the last three years of the course. There was a large number of Nigerian applicants. It materialised that the majority applied to obtain student entry permits. All students were required to attend for interview, which deterred those who were not genuine applicants.

In 1965 the Principal was approached by the National Institute for the Blind regarding the possibility of visually impaired students being admitted to the School. This was considered unacceptable as students had to be capable of conducting a full medical examination.

In 1966, due to a fall in student intake in 1964 and 1965, the total number of students in the School was only 29 compared to 40 the previous year, with a loss of income. In 1967-8, there were 34 students. four physiotherapists entered the third year. The intakes for 1968 and 1969 were again disappointing. A Local Regional Osteopathic Careers Officer (ROCO) scheme was created in 1969 to promote the profession regionally. It still exists.

The BSO: Finance and General

In the 1960s, finance, student numbers and premises again were key issues for the BSO. The School decided to launch an Appeal. In 1960 Mr Martin, who had relevant experience of appeals, joined the Board. He indicated that it needed to be nation wide, that local committees should be set up and that a brochure was needed. The BSO approached a commercial organisation that conducted appeals and employed a paid organiser. Following two unsuccessful appointments, an organiser was appointed to operate the, Extension of the Practice of Osteopathy Campaign (EPOC) from an office in Clarges Street, Piccadilly. Letters of appeal were sent to members of the profession and a monthly bulletin issued. £5,500 was raised, but in 1963, following concerns about its administration, the organiser left.

A Fund Raising Working Party considered that the EPOC did not have unqualified support from the profession and that there should be only one fund-raising body—the OEF, which was registered as a charity in 1963. Its role was to support the BSO, but in order to avoid competing with the EPOC, it had not been actively conducting an appeal for funds. The EPOC ceased in 1964 and its work was undertaken by the OEF.

A Faculty Dinner was held in the Rembrandt Hotel, London in May 1965, to commemorate the centenary of the birth of Littlejohn. The 50th anniversary of the School was marked by a dinner for graduates in July 1967 at St Ermine's Hotel, Caxton Street, London.

In 1968 the OAGB donated money to the library to be called, 'The Littlejohn Memorial Library'. The OAGB treasurer wanted the School to pay for the Incomes Survey of 1966, but it refused.

A School Bulletin was produced in 1969. 200 copies were circulated to staff, shareholders and faculty.

The BSO and the BCNO

In January 1963, the solicitors of the British Naturopathic and Osteopathic Association (BNOA) and British College of Naturopathy and Osteopathy (BCNO) that had changed titles from the BNA and BCN, respectively (see below) sent a letter to Webster-Jones regarding a leaflet sent out by the Campaign Secretary of the EPOC the previous December, making an appeal for funding, 'To extend the practice of Osteopathy'. The leaflet referred to, 'Only some 250 men and women whose professional training and competence make them eligible for membership of the Register' and that, 'All graduate Osteopaths in this country are trained and qualify at the British School of Osteopathy'. This implied graduates of the BCNO were not professionally trained and competent. It was considered defamatory and calculated to cause them considerable damage. The BSO was asked what steps it was prepared to take to remedy the situation and compensate the damage caused. The offending circular was withdrawn. The BCNO also had a nation-wide appeal for funds to improve educational facilities, provide scholarships etc at the college.

The BSO: Premises

In 1960 Webster-Jones drew attention to fact that the premises were rapidly becoming inadequate. A Premises Committee was set up to seek more adequate accommodation, or possibly temporary, additional accommodation. It reported that for 200 students 20,000 square feet was needed costing £20,000 annually. The cost of equipping the building would be £250,000. This was considered far too ambitious.

Harlow-Jones (Investments) Ltd offered to purchase the lease of Buckingham Gate for £5,000, but chartered surveyors recommended that the School ask for £20,000 and not accept less than £15,000. The landlords of Buckingham Gate wanted office accommodation and there was the possibility of leasing part of the building as a clinic.

In 1961 premises were explored in Dorset Square, next door to the BOA, of 15,000 square feet. Osteopathic Trusts, however, made a bid for it, purely as an investment.

The School considered buying a large house in Harrow Weald, with 4.5 acres of land, which Dr Lincoln Williams, a patient of BSO graduate, Leonard Wardell, used to treat alcoholics. It was offered for £60,000. It was old and needed a resident caretaker/gardener. Being so far from London, a Central London clinic was also needed. The BOA was approached with a view to a joint clinic, but negotiations were unsuccessful, though not due to lack of goodwill. £35,000 offered for the house was neither accepted nor rejected. The request of a lease was refused. In 1962 planning permission for change of usage was granted.

An offer of £45,000 was made for Ivy Lodge, North End Road, Hampstead in March 1962, but the owners decided to auction it. A freehold premises was also inspected in Battersea Rise, but was unsatisfactory.

In 1962 Webster-Jones again reported on the lack of space for clinical teaching and technique and on the lack of lecture room accommodation. Partitions between rooms were removed. In 1963, a further offer of £50,000 made on the house in Harrow Weald and accepted, but the School could not be sure of raising the money.

In 1964, Swiss property developers bought the freehold of Buckingham Gate and the need to find alternative property became critical, or to purchase a longer lease at great expense.

That year, the School was offered the lease of the Cancer Prevention and Detection Centre, Paddington Green, with the possibility of its use as a teaching clinic, but that would have involved a loss of £20,000-£25,000 over five years, before income overtook expenditure. It was therefore refused.

In 1965 a decision was made to renew the lease on Buckingham Gate, as the purchase of another building was considered 'a nebulous hope'.

There was an offer from the landlords of a 51 year lease, eventually at £60, 000 with a ground rent of £2,250. Following a joint meeting with the OEF, the owners were offered £75,000 for the freehold. They wanted £85,000. An agreement was reached at £83,000. The School needed to borrow just over £58,000. A mortgage was obtained from the PDSA, but this was for only £50,000. At a special meeting in April it was decided to proceed with the purchase of the lease and to sell the £5,000 of savings bonds held by the company.

In 1967 a Miss Gillett bequeathed her flat at Broadstairs for convalescence of patients and for, 'Weary members of the school clinic and staff'. It was sold in 1979.

An effort was made to improve the building. In 1966 the X-ray equipment was some 40 years old and needed replacing. Second hand X-ray equipment was purchased, but fused the transformer. In 1968 a new machine was purchased. In 1968 students redecorated the clinic and X-ray department. By 1969 the problems with heating and drainage were tackled. Floods in the basement had been common for many years. It had flooded four times in one week.

A request for £250,000 was made to the OEF. The revised requirement was for a building for 100 students of 11,500 square feet and within 6.5 miles of Charing Cross.

In September 1968 a policy of expansion was agreed by the Board as being the only way forward for the School. This was to be accomplished by expanding the existing building.

The BSO: Management

The School underwent changes in its senior management in the 1960s. Audrey Smith had became Personal Assistant to the Principal in 1959. In 1961 she resigned to undertake more academic work, but was asked to remain as Registrar. In 1963 she resigned from this post, but agreed to work at the School until it was reorganised.

In 1963 a working party was set up to consider the organisation of the School, consisting of Clem Middleton, Colin Dove and Commander Morris. There were concerns regarding the Board being self-perpetuating and the control that Hall had on it and hence the School,[2] particularly as he had the support of Philip Jackson, Muriel Dunning and James Littlejohn. The proposals were to have an elected Board that was accountable, to offer £1 shares, and to have a Principal and Chief Executive run the School. In April 1964 the Board met to consider the Working Party's report. In the 56 page account of the debate, James Littlejohn commented, 'I think Part 1 is probably one of the most dangerous documents ever put into circulation in the history of Osteopathy in this country. I have little confidence in the word 'Confidential''. Hall said, 'I strongly resent this long rigmarole of condemnation of people who spent many years giving the best part of their lives to the School and Osteopathy'.

The Board was split on the proposed changes. Philip Jackson's vote was critical. The Hon B. L. Bathurst (later Viscount Bledisloe, President of the GCRO in the late 1950s) invited the Board to a dinner at Kettner's at the end of which he raised the matter of the report of the working party and asked each Board member to comment. Jackson was asked outright which way he would vote. After two days' consideration he agreed to vote for the changes, but in so doing fell out with Hall. Littlejohn threatened to resign.[3]

While it was considered that a full-time Principal was needed, it seemed unlikely that an osteopath would make this commitment and a lay Principal was sought. In September 1964 two candidates were interviewed, but both were unsuitable. A Steering Group was commissioned to find a new, 'young' Principal by Easter 1965. The post was offered, but the applicant withdrew. Webster-Jones agreed to continue until Autumn 1965 and to revise the curriculum and syllabus.

As part of the changes, Heads of Department were proposed in 1964: Anatomy and Physiology, Margot Gore; Principles of Osteopathy, Colin Dove; Osteopathic Practice, Webster-Jones; Diagnosis, Audrey Smith; Technique, Middleton.

Hall was annoyed that he had not been made Head of Technique. Although on the Steering Committee to effect the proposals, he never attended meetings. He was invited to submit a report. He did not attend the Board meeting in December 1964, but submitted his resignation, in the hope, no doubt, that his friends would support him. It was accepted, 'With regret'.[2]

In 1967 Audrey Smith assisted with the educational administration. She was appointed Deputy Principal, until a full time Principal was appointed, when she became Vice-Principal and Head of Faculty.

In 1968 Philip Jackson resigned from the Board and Dunning and Proby decided not to seek re-election. Webster-Jones indicated his wish to retire as Principal. Colin Dove offered to assume the post for three days a week on a three year appointment. By September he was acting Principal. James Littlejohn apparently commented, 'My father would have been so pleased. The School has waited 60 years for you!'[2] Webster-Jones was made Chair of the Board. In the Principal's lengthy report in 1968 he indicated a need to reduce expenditure and increase income in all its respects and to increase student fees.

The BSO: The Course and Clinic

In 1960 it was recommended to the Board that the title of the course 'Minor Surgery' be dropped and 'Clinical Emergencies' be substituted, but this was not approved as it would have necessitated alterations in the Articles of Association. The teaching of tetanus and gangrene was removed from the course.

In 1960 James Canning forwarded books of Littlejohn's lectures to S. John Wernham for review. The Board required a progress report the following year.

In May 1963, Dr Tricker of the London County Council wrote to Commander Morris that the proposal for a one year preliminary course was not considered a suitable alternative to the General Certificate of Education Advanced Level entry into the second year. Tricker was concerned about the length of classes and the inappropriateness of teaching physics and chemistry as part of comparative zoology, the lack of experimental work and deficiencies in the examination. It was strongly recommended that the course be discontinued, which it was by November 1963. There were also concerns regarding overcrowding in the school, the risk of withdrawal of LEA grants and the vulnerability of the School and Register to criticism. The GCRO inspected the School in February 1963 and made 18 recommendations.

In 1963 the final examinations consisted of two, three hour papers on Practice of Osteopathy and a further two on Clinical Examination. Technique was examined by one three hour paper and a practical assessment. Applied Anatomy II, Minor Surgery and Pathology were three hour papers and there was a viva-voce examination in Pathology. In 1964 the use of anaesthetics was prohibited on the School's premises.

In 1965 all departments were reviewing curricula. Lectures on Biochemistry were given by Ernest Keeling, who had a degree in Chemistry from Cambridge. He also assisted in the teaching of Physiology. In 1966, Faculty were then paid one guinea per hour. Dietetics ceased to be examined. Minor Surgery was eventually replaced by a First Aid and Medical Emergencies course. Clinical and Technique practical work were treated as separate examinations.

In 1968 it was planned to lengthen the course to four years, beginning in Autumn 1970. Colin Dove developed a recruitment plan. All energy was devoted to revising the curriculum led by Audrey Smith. There were regular meetings of the technique faculty with revision of terminology and teaching.

In 1961 January-March there were 496-510 patients per week, the average charge being eight shillings and sixpence. In 1962, Audrey Smith recommended a reorganisation of the clinic because of the increase in new students and new graduates: there were then three sessions a day, until 7pm, and one on Saturday mornings. In 1968, there were

562 patients a week with a charge of 13 shillings per treatment. Audrey Smith provided tuition for clinic tutors.

Other Schools and Colleges

The BNA changed its title to the British Naturopathic and Osteopathic Association (BNOA) in June 1961, following which the title of its college changed to the British College of Naturopathy and Osteopathy (BCNO), 40 years later to become the British College of Osteopathic Medicine (BCOM). The change was considered important as Osteopathy had been taught as part of the naturopathic course and there was concern that if the title of osteopath became protected by law, those graduates practising Osteopathy as part of Naturopathy would be precluded from doing so. Following the death of Stanley Lief in 1963, Albert Rumfitt became Dean and Dennis Keiley Vice-Dean. In September 1964 the BCNO accepted its first intake of full-time students. In 1965 an Education Authority for the first time granted a scholarship to a BCNO student. The appeal launched by Stanley Lief in 1954 had met with little success. In the 1960s Harold and George Cotton launched a further appeal in order to raise £250,000 for a new college and residential accommodation. £229,000 was raised by 1970.[3] The BCN had a student magazine in 1961 termed *The Pioneer*.

The GNO, founded in 1949, produced the *British Naturopathic Journal and Osteopathic Review* that in 1962, under the editorship of Clifford Quick, developed a new and enlarged format. The GNO merged with the BNOA in 1964.[3]

In 1965 the Ecole Francaise d'Osteopathie, founded in 1951 by Paul Geny, relocated to the BCNO, where rooms were rented in vacations. This was because, while it was not illegal to teach Osteopathy in France, it was illegal to practise it. Geny, who had learnt his Osteopathy from a Dr Stirling, an American-trained osteopath, was faced with fines of £3000 in one year alone. 'The French School in exile' was then under the Principalship of Tom Dummer, who had been teaching at the Ecole Francaise d'Osteopathie since 1957 and who had founded the clinic at the BCNO. Marguerite Maury (who had introduced aromatherapy to the UK) introduced Tom Dummer to Geny. Initially it was only intended to provide a facility for 16 students, all physiotherapists, to complete their course, for two or three weeks for two periods a year. The course, however, remained popular and the number of students increased. Not only did French students enrol, but also French-speaking students from other European countries. At one point there was a two year waiting list. Further accommodation was required. The 'overflow' of students received seminars at John Wernham's Osteopathic Institute of Applied Technique at 30 Tonbridge Road, Maidstone Kent. As a result, in 1968, an Educational Department was formed at the Institute.[4]

In 1960 the Fellowship of Osteopaths evolved from the study group organised by Ken Basham. (See 1948). He then ran more organised courses and a 2-year Diploma course in 1961/1962. In 1966 it became the Society of Physiatricians, based on Physiatrics—the Science of Natural Healing. It was a multidisciplinary organisation, though mostly of osteopaths. This was the forerunner of the College of Osteopaths, founded in 1974.[5,6]

References

1. Daniels, B. A. (1997). A Brief History of the GCRO. Annual Report for 1997 and News Bulletin. No. 35, GCR 6/97, pp. 41-50. (Reading: General Council and Register of Osteopaths).
2. Colin Dove. Personal communication.
3. Chambers, M.M. (1995). The British Naturopathic Association. The first 50 years. (British Naturopathic Association).
4. Margery Bloomfield. Personal communication.
5. Hugh Hellon Harris. Personal communication.
6. Jane Langer. Personal communication.

Chapter 12

'To Stephen Ward, Victim of Hypocrisy'

It has been claimed that Stephen Ward (unintentionally) did more to promote Osteopathy in the 1960s than any other person. Every newspaper in Britain documented what was the scandal of the century, of which as a 'society osteopath' he was at the centre. Everybody was asking, 'What's an osteopath?' A profession familiar to only a few gained publicity worth a fortune.

Lord Denning in his report[1] described Ward as, 'The most evil man I have ever met', but there is now evidence[2] that many of the accusations against Ward were unfounded and that key witnesses in the trial had, due to police pressure, perjured themselves. Ward committed the ultimate anathema to all social classes, of crossing social boundaries, mixing with high life and low life. Irrespective of how we may view Ward's lifestyle, we should perhaps recognise his contribution to Osteopathy, not because of the media coverage of the scandal, but as a practising osteopath.

In outline, for those unfamiliar with the affair (for there are some born after 1963 who may have never heard of Stephen Ward), the scandal of which he was the centre rocked the Macmillan Government: the sexual relationship between John Profumo, Minister of War, and Christine Keeler, an alleged call girl. Profumo denied this relationship, but after Keeler's revelation and evidence provided by Ward, he was obliged to admit to the House of Commons that he had lied, and consequently resigned. The story had all the ingredients that the press and public love: sex, politics, spies, drugs and violence. Keeler also had a relationship with Yevgeny Ivanov, Assistant Naval Attaché to the Soviet Embassy, whom MI5 suspected of espionage and with good reason. She claimed that Ward had asked her to discover from Profumo, 'When the Germans would receive nuclear warheads from the US'. Ward had introduced Keeler to both Ivanov and Profumo, but he had kept MI5 and both sides of the House of Commons informed of the circumstances. By a strange turn of events, a man whom MI5 did not consider a security risk became investigated by the police without any justification.[2]

The Council Minutes of the BOA record that in February 1939 Ward applied for BOA membership. In April 1944, as a Lieutenant in the Royal Army Medical Corps, he wrote to the BOA wishing to establish osteopathic clinics in command centres. The matter was referred to the War Office, but with no outcome. By October 1946 he was a member of the Board of Directors of the BSO on the recommendation of Jocelyn Proby and the following year was an External Examiner. Greg Currie when interviewed (See Chapter 9) related an occasion when Ward examined him in anatomy. Currie was handed a skull and asked to name the foramina (holes for blood vessels and nerves). He hesitated. Ward gave him hints, much to the annoyance of the Principal, Shilton Webster-Jones. Ward was involved with John Wernham's Osteopathic Institute of Applied Technique. There is a photograph of him at the Anniversary Dinner in 1954, sitting with Wernham, Edward Hall and other notable osteopaths of that period.

Born in Lemsford, Hertfordshire in 1912, Ward moved to Torquay in 1920 with his scholarly father, the Rev Arthur Ward, and protective mother. He was educated at public school in Canford Dorset. There an incident occurred that was to be mirrored later in life. He was wrongly accused and punished for hurting another boy. Despite his innocence, he took his punishment honourably. A master later explained, 'Someone had to get whacked, that someone just happened to be you'.[2]

After working in a Houndsditch warehouse and as a translator in Hamburg and studying at the Sorbonne, he was advised by osteopath Jocelyn Proby, whom Ward's godfather knew, to study Osteopathy at Kirksville. Shortly before he died Proby mentioned at an interview with the author that Ward's interest in local girls was an embarrassment to his parents, but they considered that at Kirksville, with its Methodist leanings, he would be 'all right'. (Lights out at 10.30!). He also had a blatant affair with a married actress.[3] At Kirksville, however, he did not, change his ways and apparently nobody thought he would pass the examinations. Ward's intelligence more than compensated for the little time he spent studying compared to 'his extracurricular activities'. Proby claimed he could memorise whole paragraphs of Gray's Anatomy at one sitting.[3] Even at that stage he displayed an interest in prostitutes and susceptibility to trouble. Twice he ended up in jail, once following hilarity at a brothel that centred on his 'pinga grande'. During the War he volunteered for the Royal Army Medical Corps. He was sent initially for training at the Armoured Corps, Bovington and set up an unofficial osteopathic clinic there, but the medical officer objected and he was transferred to the medical corps, though he could not practise. In 1945 he was sent to India where he met the Maharaja of Baroda and Poona and through him came to treat the Mahatma Gandhi for headaches and a stiff neck.[2]

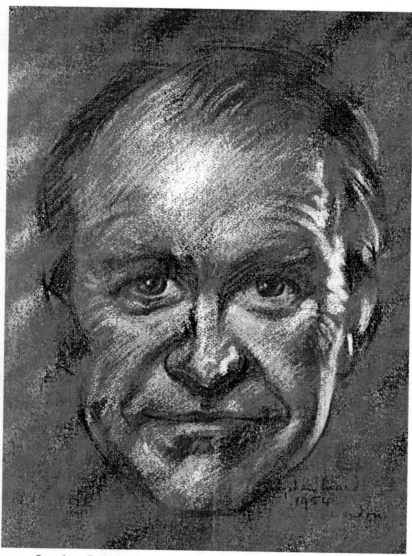

Jocelyn C. P. Proby specially drawn by Stephen T. Ward

In 1945 he suffered a breakdown and Proby considered he may have attempted suicide.[3] He returned to Torquay briefly after the war, but then worked at the BOA clinic in Dorset Square, sharing a room above the clinic with 'Sammy' Ball and acting as a locum for a Park Lane osteopath. It was at the BOA clinic that he happened by chance to answer a telephone call from the American Embassy, asking for a recommendation for a first class osteopath. Ward advised, 'You should go to our best man. His name is Dr Stephen Ward', and he arranged an appointment at the practice of a friend, whom he persuaded to lend his practice for an hour. The patient turned out to be Averell Harriman, the American Ambassador. Through Harriman, who claimed that Osteopathy was the only thing that kept him going, Ward treated Duncan Sandys and Diana, his wife. She recommended her father, Winston Churchill. When Ward treated him, Churchill was sitting up in bed wearing only his pyjama top and smoking a cigar. On learning that Ward had treated Gandhi, Churchill enquired, 'And did you twist his neck too? Evidently a case of too little too late'. He then asked Ward what he would do if his (Churchill's) head came off in his hands. Ward said he would go and practise in Moscow. Churchill unamused, responded, 'Don't you be too certain. Mr Stalin was quite a friend of mine'.[2]

Soon Ward's practice grew. His patients included Lord and Lady Astor, Sir Anthony Eden, Hugh Gaitskell, Paul Getty, Nubar Gulbenkian, Joseph Kennedy, Douglas Fairbanks Jr, Ava Gardner, Danny Kaye, Mary Martin, Frank Sinatra, Robert Taylor, Elizabeth Taylor, Sir Thomas Beecham and Sir Malcolm Sargent. The Ferriers invited him to their parties where he met Prince Philip, Jon Pertwee, Michael Bentine, Peter Ustinov and other celebrities. Ward was popular not only as an osteopath, he was amusing company and a good listener and conversationalist with a mellifluous voice and he also enjoyed playing bridge.

He was also a good artist with a distinctive style. Churchill tried to persuade him to take up painting. In July 1960, he exhibited at a West End art gallery sketches of Rab Butler, Hugh Gaitskell, Paul Getty, Nubar Gulbenkian, A. P. Herbert, Sophia Loren, Selwyn Lloyd, Harold Macmillan and Stanley Spencer, some of which were printed in the *Illustrated London News*. This was followed by a contract to sketch members of the Royal Family: Prince Philip, the Duchess of Kent, Princess Margaret, Anthony Armstrong-Jones and the Duke and Duchess of Gloucester. There are at least two sketches of osteopaths by Ward in existence: one of Edward Hall (it hangs now in the European School of Osteopathy) and one of Jocelyn Proby.

Ward's weakness was his addiction to sex, allegedly which ranged from voyeurism to sado-masochism. He seems to have been fascinated by the thought rather than the deed and revelled in the accounts of others. Allegations of homosexuality are unsubstantiated, though he had many homosexual and bisexual friends, including Godfrey Winn.[3] When he had settled in London, girls would frequently call on him for a chat. He probably had more interest in their company and their naughty stories than in their bodies. His fascination for low life and high life, as if not dangerous enough, was complemented by an enjoyment from introducing one to the other, which he frequently did at parties in Cavendish Square. That was to seal his fate.

Among the girls he befriended was Valerie Mewes, who had left home and was sharing with the later murderess, Ruth Ellis (!) He met Mewes in a doorway in Oxford Street in the rain and as a 'Professor Higgins' succeeded in transforming her from an uneducated waif into a sophisticated model. This inclination explains his interest in Christine Keeler and girls of similar background and why he introduced them to Society. Mewes appeared in a film and was befriended by the Maharaja of Cooch-Behar, before her death in a car crash in 1955.

Ward had great difficulty in close relationships. His marriage to Patricia Baines, a 21 year old actress, ten years his junior, lasted only six weeks, when she caught him associating with prostitutes. He vowed never to become emotionally attached again.

Ward met Christine Keeler, described as a physically attractive scatterbrain, when she was 'performing' in Murray's Club in London. As a girl she was well-known among local youths and men at the tyre factory and air force base near her home in Wraysbury, Berkshire. She had appeared in 'Tit-Bits' at the age of 15. She was invited to join Ward at his table in Murray's Club. He dated her and in 1959 she moved in with him. She then met Peter Rachman, the infamous property magnate, who was generous to her in return for sexual favours, but six months later she left him for a former boyfriend and moved back into Ward's flat.

The Editor of the *Daily Telegraph*, Sir Colin Coote, a patient of Ward, arranged for him to sketch the Eichmann trial in Israel. Ward then considered sketching the Politburo in Moscow, but needed a visa. Coote invited Ward and Ivanov for lunch at the Garrick Club in January 1961 with the intent that Ivanov would facilitate this. They became friends. Ward taught Ivanov bridge and introduced him to the London social scene, though he never went to Moscow.

Among Ward's patients in 1950 was Lord Astor, who after a fall from a horse was treated by Ward and valued his friendship. Ward introduced him to clubland and girls, boosting his confidence. It was Astor who helped him to purchase 38 Devonshire Street and also invited Ward to his lavish parties at Cliveden on the Thames near Maidenhead, where Ward met Royalty, the rich and famous. In 1956 he rented 'Spring Cottage' in the grounds of Cliveden, where he invited friends, including Christine Keeler.

On 8 July 1961, Keeler was staying with Ward at Spring Cottage, when they decided late in the evening to have a swim in Astor's pool. Her swim suit unfortunately being rather too large fell off and Ward threw it into the bushes. Just at that moment the guests at Astor's party emerged with brandy and cigars. Astor and Profumo joined in the fun and tried to intercept her. She drove back to London, but returned the next day, accompanied by Ivanov, for a picnic by the pool. There was a swimming race and a wrestling match in which Profumo had Keeler on his shoulders. At the end of the day Ward gave Astor osteopathic treatment, but Keeler returned to London with Ivanov. Ward was supposed to follow but he did not. Keeler and Ivanov allegedly had sex, probably the only occasion on which they did so.[2]

After Ivanov and Keeler left, Profumo asked Ward for her telephone number. During the following week he courted her and they had sex. 32 days after their meeting, Profumo was advised by the Cabinet Secretary, Sir Norman Brook, to avoid Ivanov and asked if Ivanov was for 'turning'. While he did avoid Ward and Ivanov, Profumo continued to see Keeler. He wanted her to leave Ward's flat, but she would not. The relationship ended. His final letter to her was on War Office paper—a mistake that was later to cost him dear.

It was in the Rio Cafe, Notting Hill that Keeler and Ward met Aloysius 'Lucky' Gordon, who became obsessed with and terrorised Keeler. She later met another West Indian, Johnny Edgecombe. Both were jealous and violent men. Gordon attacked Keeler in the street. Edgecombe suggested that they should confront Gordon. They met in a club and a fight ensued. Gordon's face was slashed. six weeks later, Edgecombe called on Keeler at Ward's flat at 17 Wimpole Mews. She refused to answer. He drew a gun and started shooting at the door and window and then climbed the drainpipe. This was not the kind of behaviour Devonshire Mews was used to. The neighbours called the police and Edgecombe fled. He was later charged with slashing Gordon. Ward ordered the two girls out. The papers loved the story and the link with Profumo was now leaking out.

Robin Douglas Home wrote an article in *Queen Magazine* entitled,

'Sentences I'd like to hear the end of', implying, without naming names, that as a Russian car was drawing up at Keeler's door, a Humber, (Profumo's car), was slipping away.

Keeler went for consolation to Michael Eddowes, a retired solicitor, who was fascinated by conspiracy and espionage. She told him about Profumo and Ivanov and embellished the story. She said that Ivanov was a spy and had asked her to find out from Profumo when the US would provide nuclear warheads to Germany. Ward had also met Eddowes. Eddowes asked Ward if Keeler knew Ivanov. Ward replied, 'Yes and Profumo too'.

George Wigg MP hated Profumo because Profumo had betrayed him. They were once friends both being army men, even though on opposite sides of the House of Commons. Wigg had received complaints about the treatment of troops sent to Kuwait in 1961. Wigg gave a speech in the House criticising the situation. Profumo had promised his support, but then broke the agreement.[2]

John Lewis was MP for Bolton, a successful businessman, racehorse owner and inventor of rubber substitutes vital in World War II.[4] In 1948 he married Joy who was 16 years younger. They met Ward and became part of the same social set, but their marriage began to crumble. He was arrogant, a womaniser and frequenter of night-clubs. On one occasion she walked out and sought consolation from Ward. They talked through the night, but apparently nothing sexual happened. Lewis eventually bullied her into telling him where she had been. Lewis was a man who was unremitting in obsessional hatred and malice and a seeker of vengeance. He thrived on litigation, even over trivial matters. He was convinced Ward had slept with his wife. He had him investigated by the Inland Revenue and told the police and the *Daily Express* that he was running a call girl ring. A friend of Ward, Freddy Mullally, political editor of the *Sunday Pictorial,* was similarly accused. He managed to get the *Daily Express* virtually to admit they had a tip off from Lewis. Ward agreed to withdraw a slander writ against Lewis, if the latter withdrew his intent to cite him in divorce proceedings. In 1954, Lewis succeeded in ruining Mullally financially. He also harboured his hatred of Ward and later sought vengeance.[4] So two men had related hatreds: Lewis hated Ward and Wigg hated Profumo.

Nine days after the shooting, Keeler went to a Christmas party where she met another man she could confide in. She told him everything. It was Lewis. That sealed Ward's fate. It must have been the best Christmas gift Lewis could have wanted. He invited her to his flat in St John's Wood and taped her story. She claimed it was Ward who mentioned the nuclear warheads. Lewis then asked for sex, but she refused. He gave her a gun and said shoot me! She took it and tried, but it was not loaded. Apparently Lewis went white and let her go.[2]

Ward was far from happy about the Edgecombe shooting at his flat, but the final split with Christine Keeler came at the start of the New Year. She was crammed in the back of his car with a friend. Ward had difficulty controlling the car on the icy road and asked the friend to get out. Keeler protested that if her friend had to get out she would also — and so she did. That ended their relationship.

Lewis revealed to Wigg on two January 1963 all he had learnt from Keeler, though this was 16 months after the relationship between Keeler and Profumo had ended. He did not mention his hatred of Ward. He then sought further information on Ward from anyone he encountered who knew Ward, passing it on to Wigg and, on Wigg's advice, to Wigg's friend, Commander Arthur Townsend of the Metropolitan Police. Lewis saw Townsend regularly and it was Townsend who was later to lead the investigation of Ward.[4]

Lewis also suggested to Keeler that the newspapers might be interested in her story so that they could dig up dirt on Ward. She played off the *Sunday Pictorial* against the *News of the World*. Ward got to hear of this and angrily accused Keeler of attempting to damage his career.

On 26 January, a Detective Sergeant John Burrows visited Keeler and her friend, Mandy Rice-Davies, in connection with the Edgecombe shooting, but they told him a great deal more. Rice-Davies now held a grudge against Ward. She had been the lover of Peter Rachman, who had given her a flat in Bryanston Mews, which she furnished, but which she was obliged to vacate on his death. She resented Ward having persuaded Rachman's wife to allow him to rent what she considered was 'her' flat. Keeler told Burrows that Ward was a procurer of women.

The following day Ward saw Astor and Profumo to discuss how they could stop Keeler publishing her story. There was also concern about what she would say at Edgecombe's trial. Ward managed to stop the papers by offering an alternative story.

The friendship between Ward and Ivanov was well known to MI5. Ivanov claimed in his autobiography that he photographed secret papers on Astor's desk, looked through Churchill's private papers and had secret information on the Royal Family.[5] He was using Ward to insinuate himself further into British society. MI5 had asked Ward to seduce Ivanov with the fruits of Western society, so that Ivanov would voluntarily become a counter spy—'Operation Honeytrap'—or, alternatively he might be blackmailed into so doing. Ward was an avid reader of spy novels and welcomed this new role.

Ward arrogantly was convinced that through Ivanov's connection with Moscow he could act as an unofficial line of communication between Moscow and Britain and hence America, to relieve the deadlock between the USA and the USSR during the then 'Berlin crisis'. Astor wrote on his behalf to the Foreign Office, but they were not interested. Ward then persuaded Sir Godfrey Nicholson that this role had possibilities and the latter corresponded with Ivanov. Ward requested through Nicholson a meeting with Sir Harold Caccia, the Permanent Under-Secretary of State at the Foreign Office, and offered to put him in touch with Ivanov, but Sir Harold was not interested. Ward offered, again, a line of communication with the USSR through Astor and Nicholson during the 'Cuban Crisis', but the Foreign Secretary saw this as an attempt to drive a rift between the US and Britain and refused the offer. Ivanov was very angry.

On 26 March, Ward saw George Wigg, who had appeared on *Panorama* the night before and had claimed Ivanov had expensive suits and cars and Ward wanted to correct him on this, but he also told Wigg the full story and how his practice was being ruined by the investigation and how he gained nothing from protecting Profumo. Wigg passed all the information to Harold Wilson.

Why Ward was investigated at all is still uncertain. Henry Brooke (Home Secretary) instigated a meeting with Sir Roger Hollis (Director General of MI5), Sir Joseph Simpson (Metropolitan Police Commissioner) and Sir Charles Cuningham (Permanent Under-Secretary at the Home Office).[2] It was initially to discuss anonymous letters received by Mrs Profumo, allegedly sent by MI5, but the conversation turned to Ward, particularly about him having asked Keeler to obtain secrets from Profumo. Hollis considered that it was unlikely he could be prosecuted under the Official Secrets Act, as witnesses were unreliable. It was also doubtful if he could be charged with living off immoral earnings.[2]

The decision to investigate Ward came from Brooke, who possibly considered that shutting Ward up would terminate the Profumo affair, or discredit Ward's statements on the matter. He may have been aware of Wigg's report to Wilson and that Ward was his principal source of information. Brooke received a letter from Michael Eddowes claiming that Ward and Rachman were running an espionage call girl ring.[2]

Another account[3] claims that Brooke met with Sir Dick White, Head of Security Services and Simpson. White's interest was in Ivanov and it was he who considered prosecuting Ward under the Official Secrets Act, but realised it was unlikely to be successful. Simpson felt the police might prosecute if they could get the full story.

When Simpson received a letter from John Lewis, claiming Ward was living off immoral earnings he decided there were grounds for an investigation. It was headed by Commander Arthur Townsend, a friend of Wigg and with whom Lewis had discussed the whole matter. When Lewis was arrested for drunken driving in 1963, Townsend was a witness on his behalf.[4]

Ward's investigation was conducted by Detective Chief Inspector Samuel Herbert and John Burrows who had previously interviewed Keeler. Keeler was interviewed over 20 times and told if she did not co-operate she might be charged under the Official Secrets Act. On 23 April, Rice-Davies was arrested at London Airport with a document 'resembling' a driving licence. She was jailed. The police offered to 'help' and she told them all she knew.

Another relevant incident happened. On 17 April Keeler was staying at the flat of Paula Hamilton-Marshall. She had an argument with Paula's brother, who hit her. She told the police of her injury, but blamed Lucky Gordon. She then set Gordon up by telling his friends where she was, so that he predictably would visit her. Gordon was later arrested. The two witnesses in her flat could not be found. Gordon was told that if he would help the police to convict Ward, he would be released. He refused.

Throughout April, Ward was confident that his powerful friends would protect him, but by May, some 130 witnesses had been questioned and he slowly lost both his patients and friends. Astor asked him to return the keys to the cottage at Cliveden. It gradually dawned on Ward that it was Lewis behind the accusations and that Keeler had told Lewis and the police everything, but he did not know of the connection between Lewis and Townsend.

During May, Ward made pleas to influential people in an attempt to stop the investigation. On 7 May, he saw Timothy Bligh, the Prime Minister's Private Secretary and threatened that unless the investigation ceased he would reveal the truth and cause the government embarrassment. Bligh, however, considered it a police matter. On 19 May Ward wrote to the Home Secretary regarding the damage done to him socially and professionally and related how he had shielded Profumo. The reply indicated that the police were making whatever enquiries they thought proper and were not under the Home Secretary's direction. He wrote to his MP and to Harold Wilson. On 26 May he saw Commander Townsend and followed this by a letter indicating that the allegations were false and that someone was out to get him at all costs; 'Malice was at work'. He invited the police to make as full an enquiry as possible as he considered the allegations ridiculous.

Three events on successive days in early June sealed his fate. On 5 June the trial of Lucky Gordon opened with Keeler arriving in a chauffeur—driven Rolls-Royce. Gordon was found guilty and sentenced to three years' imprisonment. On 6 June, Profumo declared to the Chief Whip that he had lied regarding his relationship with Keeler and on 7 June the Director of Public Prosecutions decided that there was enough evidence to prosecute Ward.

A friend of Ward asked Townsend if it was possible for Ward to 'get away' for a while. Townsend claimed he could see no problem, but the next day Ward was arrested at a friend's house at Watford. He asked the police to do so 'down the road', so as not to embarrass his friend. Initially he was jailed for the weekend, but then remanded for several weeks until bailed.

At a critical debate in the House of Commons on 17 June, Harold Wilson referred to, 'Clear evidence of a sordid underworld network, the extent of which cannot yet be measured and which we cannot debate today because of proceedings elsewhere'.

On 28 June 1963, Ward was charged under the Sexual Offences' Act (1956) with brothel keeping, procuring, five charges of living off the earnings of prostitutes, procuring girls under the age of 21 to have sex with a third party and abortion offences. He retained until the end his faith in British justice, despite the fact that witnesses were lying in court. (Keeler later spent six months in Holloway prison for perjury). They had either been pressurised by the police, or had a vested interest in his being found guilty, as their stories would be of lesser interest to the media if he were found innocent. The prosecution lawyer, Mervyn Griffith-Jones, with great theatrical skill painted a picture of Ward as evil and a 'thoroughly filthy fellow'. The judge, Sir Archie Pellow Marshall, a man intolerant of the 'permissive society', gave a 'hanging' summing up, biased in its tone.[6] It was not until this that Ward realised he might be found guilty. Before that he had been calmly sketching in court.

During his trial, Ward, desperate for money, particularly to pay his legal costs, saw working as an artist his only hope, now that his career as an osteopath was in ruins. His exhibition at a Bloomsbury art gallery included eleven pictures of the Royal Family. A BBC art critic, however, described him as, 'A man of tiny talent'. Even a career as an artist now seemed impossible.[2]

In late July a well dressed man bought all the sketches of the Royal Family for £5,000 in notes, removing them immediately. It is believed it was either Anthony Blunt or Roy Thomson, the Canadian newspaper magnate.

Ward spent the evening with his girl friend, Julie Gulliver, drove her home and returned to the flat of his friend Noel Howard-Jones, with whom he was staying. After writing 17 letters, he made a coffee and took 35mg of Nembutal. He wrote a farewell letter to Howard-Jones, 'I am sorry I had to do this here....I am sorry to disappoint the vultures.... Delay resuscitation as long as possible.' Howard-Jones found him the following morning on the mattress which had served as his bed on the floor of the living room, foaming at the mouth.

He died on 3 August 1963, at St Stephen's Hospital, under a police guard, unnecessarily ordered by the judge, shunned by his friends, patients and the profession which he had served, having lost everything and with a prison sentence inevitable. Keeler later wrote of the emotional bursts she had after his death, 'It was as much for me as Stephen. I had been robbed of the truth'.[7]

At his funeral six days later, at Mortlake cemetery, there was a wreath of 100 white carnations, with a card signed by Kenneth Tynan, John Osborne, Annie Ross, Jo Orton and others: 'To Stephen Ward, Victim of Hypocrisy'.[2]

Another wreath was left by three girls of Cheltenham Ladies' College on the town's war memorial. The message read, 'As a tribute to dear Dr Stephen Ward, who dared to live his life as a human being and not just as a dummy. An outraged society revenged itself upon him'. The headmistress held an investigation to discover which girls had written this.[3]

Not only did Keeler lie at Ward's trial, she had also lied at the trial of Lucky Gordon that had preceded it. Gordon's two witnesses were found and a tape of Keeler admitting the truth was handed in. Gordon successfully appealed. If Ward had bided his time, Keeler's testimony at his trial would have been deemed worthless.

Ward is best summed up in his own words, present on a tape in the possession of Knightley and Kennedy:

'I know one day the truth will eventually come out. And the truth is very simple: I loved people—of all types—and I don't think that there are very many people the worse for having known me.'[2]

References

1. Denning, Lord Alfred. (1963). The Denning Report. (HMSO, London).

2. Knightley, P. & Kennedy, C.. (1987). An Affair of State. The Profumo case and the framing of Stephen Ward. (London: Jonathan Cape).

3. Summers, A. & Dorril, S. (1987). Honeytrap. The Secret Worlds of Stephen Ward. (London: Weidenfeld & Nicolson).

4. Thurlow, D. (1992). Profumo. The Hate Factor. (London: Robert Hale).

5. Ivanov, Y. (1992). The Naked Spy. (London: Blake Publishing Ltd).

6. Kennedy, L. (1964). The Trial of Stephen Ward.(London: Victor Gollancz).

7. Keeler, C & Thompson, D. (2001). The Truths at Last. My Story. (London: Sidgwick & Jackson).

Chapter 13

The 1970s

Osteopathy and Parliament

In 1971, the Secretary of State at the Department of Health and Social Security set out the steps needed to achieve Statutory Registration of Osteopathy. These were to demonstrate that Osteopathy was valuable and that Registration was necessary to protect the public.[1] Such legislation was not without public support. The previous year, the Women's Institute agreed a resolution urging government, 'To give full recognition to the valuable work done by registered osteopaths and to aid the proper training of osteopaths so that their services are more widely available to the general public'.

In 1973 Ernest Marples MP and Joyce Butler MP invited the GCRO and nine other organisations concerned with 'natural therapeutics' to a one hour meeting in the House of Commons to discuss statutory regulation, but the GCRO refused to attend. It said, 'We are reluctant to identify ourselves with other organisations with whose therapies we are unfamiliar and whose standards of training and education are unknown to us.'[1]

In April 1976 Joyce Butler introduced a Private Members' Bill for the Statutory Registration of Osteopaths. It had tri-partisan support. The Bill read:

'The Secretary of State shall cause to be kept and shall make readily available to any person a Register....The Register shall consist of three lists:
(a) One of persons who have completed a course of training in Osteopathy at the British School for Osteopathy Ltd., or the British College of Naturopathy and Osteopathy Ltd and who have received a Certificate or Diploma from either College stating that they have reached a Standard of Competence;

(b) One of qualified medical practitioners who have completed a course of training at the London College of Osteopathy;

(c) One of persons so registered as holding Foreign or Commonwealth qualifications which satisfy the requirements of the British School of Osteopathy Ltd. or the British College of Naturopathy and Osteopathy Ltd., or the London College of Osteopathy Ltd. or any other College approved by the Secretary of State.'

BBC Radio London conducted an interview at the BSO, but it was, 'So drastically edited as to be almost unintelligible'. The Bill was to be read for a second time on 7 May, but objections were raised from the government bench. A further unsuccessful attempt was made on 25 June.

Nicholas Handoll in the *OAGB Newsletter* was critical of the Bill in that it might restrict procedures to a small range of orthopaedic conditions, the GCRO would lose its autonomy and there would be lists of BSO and BCNO graduates, separate from the medical profession and others deemed 'acceptable'.

The GCRO also was opposed to the Bill and was displeased that it had not been consulted and that legislation might be thrust upon the profession. In the August issue of *The Doctor* an article entitled, 'The Osteopaths register Disunity', quoted Joyce Butler that, 'If the majority of them do not want registration then I will not proceed with another Bill'.

A Profession Supplementary to Medicine ?

The chiropractors, having sought recognition under the Professions Supplementary to Medicine Act (1960) and refused, briefed Lord Ferrier to pursue the matter in the House of Lords. There was an Unstarred Question there in May 1976 regarding whether chiropractors and osteopaths could qualify for recognition within the Act. Lord Boothby and Lord Winstanley were supportive. The latter was a practising doctor and considered that the bulk of his colleagues would approach the subject with flexible and liberal attitudes. The GCRO received four days' notice of this debate.

The discussion was reported in '*Yesterday in Parliament*' on BBC Radio 4. Lord Platt, a former President of the Royal College of Physicians, said that the attitude of the medical profession to chiropractors and osteopaths had changed to some extent in the previous 10 or 15 years, but many processes involved in the treatment appeared to be based on the supernatural. Lord Sandys, the opposition spokesperson, told the House that Osteopathy could cure such diverse conditions as asthma, migraine and fibrositis.

Joyce Butler consulted David Owen, then Minister of Health, who was also a doctor. Owen considered that an approach should be made to the Council for Professions Supplementary to Medicine. An informal approach was made to its Registrar. A multi-disciplinary Board could be set up under the Act so that four further groups of practitioners of alternative medicine could be registered as auxiliary to the medical profession, in addition to those already so registered. Opposition was expected from the physiotherapists, who were already displeased with the Act.[2]

Raphael Tuck MP in 1977 asked the Secretary of State for Social Services whether he would institute a Register of qualified osteopaths. The latter replied that the obvious solution would be for osteopaths to become a Profession Supplementary to Medicine.

Osteopaths, however, were opposed to being recognised under this Act, as it would have prevented their undertaking diagnosis, which would be restricted to medically-qualified practitioners.

VAT, The Common Market and Other Political Matters

There was concern in 1971 that entry into the Common Market could result in legislation restricting the practice of osteopaths. After consulting the Department of Health and Social Security, it was concluded that, 'Any form of protest or lobbying by the Register at that stage would be premature'.[1]

In 1972 the GCRO attempted to obtain an amendment of the Finance Bill to extend exemption from VAT to osteopaths. 104 members wrote to 150 MPs and several members of the House of Lords. When the Bill was debated in July, one Labour MP and one Conservative MP supported exemption of osteopaths, but to no avail.[1]

When Denis Healey had been in opposition in Parliament he moved a motion proposing that osteopaths should be zero-rated for VAT. On the day he became Chancellor of the Exchequer in the new Labour government of 1974, the GCRO reminded him of this, but he reiterated the reasons given for not doing so by the previous government, that 'A line has to be drawn somewhere....The best objective criterion is that based on the Statutory Registers'.[1] The British Committee of Natural Therapeutics was also campaigning for VAT exemption.[3]

In 1974, members of the OAGB and GCRO were urged to write to their MPs concerning the 8% National Insurance contribution under parliamentary debate. A National Federation for the Self-Employed was formed. Many osteopaths were still worried that membership of the Common Market would adversely affect their livelihood.[1]

In May 1979 Barrie Darewski, Secretary to the Registrar of the GCRO, wrote to Geoffrey Howe, Chancellor of the Exchequer, requesting the exemption of osteopaths from VAT. The Queen in her speech had mentioned relief for small businesses.

In 1974 Darewski had won from the Department of Trade and Industry exemption from the 3-Day Week Act, introduced to conserve electricity.[1]

In February 1979 a debate took place in the House of Commons on a Medicines (Unorthodox Practitioner) Bill. Local osteopathic volunteers were recruited as spokespeople for the profession and were given training in media speaking.

A proposed Greater Manchester Bill in 1979 contained a clause requiring osteopathic establishments to register as massage establishments. A petition presented to the House of Lords resulted in the clause being rejected.[1]

Other Professional Issues

The 20 year old Code of Ethics of the GCRO was up-dated in 1971.

The same year the GCRO issued warning notices in the press regarding unregistered practitioners and bogus degrees.[3] In 1971, the GCRO successfully curtailed the Belfast College of Osteopathy which offered dubious courses. Newspapers were warned against accepting advertisements from the college and a dossier on its founder was compiled and sent to New Scotland Yard. The Principal, Professor Frank Anasoh, was arrested. The BNOA was concerned at the inference that as its members were not 'registered' the public might consider they had bogus degrees.[3]

In 1972, further dubious courses were identified by the GCRO: at the University of the Science of Man at Haywards Heath and the International Status Symbols at Coventry. A letter was sent to newspapers warning of the dangers. This brought to light the case of a woman with backache who consulted an unqualified osteopath and was told she had scurvy. No osteopathic treatment was given, but the patient was spending quite a lot of money, 'Buying Rose's lime juice by the crate'.[1] In 1975 William Duncan from his 'Nebraska College of Physical Medicine' sold degrees in Chiropractic and Osteopathy.

The re-opening of Article 11 of the Register was discussed in 1974, but never took place.

In 1977 a Public Relations Policy was developed by the Register and the following year a Public Relations Sub-Committee was formed.[1]

The OAGB was concerned in 1974 that of the 233 members, only 25% were women.

There was apathy within the profession at the start of 1975. Ian Smart wrote in the OAGB Journal, 'None of us can summon up much enthusiasm for 1975....Do your patients never tell you any amusing anecdotes which would give us all a laugh?'

Kim Burton, Research Officer of the OAGB, developed, 'The first real research programme'. It required each practitioner to send a random sample of case cards and to fill in a questionnaire regarding how they practised, but the response was 'abysmal'. Ian Smart wrote in March, 'For Heaven's sake will you co-operate if your conscience will allow?'

In the April 1974, supplement to the OAGB Newsletter, Bill Robertson and his wife described the techniques they developed over the previous 20 years, particularly as part of postgraduate work in the 1950s. Middleton responded listing the paper's merits, but he was critical of the 'syndrome approach' and 'corrective movements'. Kim Burton questioned the 'Desirability of a prescribed dose of osteopathic treatment' and argued the need for research into methodology.

A hospital for alternative medicine was opened in a Carmelite Friary in Hampshire by Dr Chandra Sharma in 1974, offering Homeopathy, Acupuncture, Nature Cure, Faith Healing and Osteopathy.

Second year students at the BSO conducted an opinion poll on the public's knowledge of Osteopathy, from mid March to mid April 1979, (advised by Malcolm Mather, a Director of Gallup Poll). Just over 200 persons responded to 14 questions.

Membership of the GCRO in 1971 was 279. It rose to 305 in 1976 and was 354 in 1979. In 1973, there were no new graduates from the BSO due to a change from a three year course to a 4 year course in 1970. As a consequence membership of the Register fell.

Presidents of the OAGB in the 1970s were:

1970	Arthur Millwood
1972	Mark Flawn
1974	Ian M. Smart
1976	Penny Conway
1978	Gordon Beech

The Rt Hon Earl Jellicoe was President of the GCRO in the late 1970s.

Osteopaths and the Media

In 1974 Terry Moulds treated Queen's Park Rangers Captain, Gerry Francis, and the following year Roger Uttley, England's rugby Captain. *The Guardian* ran an article on 28 August entitled, 'How the manipulators put new backbone into sport'.

James Scott-Robinson, an osteopath, received a three year prison sentence in 1976 for a bomb hoax to Harrods with a demand for £500,000.

Therapy in November 1978 carried an interview with Dr Cyril Pragnell, 'A leading medical osteopath', and former President of the BOA, who ran a clinic in a North London hospital. He was a member of the government's Back Pain Committee, which planned a trial into the value of Osteopathy. He suggested that Osteopathy, 'Could herald the end for orthopaedics....physiotherapists would be well advised to study Osteopathy'. Not surprisingly it evoked a reaction from readers, many of whom were physiotherapists. In a response in March 1979 in *Therapy*, he claimed that, 'It produced a mass of personal comment amounting almost to abuse' and that he did not choose the title and that he was not familiar with the paper in which the article appeared. 'Had I known the readership, I would have been more tactful.'

Brian Inglis wrote an article in the *Spectator* in 1976 in which he suggested that more independence could be given to professions supplementary to medicine and to embrace osteopaths, but that the BMA would object as some therapies are not scientifically proven.

> 'There is little doubt that most of those practitioners of alternative medicine mentioned by Mr Inglis would not be happy if they were so embraced. Furthermore, they would all consider themselves adequately qualified for their chosen professions, and satisfied with their training without assistance from any sector of the NHS.'[2]

In 1978, Inglis published *'The Book of the Back'* (Ebury Press) and Polly Toynbee wrote an article relating how she had been treated by an osteopath, but also wrote:

> 'The most serious complaint about the osteopathic approach is that osteopaths cannot explain in a clear medical sense what the ailment is that they are treating, or what exactly they are doing when they cure someone. The cracking of bones has been regarded as a piece of showmanship. The founder

of Osteopathy had a somewhat cranky view that almost all diseases and symptoms could be cured by adjusting the spine to ameliorate the flow of blood....Can the strength of opinion amongst humble patients, desperately seeking a cure that works break the cartel of the monstrous regiment of doctors?'

An article in the 'Book of Life' The Marshall Cavendish Encyclopaedia of the Human Mind and Body of 1969 was republished under the title, 'The osteopath his work and training'.

In 1974 Hewitt and Wood in Volume 14 of *Rheumatology and Rehabilitation* argued that the time had come for the medical profession to co-operate with chiropractors and osteopaths.

A 1974 edition of *'Osteopathy Explained'* was produced. By 1978, it had sold out. Leslie Korth published, *'The Power of Creative Imagination'* and in 1977, 'The Mysterious Odic Force' and in 1978 (aged 91), in the *OAGB Newsletter*, articles on, 'The Hidden Purpose Behind Diseases' and, 'Analysis of a Stammerer's Dreams'.

In 1976 Cyriax wrote a letter in *the Sunday Times* supporting the need for spinal manipulation in the NHS and ending, 'Meanwhile the osteopaths remain jubilant at a situation that, at my age, time must eventually resolve in their favour'.

In January of that year *Homes and Gardens* carried an article on Osteopathy.

Deaths

In 1976 Commander Morris the first full-time Secretary of the GCRO (1967-72), died. From 1962 he had spent over 12 years working for the GCRO and OEF, following a distinguished career in the Royal Navy. His obituary in the OAGB newsletter of August 1976 referred to, 'Long hours spent at Broadcasting House with corned beef sandwiches and gin'.

There were several deaths in 1977. Vivian Barrow practised with his brother, George Curzon Burrow, first in Park Lane and then after the war in Maidenhead. He was a nephew of the bone-setter, Sir Herbert Barker. Elizabeth Page was a physiotherapist who became an osteopath and included dietetics and homeopathy in her practice. She had helped with the children's clinic at the BSO.

Parnell Bradbury died aged 73. He started as a chiropractor and was a member of the European Chiropractors' Union in 1936, later joining the Register of Osteopaths and the British Naturopathic Association. As a close friend of Tom Dummer he taught at the European School of

Osteopathy (ESO) in its early days. He had written many novels, plays and books, including, *Healing by Hand* (1957) and *The Mechanics of Healing* (1967). His essay on stress was published by the British Osteopathic Journal in 1963.

In 1978, the death occurred of James Terry-Short who had practised for over 50 years in Wolverhampton and Stafford and was a Looker graduate.

Muriel Dunning died in November 1978. She joined the BSO as Muriel Higham and graduated with the Gold Medal from the BSO in 1939. During the war she took over radiography on the death of the radiographer. She took over the running of the BSO children's clinic in the late 1930s. 'Her firm handling and understanding of the patients (and their parents), and her use of very specific short leverage techniques proved of inestimable value and a lesson to us all.' She organised a regular Christmas party in the late 1940s and early 1950s for children, with her husband and daughter. It was an enormous undertaking as some children were handicapped and all ages had to be catered for.

She was a President of the OAGB (1953-4) and a Member of the Board of Directors of the BSO. She gave the Littlejohn Memorial Lecture in 1959 on anatomical variations of the sacrum, assisted by her husband, Gerald, who was a distinguished archaeologist. He received the 'OAGB J. Martin Littlejohn Memorial Award' in 1970, 'In Honour and appreciation of Outstanding Services to Osteopathy', and died the same year as his wife.

Henry Dean Foggitt died in 1979. He was nearly 95 and had only recently retired from practice. He graduated from the BSO as student number 12 in 1928. Before the war he practised in Sheffield and London. He founded the Sheffield Osteopathic Clinic with Harold Mather, Arthur Booth and Margaret Brougham, but moved to Chesterfield in the early 1940s. He worked from 8am until 7pm, six days a week, but decided at the age of 80 to cut back by one day a week.

On 24 March 1979, Edward Hall died after a long illness. He became interested in Osteopathy after having met Nettie Bowles, who taught anatomy at Kirksville, on a transatlantic liner bound for Montreal, when he was a jazz musician. He played international hockey as goal keeper and was impressed at the treatment of his injured knee. He graduated from the BSO in 1929 as student number 19. He expanded upon Littlejohn's long lever techniques after working in the US with Fryette and Downing. Hall was very influential at the BSO from 1943 until his resignation in 1964. The *OAGB Newsletter* carried several obituaries of him.[4] The President of the OAGB, Gordon Beech, described him as,

'One of Osteopathy's finest technicians...who remained to the last a colourful character'.

Middleton wrote:

'Every graduate of the BSO owes a debt to Edward Hall for the pioneering work he did in promoting technique teaching in the School. He was the originator of our classroom teaching system under which the practical details of osteopathic technique, its principles, and the methods of patient handling were demonstrated tutorially, each student receiving individual attention. Prior to this, technique had been demonstrated on clinic patients, but not taught in the form of an organised syllabus. Edward Hall's efforts laid the foundation of the highly successful technique tuition of the post war years. His personal interpretation of the writings of Downing and others put the technique theory and practice into easily understandable terms for the benefit of the undergraduate.

His skill at manipulation was extraordinarily brilliant. I doubt if there has ever been, or will be, any osteopath possessing the same almost uncanny ability.

I knew him well, we had many differences of opinion on matters of policy, but remained good friends. I shall remember him with personal affection, and for the work he did.'

Barrie Savory treated patients in the same practice as Hall for the last few years of the latter's working life. He wrote:

'We would often sit of an evening at Cumberland Mansions musing over the trials and tribulations of life. Amidst a vast array of acquaintances he was yet a lonely man, as he was capable of a professional vision that few of us could comprehend. His, somehow, was the genius that defied the channels to explain. He could do things with his hands that other mortals before or since cannot hope to emulate; and all done with an incredible love for the task in hand. As with all individuals he was frequently misunderstood, and sadly in his latter years his unique abilities were lost to the profession. A situation which he regretted deeply. When he retired to Hove I continued to visit him at regular intervals and take him out to lunch, until eventually he became so bedridden that he was

unable to move from his home....Eventually he moved in and
out of coma.

...It is now rare to find one such man who could rise so far
above his contemporaries. We will not see again his spanning
of the very foundations of our profession and neither will we
see any with his vast fund of techniques. A great force has gone
from us, and many of his skills have died with him. We should
all pause a moment to thank him for enabling us to work as we
do today, and hope to gain a little of the spirit that he had.'

Other Registers and Associations

The Guild of Osteopaths was formed in 1971. Its purpose was of,
'Enhancing, promoting and unifying the profession of Osteopathy world-
wide and to provide a range of educational and professional services
for its members'. Under the leadership of George Palmer and Dennis
Cox, assisted by Robin Fairman and Leslie Rice, the Guild, 'Succeeded
in bringing together a nucleus of highly successful osteopaths prepared
to share their knowledge and experience with younger members of a
growing profession'.

The British and European Osteopathic Association (BEOA) was
founded in 1976 (initially as the British Federation of Osteopaths), 'As
a voluntary body, for the purpose of uniting all qualified osteopaths,
regardless of the school of training or primary professional association'.
It changed its name following its growth in Europe. Dennis Brookes
was the President and Michael Knightingale the Secretary. It had over
200 members.[5]

The Natural Therapeutic and Osteopathic Society was
reconstituted and registered with the Charity Commissioners in 1977.

The Andrew Still Association of Licensed Osteopaths and Register
was incorporated in 1977 and provided osteopathic education as the
Andrew Still College. The first Principal was Bill Graham who left in
1984. The first graduates were in 1983.[5]

The BSO: The Building and Relocation

In 1970, the mortgage of £50,000 obtained from the PDSA in 1965
to purchase 16 Buckingham Gate was due for redemption. The OEF
agreed to support the School, but this would temporarily empty its
coffers. In 1972 the OEF felt that £29,000 would be better spent on
a new building, but in October 1972, Lord Cullen of Ashbourne, the
Chairman of the OEF, offered an interest free loan of £30,000 (rather
than a gift), repayable over 25 years.

The library was reconstructed and redecorated in 1970. By 1973 the lengthier Diploma course and successful recruitment required an expansion of the clinic. A first floor extension of the clinic annexe was planned for 1973 to provide an extra 1,500 square feet. The OEF was asked to fund the major part of this. In 1971 Lord Cullen refused to do so, as he considered there was no evidence of overcrowding and they did not have the money. He considered it only a temporary solution and the School should consider moving to larger premises. 39 questionnaires were sent out to canvas opinion as to where to relocate. Relocation from Central London was rejected. It became apparent that relocation would cost £2 million to £7 million, so the OEF reluctantly agreed the £30,000 loan as Lord Cullen declined to support purchasing a larger building.

In 1977 Colin Dove retired from the position as Principal and Stanley Bradford, an educationalist with business experience, was appointed full time with a brief to relocate the School into larger premises. Margot Gore became Chair of the Board on the resignation of Webster-Jones in 1978. Several lay members were appointed to the Board including Kenneth Rush of Rush & Tomkins, Building Contractors and John Hughes, the Managing Director of an advertising agency that administered *Nature* and *The Lancet*.

In May 1978, an offer was made for the lease of St Mark and St John, King's Road, Chelsea, with a plan to set up special clinics and provide preventative medicine, but the site was put up for auction. The OEF were unwilling to assume responsibility for raising the money.

There were also plans that year to purchase the Helen Grace Clinic at St Leonards-on-Sea and also to set up subsidiary English language and secretarial schools or colleges on a profit-making basis.

In 1979 an intake in the first year of 84 students required temporary accommodation in Westminster Central Hall.

Negotiations began for the purchase of the Kingsley School, Chelsea and then an offer was made to purchase Jews' College, Montague Place for completion by October 1979. However, the college was unwilling to vacate before December and more likely March 1980 and they required £1.25 million. An offer was made in July, but by December outstanding problems were not resolved and there were difficulties in raising the sum required. There was renewed interest in the Kingsley School, but the bid in November was not acceptable to the Greater London Council (GLC).

By December, 1-4 Suffolk Street, off Trafalgar Square, was of interest as a rented property on a 99 year lease. An application was made to Westminster City Council for planning consent to develop Buckingham Gate for office use, as a prerequisite for its sale, but this was refused and much political lobbying was needed. Arthur Latham MP, who had friends on the Planning Committee of Westminster Council, helped, but being Labour they were expected to be opposed to private medicine and needed convincing of the value of Osteopathy. Consent was eventually obtained in October. This change of usage more than tripled the value of the Buckingham Gate building.

The BSO: The Curriculum

In 1970, a 4 year course and new syllabus were delivered. In September the Principal, Colin Dove, presented a paper on the teaching of Cranial Osteopathy and a policy statement was issued by the School in November:

'After careful consideration of the suggestion in all its aspects, the Board has decided that at the current stage of its development it is wiser not to include it in the syllabus for undergraduates....The Board of Directors will, however, continue to keep the matter under review.'

In 1972 he wrote that, 'So far the theories of cranial movements, whilst highly ingenious, are unconvincing'.

However, he investigated further the teaching and practice of Cranial Osteopathy in the US, attending in 1973 a course and conference at Colorado Springs. He became a convert and in 1974 lectured at the Cranial Academy Conference and visited Kirksville College of Osteopathic Medicine (previously the ASO). He developed a growing relationship with the Sutherland Cranial Teaching Foundation (SCTF), the Cranial Academy and the American Academy of Osteopathy. The first cranial course in the UK held under the auspices of the SCTF took place in the UK in September 1974, at the Eccleston Hotel, under the direction of Dr Tom Schooley. Greg Currie encouraged American osteopaths to participate by holding it in Ascot week. Mrs Pamela Brown, clinical assistant, researched cranial rhythms at a hospital in St Albans in 1976.

In 1972 it was decided that clinic training should not be less than 1,000 hours. Stuart Korth and Joyce Vetterlein proposed a scheme to re-establish a children's (cranial) clinic in June 1979. There had been no children's clinic since 1966. Most of the patients then had poliomyelitis or cerebral palsy, but the former became rare following vaccination and children with the latter received considerable provision in the NHS. The Board agreed to the clinic, as a pilot scheme, under the supervision of Colin Dove.

In 1979, a business studies course was introduced by the new Principal, Stanley Bradford, in the Summer Term of the fourth year.

The BSO: Recruitment of Students

There were still concerns regarding student recruitment. The entry requirements were made more flexible. A recruitment campaign was launched by the Principal.

In 1971 there was a fall in student intake to 13 and fewer graduates were retained as clinic staff, thus clinic income decreased, despite an increase in fees. The refusal of the OEF to support the clinic extension set a limit of 16 on the intake for the following year, as overcrowding with the four year course was predicted.

In 1979 an attempt was made to obtain designation from the Secretary of State and Department of Education and Science to enable students to obtain mandatory grants, supported by Lord Jellicoe and Lord Cullen. Of the student intake only 35 (40%) received discretionary grants. In previous years it had been 80-90% of students. It was considered that while the DHSS might not oppose it, the government might in view of its stringent monetary policy. The DES turned down the application as osteopaths were not employed by the NHS.

Negotiations began with the Open University (OU) for credits for BSO diplomates. Following a visit to the school, a study of the revised syllabus and references from seven 'external' referees, the OU Committee on Advanced Standing agreed that applicants for OU degrees would receive the maximum award of three general credit exemptions if they had successfully completed the Diploma course. This would provide a clear recognition by an independent educational body of the academic standing of the course.

Preliminary negotiations began with the Council for National Academic Awards (CNAA) regarding converting the Diploma course to a Degree course. A meeting took place in February 1979. They advised the School to seek initially some association with an already accredited institution. To this end discussions occurred with the Polytechnic of Central London (PCL) School of Paramedical Studies, in July. It was agreed to set up a working party to prepare a submission to the CNAA for a combined degree course, to begin in 1982. PCL agreed to deliver a preliminary 'Bridging' course in Chemistry for students without the appropriate science background, in the Summer term of 1981.

Student numbers at the BSO in the 1970s increased as follows:

1971	32	1976	84
1972	43	1977	87
1973	66	1978	98
1974	78		

The BSO: Other Developments

Between 1973 to 1976 there was sharply rising inflation due to the oil crisis, which put the School at risk. The rising costs resulted in the loss of faculty and support staff as the School was unable to afford increases in salaries. Anatomy and Physiology lecturers were paid £5 per hour, others £1.75. Because of the chronic staff shortage at the BSO, it was necessary to form teams in the clinic. In 1973-4 there were 44 faculty. This number fell to 41 the next year and 35 the following year, at a time when student numbers were rising.

In 1971, after agreeing to defray the cost of books for the Anatomy and Physiology Prize, T. E. Hall refused to pay for one of which he disapproved. It was suggested that as the Board chose the prizes, Hall might choose to withdraw from the list of donors. In 1972, Blagrave, not Hall, donated a prize.

The absence of graduates in 1973 (see above), made it difficult to find assistants in 1975. To maintain his practice, the Principal, Colin Dove, was only at the school two days a week.

The School's 'Centenary of Osteopathy' dinner in 1974 took place at the St Ermine's Hotel.

In 1974 the Postgraduate Department admitted graduates of other Schools/Colleges onto its courses.[6] In 1975 a postgraduate course was held at the Eccleston Hotel at which Irwin Korr lectured. 104 people attended (including students). The one in 1977 was on, 'A Cavalcade of Technique'. Lecturers included Edward Hall and Martin Pascoe. BOA and British Association of Medical Managers (BAMM) members were invited. MROs attended the BAMM Annual Symposium in April. It was considered that, 'There was a considerable gulf between their ideas and our own, but it was useful to have the opportunity to try and identify this'.

There were 20 new students in the first year in 1976, and it was close to its physical limit. There were 38 members of Faculty, but there was still a problem regarding departures and recruiting replacements. In October 1976, Middleton resigned as Head of Technique, having served the School for over 40 years. Laurie Hartman replaced him.

In a letter to the OAGB dated 3 November 1976, Webster-Jones notified the profession of Colin Dove's resignation as Principal, as Mr Dove found the tasks, 'Too onerous to be filled by one person in a part time capacity' and that he had resigned to allow the Board to set up the type of administration that was needed. In May 1977 Stanley Bradford was appointed as Principal designate, which was confirmed in November.

In 1974 there was a proposal to initiate a higher degree. In 1976 Dr James Littlejohn and Audrey Smith presented papers on the matter. In July, an Honours pass was instigated in the final examination — DO (Hons), was to be used from 1977 and a Fellowship of the BSO was also introduced.

Although OEF fund-raising fell from £6,000-£7,000 pa to £2,000 in 1976, it made £300 available to the BSO library, paid for Colin Dove's trip to the US and for the redecoration of the BSO building inside and outside.

In 1977 the BSO Diamond Jubilee and Annual Prize and presentation took place at St Ermine's Hotel on 23 September. 183 osteopaths and guests attended, including the American cranial osteopaths, Roland and Alan Becker. A Diamond Jubilee Yearbook was published in October, 1978 price £6.

In 1977, a five term course for registered medical practitioners was developed. Two students enrolled in 1979. A short course was proposed for qualified physiotherapists, naturopaths and chiropractors. In 1978, Middleton and Webster-Jones retired from the BSO Board, but Audrey Smith was re-elected. The Littlejohn Trust, set up in 1940, was wound up and the 94 shares sold. Middleton by then was the sole Trustee.

In 1978 four Departments were designated at the BSO: Anatomy and Physiology; Applied Anatomy, Physiology and Pathology; Osteopathic Technique and Clinical studies. A Postgraduate and Research Department was to be set up with Colin Dove as Head, as from September 1979, but he indicated that the Research Department should be separate.

In 1979 'Limited' was dropped from the title of the BSO.

BSO patient numbers in 1973-4 were 15,350 and in 1974-1975: 17,600. 25,000 were seen in 1978.

Stanley Bradford in 1979 made a plea for unity among BSO graduates (e.g. those who practised Cranial Osteopathy and those who did not) and in the profession between LCO and BSO graduates. It created much debate.[7]

Other Colleges

To enhance greater unity within the Profession, Colin Dove lectured to a conference of the BNOA in 1974 and on 6 October he dined with Brian Youngs.

Barrie Darewski, Secretary to the GCRO, and Colin Dove were invited by John Wernham to the European School of Osteopathy (ESO) (see below) in September 1974. The School then occupied two large houses at 28 and 30 Tonbridge Road, Maidstone. Present were: the Principal, Tom Dummer, Douglas Mann, J. Keith Blagrave, Barry Savory, John Wernham, Edward Hall, Colin Winer and Peter Blagrave. BCNO graduates present were Steven Pyrie and Brian Youngs. Lectures were given by David Gilhooley and John Wernham.

By 1971, legal rights had been transferred to the Board of Governors of the BCNO from the BNOA to ensure the financial independence of the former.[3]

The 'French School' (See Chapter 11) was only present in vacations, but the numbers of students resulted in it being a significant activity at the BCNO. Not all the BCNO faculty were supportive of this shift of emphasis. By 1971, there were so many French-speaking students from European counties in addition to France attending the Ecole Francaise d'Osteopathie that it changed its name to the Ecole Europeene d'Osteopathie. Due to the large student numbers, some tuition was provided at the Osteopathic Institute of Applied Technique at Maidstone. There was concern at the BCNO of the growth of this French course as it had become a major activity of the School.[11] The casualness of the French students, particularly their smoking was an irritation to some. The BCNO withdrew the award of an External DO. In 1971, the Ecole Europeene d'Osteopathie moved entirely to 28 Tonbridge Road, Maidstone with Tom Dummer as Principal. John Wernham ran the clinic and owned the building.

In 1973 some members of the BNOA considered that the BCNO was not sufficiently accountable to it. It had recommended that the college accept an offer of Associate Membership of the International Federation of Practitioners of Natural Therapeutics founded in 1965, but the Board of Governors of the BCNO was not prepared to do so as it considered this would align the college with practitioners of a lower standard of training.[3]

A group at the BCNO planned to take over the college and to make it more eclectic, to oust out the Dean and a Board member. This failed. Some 25% of the Faculty left as a consequence and took with them half of the students.

A contributory factor may have been the Board of Governors' refusal to make the college an affiliate of the International Federation of Practitioners of Natural Therapeutics[3], but there was possibly a, 'Much deeper resentment over what was described as the ultra conservative policy of the self perpetuating Board of Governors and the impotence of the BNOA to influence their college'. Some BCNO faculty transferred to the Ecole Europeene d'Osteopathie. About 16 students transferred to the ESO. One student transferred to the BSO. This exodus benefited the BCNO as the course became more narrower and professional. At this time Ian Drysdale was appointed as a full time lecturer at the BCNO. In 1975 Dennis Keiley became Dean at the BCNO and Ian Drysdale Vice-Dean.[8]

The Ecole Europeene d'Osteopathie changed its name to the European School of Osteopathy (ESO) as by 1974 English-speaking students were admitted onto the course.

A Research Society for Naturopathy was in existence at that time.

In December 1971, the Society of Osteopaths was founded. This became the professional association for graduates of the Ecole Europeene d'Osteopathie and others. It sent a letter to the BNOA, hoping for close relations with it, but the latter feared if members belonged to both they may have divided loyalties.[3] The Society of Osteopaths had an AGM and Conference in 1976 at which Colin Dove had lunch with Tom Dummer. Barrie Savory was President. Dennis Brookes was the principal speaker. Others present were, T. Edward Hall and S. John Wernham.

In 1973 Tom Dummer wrote to Colin Dove asking the BSO to nominate an External Examiner at the Ecole Europeene d'Osteopathie. Barry Savory, a graduate of the BSO, was working at the college which provided almost 3,000 hours of training. 'We are most keen to ensure that the end product, the graduate osteopath, compares equally with the graduate of the full time school such as the BSO who start their studies virtually from scratch.'

By 1978, the ESO had outgrown its accommodation with John Wernham at 28 Tonbridge Road and purchased its own property, moving to 104 Tonbridge Road in 1979. Clinical education was still provided at 28 Tonbridge Road and John Wernham provided the mortgage for the new building.[9]

Due to insufficient numbers, the London College of Osteopathy ceased to operate in 1975, but recommenced in 1978 as the London College of Osteopathic Medicine, though with a limited number of students. The premises in Dorset Square were sold by Osteopathic

Trusts Ltd and the money used to modernise the clinic in Boston Place.

The College of Osteopathy and Manipulative Therapy emerged from the Society of Physiatricians Diploma course in 1974 and acquired charitable status. It became the College of Osteopaths in 1979. Ken Basham was a leading figure, but then he moved to Jersey and then to the USA. Donald Upton from Surbiton was President for many years. Hugh Hellon Harris was Secretary and for a short spell President. Joe Goodman was Dean from 1977-1993.[10,11]

In 1977 the Croydon School dropped the teaching of Naturopathy to concentrate solely on the teaching of Osteopathy.

References

1. Daniels, B. A. (1997). A Brief History of the GCRO. Annual Report for 1997 and News Bulletin. No. 95, GCR 6/97, pp. 41-50. (Reading: General Council and Register of Osteopaths).
2. Bloomfield, R. J. (Undated). <u>The Time bomb under Alternative Medicine</u>. (Information and Study Centre for Alternative Medicine).
3. Chambers, M. M. (1995). The British Naturopathic Association. The first 50 years. (British Naturopathic Association).
4. *Newsletter.(1979)*. The Osteopathic Association of Great Britain. May: 1-3.
5. David Dyer & Malcolm Mayer. Personal communication.
6. Colin Dove. Personal communication.
7. *Newsletter.(1979)*. The Osteopathic Association of Great Britain. December 1978/January 1979:2-3.
8. Dr Ian Drysdale. Personal communication.
9. Margery Bloomfield. Personal communication.
10. Hugh Hellon Harris. Personal communication.
11. Jane Langer. Personal communication.

Chapter 14

The 1980s

General

The Healing Research Trust in 1980 met representatives from the Society of Osteopaths, the BSO and other osteopathic practitioners. At a follow-up meeting in 1981 representatives of Chiropractic, Oriental Medicine and Acupuncture and Medical Herbalism, met Stanley Bradford, Colin Dove and Tom Dummer representing Osteopathy. Colin Dove suggested that the next step should be for them to get to know each other better and a further meeting was held in April. Gordon Beech of the BSO Board of Directors expressed concern to Stanley Bradford regarding the involvement of the BSO. He stated, 'I feel that any liaison will be detrimental to our quest for improved status and I certainly do not think that the BSO should become the focal point for BFNT activities', and objected to the meeting taking place at the BSO.

The Healing Research Trust became the British Foundation for Natural Therapies (BFNT) in 1984 and was officially launched in February 1985 at the House of Commons. It aimed at a single Register, common ethics and disciplinary procedures and a high standard of education. An Honours Degree was planned with the Polytechnic of Central London (PCL). Its patrons included the Hon Angus Ogilvy and Katie Boyle. It later became the Council of Complementary and Alternative Medicine.

A survey was published in October 1981 by the Threshold Foundation on, 'The status of Complementary Medicine in the UK', which showed for the first time the extent to which unconventional medicine was being used by the public and its 'fragmented nature'. The survey was presented at a conference on Conventional and Alternative Medicine held at the Charing Cross Hospital in November, convened by Dr Peter Nixon, a consultant cardiologist, who had for several years been exploring non-invasive therapies in managing cardiac patients. It was the first of its kind in an NHS hospital. At the conference, Richard Tonkin, the Chairman, and Harold Wicks, its Secretary approached the Director of the British Postgraduate Medical Foundation, John Heron, to set up a working party to explore research into complementary medicine.

This was the forerunner of the Research Council for Complementary Medicine (RCCM),[1] which received charity status in July 1983. Richard Tonkin and Harold Wicks were the Chairman and Secretary respectively. John Heron was the Chairman of the Research Policy Committee.[1] Its purpose was, 'To encourage and fund research into long-standing and well structured therapies, as well as various techniques that use meditation, biofeedback and dietary programmes. In this respect, the Trustees have come together, not to represent specific interests or organisations but, by providing relevant expertise and insight, to contribute towards building bridges between orthodox and complementary medicine.' The Council was quite independent of any particular viewpoint or therapeutic technique, but aimed to encourage the incorporation of what was best in complementary medicine into the mainstream of modern medical practice.[2]

The RCCM held its first conference on research methodology in 1985 at the BSO.[3] Richard Tonkin gave the opening address. It, 'Aimed to take forward the development of research methodology appropriate to complementary medicine with the maximum participation of those active in therapeutic practice.'[2] Further annual conferences followed. The RCCM attempted to widen its range of support and embarked on research projects of greater depth, as the majority were initiated by orthodox practitioners and were hospital based. A Newsletter was published.

A seminar was held in February 1982 on the developing relationship between Osteopathy and Medicine, attended by medical practitioners and the medical press and again in 1983 at the Medical School of Southampton University. 60 delegates attended the latter.

In 1987 the Medical Care Research Unit of the Department of Community Medicine at Sheffield University began a national study of the utilisation of alternative health care delivered by professionally qualified practitioners in the UK, funded by the Nuffield Provincial Hospital Trust. It investigated the scale and scope of six established disciplines, including Osteopathy, as practised by non-medically qualified practitioners, whose qualifications were endorsed by a professional organisation.

In the 1980s, membership of the Register progressively grew:

1980	369	1986	842
1981	390	1987	936
1982	416	1988	214
1983	576	1989	1308
1984	655		

The Earl De La Warr was President of the GCRO in the late 1980s, followed by the Rt Hon The Lord Cullen of Ashbourne.

Negotiations took place between the GCRO and the Society of Osteopaths. Following the successful accreditation of the ESO in 1983, 97 members of the Society were elected onto the Register.

In 1986 an investigation was conducted regarding the government's position regarding VAT exemption for osteopaths. John Barkworth represented a test case, backed by the GCRO. After his appeal to the VAT Tribunal was dismissed, he took the case to the High Court, backed by the GCRO, but as reported in *The Times* in September 1988, he lost the case there as well.[4] The Legal Department of the European Commission were not prepared to intervene.

When the BSO moved in 1980 (see below), the GCRO, which previously occupied the basement of Buckingham Gate, moved to the attic of the new building. Rooms were also rented by the OAGB and OEF. In 1986 the GCRO moved to 21 Suffolk Street, (opposite the BSO), but in 1989 it took a 25 year lease at 56 London Street, Reading.

The BSO held an International Conference, 'Osteopathy in Three Continents' in April, 1980 at the Mount Royal Hotel at Marble Arch. Speakers were from the USA, Australia, New Zealand and Britain.

In 1986 a colloquium on Conventional and Complementary Medicine was instigated by Sir James Watt, Past President of the Royal Society of Medicine, attended by both orthodox and complementary medical practitioners, at his personal invitation.

It was reported in an article in the *British Naturopathic Journal and Osteopathic Review* in 1986 that the Council of Complementary and Alternative Medicine and the GCRO had 3,000 members between them and that there were a further 4,000-5,000 practitioners who were not members of either. Market research indicated that about 25% of the population had an interest or positive attitude towards complementary medicine and there was an increasing interest from GPs.[5]

There was concern in 1984 that the avoidance of commercialism disadvantaged osteopaths compared to chiropractors, who it was considered engaged in aggressive commercialism. A joint working party was proposed with the British Chiropractic Association to consider common standards.

Advertising was also a concern of the GCRO in 1986. New graduates needed to build a practice; established ones were concerned about a decline in ethical standards. The Office of Fair Trading published a report in October on advertising in the three paramedical professions, advocating lifting restrictions in order to stimulate competition. In July 1987 the GCRO wrote to the Office stating it was unable to accept its recommendations. In 1988 the GCRO was required to appear before the Monopolies and Mergers Commission regarding restrictions on advertising. It wanted to relax restrictions at its own pace, rather than abandon them immediately. In 1989 the Commission published its findings. The restriction was lifted on the grounds that it hindered patients and doctors from making an informed choice of osteopath.

Professional Indemnity Insurance became compulsory in 1989.

A survey of osteopathic schools in the United Kingdom, conducted by the British Accreditation Council in the Spring of 1988, was published in 1989, commissioned by Baroness Lane Fox and sponsored by Lord Brougham and Vaux. 14 establishments were asked if they wished to participate in the survey, nine agreed, but one withdrew. Its terms of reference were:

'Having particular regard for criteria which clearly safeguard the interests of the public and ensure the safety of patients, to... assess the efficiency of institutional provision for osteopathic education...recommend in the light of consultations with the providers of osteopathic education, appropriate minimum standards for osteopathic education.'

Presidents of the OAGB in the 1980s were:
1980   David Wainwright
1982   Michael Tyrie
1984   Christopher Dyer
1986   Donald Norfolk

At the 150th anniversary of the BMA in 1983, Prince Charles spoke in favour of complementary medicine. A BMA working party was set up that year, 'To consider the feasibility and possible methods of assessing the value of alternative therapies, whether used alone or to complement other treatments and to report to the Board of Science and Education'. The Principal and Vice-Principal of the BSO met representatives in November and argued that Osteopathy was complementary to medicine and not alternative. The Board produced its report in 1986, including a distinction between Orthodox Medical Manipulation, Chiropractic and Osteopathy, which received an appropriately scathing attack by Nicholas Handoll in the *OAGB Newsletter* of August.

The road to statutory recognition was re-opened in 1985. In a debate in the House of Lords, Lord Glenarthur, Under-Secretary of State to the Department of Health, outlined the essential criteria which any health care profession would have to fulfil before it could be considered suitable for statutory regulation, namely that:

a) There should be in existence a recognised and workable system of voluntary regulation;

b) The therapy was founded on a systematic body of knowledge;

c) There was in existence an appropriate and acceptable code of professional conduct;

d) The profession could secure the support and acceptance of the medical profession.

The Junior Health Minister said that he was encouraged to hear about the progress that the osteopaths had made.

In July, 1986 under a 10 Minute Rule, a Bill was presented for the statutory recognition of Osteopathy. It assisted in establishing strong, all-party support, but it never proceeded beyond the First Reading. It proposed a two-tier registration, those who graduated from colleges approved by the GCRO being, 'Registered osteopaths' and the others being 'enrolled' on a lower tier. Because of the divisiveness this caused and a shortage of parliamentary time, the Bill did not proceed.[5] It provided the basis for a major lobbying campaign. Over 350 MPs were visited by osteopaths in their constituencies.[6]

In 1987 Lord Skelmersdale, then Under Secretary of State for Health, stated that osteopaths had reached a sound basis for seeking statutory regulation. In the debate in the House of Lords on complementary medicine on 11 November, he said that whilst the government welcomed tighter regulation if this achieved common, recognised standards and claimed, 'A system of registration would...require the force of law if the desired aim of providing protection for the public is to be achieved'.

In 1988, to ensure the full support of the medical profession, HRH The Prince of Wales hosted a luncheon meeting of two Health Ministers, Presidents of the Royal Colleges of Physicians and Surgeons and the GMC, which encouraged Osteopathy to proceed with its proposals for statutory regulation.

In 1989, following discussion with Ministers, a Working Party was established by the King Edward's Hospital Fund of London (a respected independent medical foundation), to consider the scope and content of legislation to regulate the practice of Osteopathy. It was chaired by the Rt. Hon Sir Thomas Bingham (a Lord Chief Justice at the Court of Appeal, then Master of the Rolls) and had the following terms of reference:

> 'Having regard to the growing public demand for osteopathic treatment and increasing support, both professional and political, for early legislation, to establish a statutory register to regulate the education, training and practice of Osteopathy for the benefit and protection of patients, to consider the scope and content of such legislation, to make recommendations and to report.'

It consisted of leading members of the osteopathic and medical professions together with two representatives from the Department of Health and consulted widely, including with the GMC, BMA, the Royal Colleges of Physicians and Surgeons, consumer organisations, professions allied to medicine and the Departments of State.

Publications

Several publications appeared in the 1980s. In 1980 Philip Latey published *The Muscular Manifesto. A revolutionary study of people, illness and change*, discussing emotio-somatics. In 1982 Nicholas Handoll published, *'Osteopathy—Your Questions Answered'*. In 1983 Laurie Hartman's *Handbook of Osteopathic Technique* was published. On 22 July 1986, the Golden Jubilee Day of the GCRO, Nicholas Handoll published *Osteopathy in Britain: its development and practice*. In 1987 *'Osteopathy'* by Stephen Sandler was published by Macdonald Optima, and Jocelyn Proby published *'The Integrity of the Pelvic Girdle'*.

The *Daily Telegraph* in March 1982 carried a feature on the BSO Children's Clinic. Cynthia Tucker in 1983 treated John McEnroe and appeared in the television programme, 'Wogan'. In the spring of 1985 the British Broadcasting Corporation published, *'An Alternative Way of Healing'*, written by Anthea Courtenay, which included a chapter on 'Osteopathy and Chiropractic'. In May 1986 the *New Scientist* reported the claim of the OAGB that British shoppers strain their spines by carrying groceries in bags with handles, rather than the American way in a tough paper bag held close to the body.

The BSO

After 50 years at Buckingham Gate the BSO relocated in 1980 to 1-4 Suffolk Street, London SW1, a prestigious building in a prestigious location, a stone's throw from Trafalgar Square. It was a fraught time, when there was uncertainty as to whether the School would go into liquidation. Two public announcements were prepared to be made at the OAGB convention at Cambridge in 1979: one to state this; the other to declare the relocation viable. (Audrey Smith, Personal communication). The building was constructed for the United University Club, which ran into financial problems and the building was taken over by Coutt's Bank, until leased to the BSO.[7]

In February, the Crown Commission agreed to a 99 year lease following intense lobbying by Lord Jellicoe, Sir Hugh Casson and Merlyn Rees.

A total expenditure of £700K was approved by the Board, but the eventual total cost of the conversion came to over £930K. No agreement had been signed with the Crown Commissioners and the potential buyers of Buckingham Gate were slow in agreeing the terms.

As a registered charity the School could not borrow money without permission of the Charity Commission, nor sell its capital asset at Buckingham Gate without its consent. The Charity Commission withheld consent of the sale to Rush and Tompkins, as the School had received nine higher offers. At a Board meeting the Chairman indicated that the School could not afford the extra money and would have to go into liquidation. Compensation would be made to students. The School would be put on the open market, but the sale would take time. The alternative was for Rush and Tompkins to agree to purchase Buckingham Gate at a figure in excess of the debt. They were prepared to offer £900K, but no more.

One million was offered for Buckingham Gate by Imperial Life Insurance of Canada. A 'Farewell to 16 Buckingham Gate' party took place in September. The move in October was followed by a series of open days. On 25 October, the building, designated (wrongly) 'Martin Littlejohn House', was dedicated at a service in St Martin-in-the-Fields, when the diplomas and prizes were presented. *The Daily Telegraph* visited in November and published an article as did *The Times*. Anna Ford of *Independent Television News* visited the School in December.

While there was concern regarding the extravagance of the refurbishment by some members of the profession there was a need to ensure that facilities were appropriate for a Higher Educational Institution.

An independent quantity surveyor was commissioned to investigate the contractual cost of refurbishment of Suffolk Street, but the matter was settled amicably. An Appeal Fund was set up, 'A Major Step Forward', with Lord Jellicoe as its President.

Lord Jellicoe led a deputation of Stanley Bradford, Audrey Smith and Professor John Marsden of the PCL in June, to see Dr Rhodes Boyson regarding designation of the course for government funding. The meeting was positive and it was indicated that when the economic climate permitted, designation would be granted.

The new building enabled a first year student intake to grow to 100 a year, giving a total student population of 400 and an enlarged clinic capable of treating 1,100 patients a week.

In 1981, a meeting took place between the BSO, PCL and the CNAA with a view to the BSO and PCL starting a joint degree course in Osteopathy. The Inner London Education Authority (ILEA) would not support it because of insufficient input from PCL and objections from the Medical Officer of Health for the GLC.

In the joint degree PCL was to provide 40% of the tuition. As from September 1981 a 'Bridging Course' in Chemistry for prospective BSO students with limited science background was taught by PCL. First year BSO students visited PCL for physiology tutorials and practical work, two half days a week, to supplement lectures given in Suffolk Street.

In December 1981 a decision was made to proceed with a proposed affiliation with Columbia Pacific University (CPU) and they inspected the School. in 1982 seven members of the BSO staff became UK Faculty members of the University, including the Principal, Vice-Principal, Head of Postgraduate Studies and Head of Anatomy and Physiology. Stanley Bradford received an Honorary Fellowship and a Doctorate from CPU in History and Educational Administration, based on previous works published. CPU Degrees were offered to BSO students for 2,000 dollars and on submission of some original work. But as Peter Gibbons wrote in the OAGB Newsletter in April, 'This afternoon I telephoned the University of London and enquired about CPU. They could not find CPU on their list of accredited universities, nor anywhere else, until they looked under their list of "Bogus Universities"'. He considered that the BSO should disaffiliate as soon as possible as it could seriously jeopardise the chances of CNAA accreditation. His advice was followed.

Stanley Bradford resigned as Principal in July 1981 to join Exeter College of Technology. Stephen Humphrys, a member of the Board of Directors, recommended as a replacement Sir Norman Lindop, who was a patient and neighbour. Sir Norman had a background in chemistry and was a lay member of the GMC, Director of Hatfield Polytechnic and a significant figure in the foundation of the CNAA. He was appointed Principal designate in March 1982. Margot Gore managed the School until Sir Norman took over on 1 May.

In 1982, meetings between the BSO and the ILEA took place in County Hall, London. The ILEA agreed to re-examine the proposal and its policy with regard to supporting an Osteopathy course, but starting the degree course that year was not possible. An inspection of the School took place. By December it was also evident that having so many part-time teachers was a block to CNAA accreditation and there was a need to appoint a full-time Academic Co-ordinator. In September 1983 Derrick Edwards was appointed to this position. The Academic Board was also revised and enlarged.

By 1983 stricter national controls on course provision in Polytechnics precluded the possibility of a joint degree with PCL. The BSO received notification in July from the Department of Education and Science that they could consider validation by the CNAA of the Diploma course as a Degree, but if this was to be in conjunction with PCL there would be administrative complexities. The BSO decided to proceed with its own degree course for CNAA accreditation, though with support from PCL. A degree submission was made to the CNAA in 1984. Representatives of the School met with the CNAA, but its Health and Medical Sciences Board did not consider the course proposal was sufficiently developed to justify a visit. The CNAA did not have much experience of institutions such as the BSO. The reliance on part-time staff was still a problem. Sir Norman Lindop, the then Principal, considered their negative response, 'A sweeping condemnation with little or no experience as a Board in evaluation of courses in the primary health field and who were not sufficiently informed about the School'.

In 1983 a part-time Osteopathy course was discussed, of three evenings a week, with clinical training on Saturday mornings and evenings during the vacations, two or three years longer than the full-time course.

The BSO produced a revised degree submission in June 1987. In preparation for this, a decisive Faculty Weekend took place on 28-29 March 1987 at Canterbury, when the curriculum was discussed in detail.

In 1981 Dr Ann Woolley Hart was researching into Osteopathy and respiration. In 1982 a Research Advisory Board was set up consisting of Kim Burton, Colin Dove, Ken Kingsbury, Sir Norman Lindop, Dr Philip Wood, Dr Ann Woolley-Hart, Dr Richard Tonkin, Professor Irvin

Korr and Professor John Marsden. A working party was set up led by
Ernest Keeling to discuss the introduction of Cranial Osteopathy into
the Diploma course. It produced a report but the Board was undecided
about the matter. The working party met again in 1983 to consider
an optional course. Philip Latey wrote to the Board condemning the
teaching and practice of Sutherland's cranio-sacral method. 'I do feel
that we must sever our relationship with the Sutherland Cranial Teaching
Foundation immediately and definitely.' The Board was still undecided
on the matter and a further meeting took place the following July.

In 1983 HRH The Princess Royal became Patron of the BSO,
following an initial approach from the Marchioness of Bute and an
invitation from Sir Norman. A press statement was prepared in October.
The Princess Royal visited the School on 8 March 1984 and the Prince
of Wales visited on 18 October.

Other events in 1983 were the opening of the Expectant Mothers'
Clinic at the BSO, which attracted much press coverage. *The Daily
Telegraph* carried an article on 23 April and the *Sunday Telegraph* the next
day. The old prospectus of the BSO was replaced by 'Osteopathy Today'.
The BSO established a Board of Postgraduate Studies to develop the
programme of postgraduate education. A BMA working party visited
in April.

The BSO needed a larger lecture theatre. The art gallery next
door at 1 Hobhouse Court was obtained and a doorway made from the
rest of the BSO building. The 'Gallery Lecture Theatre' was opened
in January 1986 by HRH The Princess Royal. Alan Stoddard gave the
John Martin Littlejohn Lecture. The 'Learning Resources Room' was
also opened, through a bequest from the estate of Dr William Charles
Minifie (See Chapter 2) and formally designated 'The Minifie Room'.
On the 4 March the Lord Mayor held a reception in the Mansion House
to launch the School's development appeal.

Audrey Smith resigned from the Board and also as Vice-Principal
in July 1986, due to family circumstances, but continued to organise the
student selection programme.

In 1987 an Active Research Group and a new Research Advisory
Group was formed at the BSO, under the leadership of Dr Martin
Collins, who was seconded half-time from PCL as Senior Research
Fellow, to develop research at the BSO. The research group started in
a small way in the attic room of Suffolk Street, vacated by the GCRO.
Martin Collins was joined by osteopath Alan Szmelskyj and they began
to explore the measurement of leg length inequality using equipment
on loan from Guy's Hospital Medical School. The undergraduate

dissertation, which previously had been a 'Principles Project' was developed as an independent piece of work and it was hoped through this to encourage research within the profession, particularly through the training of supervisors of the dissertations.

In the summer of 1988 the BSO Board accepted the Principal's proposal that two Vice-Principalships be created. Clive Standen was appointed Vice Principal, Professional and Derrick Edwards Vice Principal, Academic.

The CNAA institutional visit occurred in May 1989 and the course validation visit in July. The course started in September 1989, but approval was backdated to October 1988.

Other Schools and Colleges

In 1981, the ESO divorced itself completely from John Wenham's accommodation at 28 Tonbridge Road where the course had developed, to include visceral and cranial Osteopathy, which were unacceptable to Wernham's 'Littlejohn' approach. The mortgage was transferred from John Wernham to a bank. Another clinic was sought.[9] From May, ESO students worked in the BSO clinic, tutored by their own staff. Private discussions had taken place between Colin Dove, John Upledger and Tom Dummer regarding accreditation of the ESO by the GCRO. Given that the GCRO was composed largely of BSO graduates, there were concerns that it would be biased against the accreditation of another School. Colin Dove advised the ESO to work with the GCRO to reach an appropriate standard before a formal application for accreditation was made.[8]

Following inspection of the ESO by the GCRO it gained accreditation in 1983 and opened up its own clinic at 104 Tonbridge Road the same year.

John Barkworth, President of the Society of Osteopaths, questioned the future of the Society, as members joined the GCRO in 1993. It considered that it could give up its political activities and the financial costs involved and by ceasing to be a limited company it would also be able to cut costs. By June 1984 it had decided to continue as a postgraduate body or alumnus of the ESO, participating in research, holding conferences and refresher courses.

In 1987 the ESO decided to run down its six year course in the French language (the 'Cours Francophone'), but was approached by some of the early graduates to run a comparable course in France, the College Internationale d'Osteopathie (CIDO), with one seminar a year at Maidstone. Tom Dummer retired as Principal of the ESO and Peter

Blagrave took over, but was replaced by Barrie Savory in 1988, due to Peter Blagrave's ill health. In 1989 Paula Fletcher joined the ESO.[9]

In 1983 negotiations began between the GCRO and the BCNO regarding accreditation. The latter was achieved in October 1987. In 1986 and 1988 Frazer House, the BCNO building, was extended and 32 students enrolled in the first year in 1986, such that the total student numbers was 121. A free children's clinic opened in December. Dr Ian Drysdale was appointed Dean in 1989.[10]

A review of the osteopathic curriculum at the Croydon School of Osteopathy, was undertaken in 1982. Michael Cummings was appointed Principal. The School became the London School of Osteopathy and moved to Whitelands College, Putney in 1987. In 1988 it opened a clinic and began work on an Honours Degree programme to be validated by the University of Surrey, but there were insufficient resources at Whitelands College to achieve this and so alternative premises were sought.

In 1987 Jane Langer became President and Chairman of the Board of the College of Osteopaths Educational Trust (COET), retiring in 1998.[11]

The Andrew Still College of Osteopathy and Natural Therapeutics became the official teaching institution of the BEOA in 1984. A 5-year part-time course led to the award of the Diploma in Osteopathy and full membership of the BEOA. Carlo di Paoli was Principal until 1988 and the course increased to 27 sessions a year.[12]

Deaths

By the 1980s many of those who graduated from the BSO in its early years and contributed so much to Osteopathy in the UK had reached an age when departure from this world was inevitable.

Ida Foggitt, who died in 1980, was born in 1896 and educated at Leeds University from 1907-1912. After obtaining a BA and Diploma in Education and becoming a teacher, she followed her brother, Dean Foggitt, into Osteopathy. She entered the BSO in 1924 and graduated in 1928 (Graduate number 10), having undertaken the Basic Sciences first year at Leeds. She initially practised with her brother and James Canning in Portland Place, before Dean extended his practice to Sheffield. She lectured on gynaecology at the BSO. She was a vegetarian and she prescribed homeopathic remedies. She retired from the BSO in 1976. She received the OAGB Littlejohn Award in 1969 in token of services to Osteopathy and the BSO. Her last few years were spent in a nursing home, 'Recognition and memory having gone'.

Robin Oakshott won the BSO Gold medal in 1939, as had his wife Margaret Adam in 1941. He lived in Australia for two to three years, returning to England in 1951. He became School Secretary and Secretary to the GCRO (1958-1966) and practised at Bickenhall Mansions, close to Baker Street, London and at Epsom, Surrey.

Keith Blagrave had lectured in applied anatomy in the 1960s and had an expertise in foot techniques. He invented unusual treatment schemes and mechanical gadgets to aid treatment. He was noted for his wry humour and his motor bike gear.

Leslie Korth, born in 1887, ran one of the earliest in-patient establishments in Bexley, Kent in the early 1930s and a further one after the war at Tunbridge Wells. He specialised in manipulation of the feet and wrote on medical psychology and forces of universal energy.

In 1981 Dr James 'Jim' Littlejohn, the second son of John Martin Littlejohn, died. He had studied medicine at St George's Hospital and became an ENT specialist. He taught for 45 years at the BSO: anatomy, principles of diagnosis in medicine and surgery and served on the Council of Education and the Board. During the war he was a Major in the 8th Army Royal Army Medical Corps and was awarded a MBE. He lived with his younger brother, John 'Jock' Martin Littlejohn Jr.

Tom Mitchell-Fox died in 1981 aged 83. He studied at the Looker College for four years before going to the USA. In 1926, he returned, set up the first osteopathic practice in the Western Counties and participated in moving the British College of Chiropractic from London to Plymouth and affiliating it with the Western Osteopathic School. (See Chapter 2). This proved unsuccessful and so he chose to enrol at the BSO and, like others who transferred at that time, he graduated in 1928. He was still paying squash at age 80.

In 1982 R. ('Bob') Atkinson Reddell died. He graduated from the BSO in 1940 and was noted for his eclectic approach to treatment. He had studied and practised natural therapeutics in New Zealand, USA and the UK and worked with Stanley Lief at Orchard Leigh and then Champneys, before starting Enton Hall in 1949 as a dietetics and osteopathic health retreat. It provided organic food grown on organic compost and had its own pedigree herd of cows. In 1984 Enton Hall was taken over by the Seventh Day Adventists, of which Reddell was a member.

Harold Banbury died aged 75 on 1 April 1987. Ian Smart wrote, 'The date of which if he had the choice as a humorist, could not have been better'. At the age of nine he spent nine months in a wheel chair with polio. In 1928 he was treated by Mitchell-Fox and started training at

the BSO the following year, when it was still at Abbey House, Victoria
Street and helped it move to Buckingham Gate. After graduating in 1933
he went to Cornwall to join Mitchell-Fox, Stanley Holdich, Henry and
Conrad Barber, all founder members of the Western Counties Society.
At the BSO he had lectured on 'Principles'. He was on the Council of
the Incorporated Association and President of the OAGB in 1952.

In 1988 Trenear Michell died aged 84. He was the brother in law
of Tom Mitchell-Fox. He studied initially in the Western Osteopathic
School in Plymouth before transferring to the BSO and after graduating
in 1929, he practised in several towns in the West Country and in
Weston-Super-Mare, treating dogs as well as people. He ceased to
practise in 1972 due to illness.

W. Hargrave-Wilson who had studied at Kirksville and later St
George's Hospital died in 1983. He was co-author of 'The Osteopathic
Lesion', with Dr George MacDonald, with whom between 1945 and
1947 he started the London College of Osteopathy. A man who enjoyed
the outdoor life and polo, he then emigrated to Kenya, returning to
London from 1957 to 1963, before emigrating to Hobart, Tasmania,
where he died.

Profile: Clement ('Clem') H. Middleton (1906-1984)

In February 1984 Clem Middleton died. Following schooling in
Dublin, he moved to Brighton in 1920. As a result of pushing a bead
in his ear, the ear drum burst resulting in infection, deafness, a Bell's
palsy and speech impediment that persisted for the rest of his life. He
enrolled on the BSO course, studying Basic Sciences at King's College
and graduated in 1934.

He practised in Portman Mansions before moving to Bickenhall
Mansions, Baker Street, London. He also had a practice in Crawley. In
1962 he became Head of the Technique Department, teaching in a clear
and precise way, breaking the techniques down into their individual
components. This complemented Audrey Smith's developments in
teaching diagnosis, but he acknowledged that, 'Attempts to copy the
techniques in outline will only meet with limited success.' He wrote
a number of witty osteopathic articles under the name of 'Simon
Simplex' and 'Nelson's Column', some collected as 'A Day in the Life of
the Spine'.

His obituary records that he was a true gentleman, immaculately
dressed, who never took himself too seriously and with a sense of
humour. He had an interest in metaphysics, the occult, wood carving
and vintage cars and was famous for his after-dinner speeches.

As *Simon Simplex*, he claimed to be, 'A quasi teetotaller who drinks alcohol only for the purposes of experiment and research, who is always happy to participate in such research with any serious enquirer seeking further enlightenment'.

He once commented that at Buckingham Gate, due to the shortage of lavatories, 'An osteopath learned to be a gentleman who can not only hold his drink but also his water.'

In an obituary, Billy Naidoo related an anecdote of how Clem called one evening when Billy was listening to the 6 O'clock News. On seeing the radio, he said, 'Ah, I see you've had the operation'. (The Indian government at that time were giving portable radios to male citizens who were prepared to have a vasectomy. Billy Naidoo is of Asian descent.)

In 1981 he encouraged students to undertake a career in Osteopathy, 'As rewarding as those of a bookmaker, top jockey, top racing driver, tennis or golf star, oil magnate, drug pusher or chartered accountant allowing them to rub shoulders with sheikhs, bishops, actresses, trade union leaders, diamond cutters, long distance lorry drivers, politicians, pornographic booksellers and lots of other very nice people'. He died from a heart attack at the wheel of his car, following a lecture to the Southern Counties Society.[13]

Profile: Shilton Webster-Jones (1899-1986)

Shilton Webster-Jones ('Webber') died in January 1986 from renal failure. The obituaries of him by Colin Dove and Audrey Smith in the *OAGB Newsletter* of March 1986 reflected upon his many contributions to Osteopathy. Born in 1899, he studied Pharmacy at Liverpool University. Following successful osteopathic treatment he became a student at the BSO in 1931, qualifying three years later as graduate number 83. He joined the Faculty and was Assistant Registrar. He became Principal in 1948, following the death of Littlejohn and remained so for 20 years. Following his retirement aged 69, he became Chairman of the Board. He received an Honorary Fellowship from the School and the Littlejohn Award from the OAGB of which he was President.

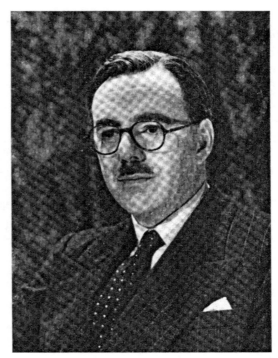

Shilton Webster-Jones ('Webber')

A memorial service of thanksgiving for his life and work took place at St Martin-in-the-Fields. As he was a keen morris dancer, the service concluded with a performance by the London Pride Morris Men.

In 1986 Arthur Millwood and Willis Haycock also died. Millwood, with Pat Saul of Liverpool, was a founder member of the Northern Counties Society of Osteopaths and helped create the OAGB and also was the first editor of *The Newsletter*.

Willis Haycock died aged 87. He was a 'Looker Graduate', who transferred to the BSO and graduated in 1929. After practising in Sheffield, he moved to Bradford. He frequently wrote articles, some of which were published in the Osteopathic Institute of Applied Technique Yearbooks: 'The expanding concept of Osteopathy', in 1956; 'The Osteopathic Lesion and Body Unity in Relation to Diagnosis, Prophylaxis and Therapeutics' in 1959 and 'Osteopathy and the Problem of Stress' in 1961. He was an exponent of functional and muscle energy techniques. A friend of Pat Saul and Herbert Milne, he was an active member of the Northern Counties Society of Osteopaths. He was also a member of the Maidstone Osteopathic Institute of Applied Technique. He gave the Littlejohn Memorial Lecture in 1955 on the Exanding concept of Osteopathy.

References

1. Research Council for Complementary Medicine. The first 5 years 1983-1988. (London: RCCM):pp 5-6.
2. *Newsletter*. (1985). Research Council for Complementary Medicine. January, No. 5:1.
3. Tonkin, R. (1986). *Complementary Medical Research*, 1(1):1.
4. *The Osteopath*. (1997). VAT Exemption for the services of osteopaths. November, 1(1):8.
5. Chambers, M. M. (1995). The British Naturopathic Association. The first 50 years. (British Naturopathic Association).
6. Daniels, B. A. (1997). A Brief History of the GCRO. Annual Report for 1997 and News Bulletin. No. 95, GCR 6/97, pp. 41-50. (Reading: General Council and Register of Osteopaths).
7. Leaflet produced by the University of Notre Dame, London. (1997).
8. Colin Dove. Personal communication.
9. Margery Bloomfield. Personal communication.
10. Dr Ian Drysdale. Personal communication.
11. Jane Langer. Personal communication.
12. David Dyer & Malcolm Mayer. Personal communication.
13. Kyria, S. (1993). Clem Middleton 1906-1984. *The British Osteopathic Journal*, X: 40-42.

Chapter 15

The 1990s

Writing a history of Osteopathy in the last decade of the 20th century is as difficult as writing that of the first decade, but for opposite reasons. Obtaining information on the first decade was difficult as so little exists, but there is nobody alive today who can from first hand experience dispute its accuracy. For the last decade there is a surfeit of information and interpretations of what took place and why, by the many who have lived through that period.

The 1990s was decade of rapid change in the profession, welcomed by many osteopaths but certainly not by all. At the beginning few could have envisaged the impact and ramifications of the Osteopaths Act of 1993 and Statutory Regulation.

Legislation

The government welcomed the initiative of the King's Fund (discussed in the previous chapter). Baroness Hooper, in the House of Lords in May 1990, stated that government awaited the report with interest and hoped that it would point the way to Statutory Recognition and that, 'The osteopaths have clearly shown the way forward and it is for others to follow'.

Given the support for it, the King's Fund commissioned a draft Osteopaths Bill appended to the final report, which was launched at a press conference on 3 December 1991.¹ Present were HRH The Prince of Wales, President of the King's Fund, the Under-Secretary of State for Health, members of both Houses of Parliament, leaders in orthodox medicine, officials of the Department of Health and representatives of osteopathic bodies. HRH The Prince of Wales said that, 'For many years the osteopathic profession has provided high standards of responsible care and conduct which are of real value to a large number of people. I have long believed that Osteopathy deserves greater public recognition provided the appropriate professional regulation goes along with the recognition. The report on Osteopathy by Sir Thomas Bingham and his colleagues shows how this can be done.'[2]

The Act established the General Osteopathic Council, the GOsC, (the 's' avoids confusion with the General Optical Council), with the statutory duty to develop, promote and regulate the profession,'Including making provision as to the registration of osteopaths and as to their professional education and conduct; to make provision in connection with the development and promotion of the profession; and for connected purposes.'[3] The Privy Council, appointed the first professional and lay members of the Council.

Potential applicants for registration had a period of two years to apply for registration as osteopaths. After this transition period, only graduates holding a Recognised Qualification from an institution accredited by the GOsC would be eligible for registration, after which it would become an offence for those not registered to call themselves osteopaths.

Perceived benefits of the Act were considered to be:

a)   A guarantee that in future all osteopaths will be trained to the same high standards.
b)   Patients will be provided with the safeguards they expect when consulting an established health care professional.
c)   A guarantee that all practitioners will be covered by professional indemnity insurance.
d)   Recognition that Osteopathy is part of mainstream health care.
e)   A closer working relationship with the medical profession.
f)   Increased ability to attract funds for research.
g)   More patients may consider Osteopathy as a treatment option.
h)   Freedom to develop Osteopathy.

It also recommended a pre-registration year of supervised clinical practice for all new graduates, as a future option and a system of compulsory professional training as a prerequisite of continued registration, ensuring the maintenance of high standards of clinical practice. There was no definition of Osteopathy in the Bill.

On 17 December Lord Walton of Detchant, former President of the BMA, introduced the Osteopaths Bill into the House of Lords where it received its First Reading. A second, unopposed Reading occurred on 31 January 1992. The Health Minister, Baroness Hooper, stated that, 'The government supports the Bill in principle and they hope it will receive the support of this House'. It attracted strong all-party support and successfully completed its Committee Stage on 11 March and began its Report Stage. In redrafting the Bill, attempts were made to set a pattern for all up-to-date medical legislation.[4]

All 68 amendments were agreed in 36 minutes, before falling when Parliament was dissolved just prior to the General Election. The Bill generated an enthusiastic response from the medical profession, including the President of the GMC. On 10 June 1992 Malcolm Moss MP introduced it in the House of Commons as a Private Members' Bill. It again received all-party and Government support.

As the Bill progressed through Parliament there was a call for greater unity in the profession, to end long-standing animosities between the Schools/Colleges, particularly between those accredited by the GCRO and those that were not.

On 15 January 1993,[5] the Bill received its Second Reading in the House of Commons and was carried unopposed. Health Minister Tom Sackville stated that he, 'Looked forward to a time when the profession could hold aloft the long-sought prize of the Osteopaths Act, 1993'.

The Bill completed its Committee Stage and began its Report Stage in mid-March.[4] A Third Reading took place on 7 May. It then moved on to the House of Lords, where it was steered through by Lord Walton. It received a First Reading on 10 May.[6] Royal Assent was given on 1 July 1993.

The Chiropractors Bill received Royal Assent on 5 July 1994.

The GCRO and OAGB

The GCRO's Code of Ethics was re-published as 'The Handbook of Professional Conduct' in 1991, with what was considered a fairer set of disciplinary procedures. The Journal of Osteopathic Education was launched. Osteopathy and Medicine Today was published for osteopaths to send to their local GPs. The Public Relations Committee organised regional road shows to increase communication skills in the profession in dealings with orthodox medicine and the public.

In October 1991 a resolution was put forward at the AGM of the OAGB for a merger with the British Naturopathic and Osteopathic Association (BNOA), supported by the OAGB Council and the Presidents of the BNOA and BOA. A draft agreement was published in December,[7] advocating integration between professional associations, while establishing close liaison with the GCRO.[8] The merger occurred following a meeting in March 1992. The OAGB then had 936 members and the BNOA over 200. Some members of the BNOA, however, wanted it to retain its identity.[7] A new British Naturopathic Association (BNA) was formed, with Wendy Arnheim as President.[7]

In 1991 the relationship between the OAGB and GCRO became strained. There were rumours that the GCRO intended to set up as a separate professional association in competition with the OAGB, in that they had been given a mandate in 1961 to oversee professional activities, as well as the function as a Register.[7,9,10] Some thought the profession was too small for more than one body. The OAGB and the BNOA, however, jointly considered that the GCRO was not the appropriate body to co-ordinate professional activities of osteopaths and that it was incompatible for a body to be responsible for both the interests of the public and osteopaths.

In July-August 1992 antagonism between the OAGB and the Register worsened, but then the 'Langham Group' was constituted to discuss differences, so named because meetings took place in the Langham Hilton Hotel, London. Collaboration in shaping the profession was discussed.[11,12]

In December 1992, Simon Fielding replaced Barry Lambert as Chairman of the GCRO Council. David Weeks joined the GCRO to provide support for the central administration and management, which later became the Professional Affairs Department. He then became Assistant Secretary and then Secretary in 1995, after Peter Blaker, who had been Secretary since 1986, retired.

The GCRO re-defined its objectives and published them in July 1992. A reception was held in Honour of HRH The Princess of Wales, who became President of the GCRO in 1991, on 5 February 1992, at the Royal Pharmaceutical Society. The following day the *Evening Standard* carried a photograph of her with Simon Le Bon, Duran Duran's lead singer, and his brother Jonathan, who was then a student of Osteopathy at the BCNO. Jonathan Le Bon talked about Osteopathy and how useful it was.

Another reception took place on 30 November 1993 in the State Apartments of Kensington Palace, in the presence of HRH The Princess of Wales, to mark the 50th AGM of the GCRO.

In March 1992 in a new format, the *OAGB Newsletter* replaced *The Newsletter*. Associate Membership of the OAGB was offered to graduates of Schools and Colleges not accredited by the GCRO. In May, 1993 the GCRO *Reading Matters* combined with the *OAGB Newsletter* as a coloured insert.

In March 1993 the GCRO produced, '*Guidelines on Presenting Osteopathy to the Medical Profession*', particularly to present it to General Practitioners. The report, '*Competences Required for Osteopathic Practice*' (CROP), begun in 1991, was published in October 1993, which was a unique and admirable attempt to define such competences, probably the first of its kind for any health care profession. The GCRO commissioned

Martin Collins to produced '*A Guide to Audit in Osteopathic Practice*', included in '*Your Osteopathy. Getting Your Professional Message Across.*'

The first Osteopathic Congress for all members of the profession, 'Osteopathy 2000', took place in February 1993 at the Royal Postgraduate Medical School, Hammersmith, London.[43] The theme of the 1994 meeting was 'The Way Ahead. Osteopathy and the Community'. In 1995 it was held at the Commonwealth Institute in London, entitled, 'Osteopathy: Taking its Rightful Place'. The keynote speaker was Dr Irvin Korr. It was followed by a one day course on 'Presenting Osteopathy to the Medical Profession.'[44] Further annual Congresses followed (see below).

In November 1995 *Osteopathy Today* replaced the *OAGB Newsletter*, to serve the needs of all practising osteopaths and to draw all osteopaths together into one family, ahead of statutory regulation.[13] The GCRO and OAGB decided to support jointly the initiative, by sharing the start-up costs. The pink insert of '*Reading Matters,*' a feature of the *OAGB Newsletter*, ceased.

In October 1997 the OAGB Council voted unanimously to open membership to all osteopaths. A new mission statement was drawn up. In the same month, Michael Murray was appointed the OAGB's first Chief Executive. In October, the BOA invited each of the five professional associations to send two members to a meeting to discuss the future needs of the profession once regulation by the GOsC was in place. Three groups attended: the OAGB, the BOA and the Guild of Osteopaths, which in December decided to form a single professional association.[14] The merger and first joint meeting took place in April 1998. The title BOA was adopted though this proved difficult as 'British' was a protected name under Company Law and the new company had to prove it was prominent in the field.[15] The new BOA Council redefined its membership rules and introduced a free and comprehensive legal service, 'First Assist', in July 1998.

Presidents of the OAGB in the 1990s were:

1990	Dorothy Griffiths
1992	James Miller
1995	Joanna Hyne
1997	Catherine Hamilton-Plant

At an Extraordinary General Meeting in February 1998, members of the GCRO passed a special resolution to transfer the GCRO's remaining assets of about £340,000 to the General Osteopathic Council. A further meeting in April placed the Company in liquidation. Its headquarters in London Street, Reading closed on 31 April.[16]

The GOsC

The intent was to have the General Osteopathic Council operative by January 1995, but it was not until 1996 that Members were appointed to a GOsC designate. The Council could not formally come into being until a Commencement Order the following year.[17]

On 1 February, a press conference was held at Richmond House at which the Health Minister, Baroness Cumberlege, announced the names of the Chairman and first members of the General Osteopathic Council.[18,19] Members designate met for the first time on 29 February 1997 at the Department of Health.[20] The next meeting took place on 30 April, at which Baroness Cumberlege made a speech.[21]

The Commencement Order to appoint formally the membership of the GOsC and establish Statutory Committees took place on 14 January 1997. It enabled the GOsC to obtain funding, employ and remunerate staff, engage lawyers and auditors, acquire premises and begin constructing the legal framework for registration and fitness to practice.[22] On the same date, a small reception was held at the Royal College of Physicians, attended by many past and the then current members of the GCRO, to mark its Jubilee Year.[23]

On 1 April, 1997 Madeleine Craggs took up her position as Registrar and Chief Executive of the GOsC.[24] The Educational Directorate was established formally on 1 July, with the appointment of Derrick Edwards, previously Vice-Principal of the BSO, as Director of Education.[25] A Recognised Qualification (RQ) Sub-Committee was set up as a sub-group of the Education Working Group. It drafted documents for the process leading to RQ status, and finalised procedures for the regulation of institutional osteopathic qualifications. The first Osteopathic Institutions Liaison Conference took place on 8 October 1997, at which 13 institutions wishing to be recognised as providers of osteopathic education, together with representatives from their academic validation bodies, discussed the process of application for RQ Status.[26] These were:

    The Allied School of Osteopathy
    Andrew Still College of Osteopathy
    British College of Naturopathy and Osteopathy
    British School of Osteopathy
    College of Osteopaths Educational Trust
    European School of Osteopathy
    The Faculty of Osteopaths
    London School of Osteopathy
    Oxford School of Osteopathy

University College Suffolk
The SMAE Institute
London College of Osteopathic Medicine
John Wernham College of Classical Osteopathy

In October1997, at a reception at St James's Palace, it was announced that HRH The Prince of Wales was to be the Patron of the GOsC. *'Pursuing excellence. Good Practice for Osteopaths'* was launched at the event.

In November 1997, the GOsC invited applications for registration and launched *The Osteopath.* The first edition contained information on *'Registration—Your Questions Answered'* and information regarding VAT exemption of registered osteopaths. In November, Robin Kirk became editor of *Osteopathy Today* and introduced the 'Hello' column, a series of outrageous and witty comments regarding members of the profession. The profession then had two very different journals.

On 9 May 1998 at the 'Osteopathy 2000' Conference, the Statutory Register was opened. Following a speech by Simon Fielding, an actor impersonating A. T. Still appeared.[26] Thus began the 'transitional period' until May 2000 for osteopaths to register. They were required to complete the Professional Profile and Portfolio (PPP), produced by the Education Working Group, under the Chairmanship of Brian Jolly, the Secretary of State's appointee on the Council, and approved by the GOsC as a means of entry onto the Register. While printed early in 1998, dissemination was compromised by the lack of approval of the Department of Health until late spring. The *'Standard of Proficiency'* was published by the GOsC early in 1998 and a revised version in the autumn used for evaluation of the PPP. Training events were required for PPP evaluators.

For those who were recent graduates, this was a relatively easy process, but for others less so. Some older osteopaths decided to retire, others were embittered that they were required to submit themselves to this process only a short time before retirement. A few dissenters preferred to opt out of the process and become 'osteomyologists'. As Simon Fielding commented at 'Osteopathy 2000' held in May, there was, 'Real sadness and concern for those of our colleagues who are experiencing anxiety or difficulty with the registration process'.

The GOsC began a series of 'Registration Roadshows' in 1998. The first was held in February in London with over 130 practitioners attending. Others followed in major UK cities. By January, 1,375 osteopaths (about half the known profession) had paid the £150, as an indication of their intent to register. By August, 128 had registered and 630 profiles and 280 portfolios had been received. However, by the end of the year, only 25% of the members of the BOA had actually registered.[29] In April 1999, the first GOsC Register was published with 784 entries.

At the start of 1998, Catherine Hamilton-Plant, as President of the BOA, raised concerns regarding the cost of the registration process with Madeleine Craggs.[30]

In January 1988 Jonathan Hobbs was appointed Deputy Director of Education of the GOsC. Following the second commencement order on 1 April 1998, the statutory Education Committee replaced the Education Working Group of the GOsC.[28]

The second Osteopathic Institutions Liaison Conference was held in January 1988 to explore further key issues of mutual concern between the GOsC and providers of osteopathic education.[27] A meeting took place between the Schools and Colleges and the Educational Directorate in September 1998.

In March 1999 the final version of documents and procedures associated with the RQ process was distributed to providers of courses of osteopathic education seeking recognition at that time. Several institutions completed the appropriate documentation and were inspected by teams appointed by the GOsC.

The GOsC moved from Premier House, Greycoat Place, Victoria to 126 Tower Bridge Road, London SE1 in November, made possible by the money received from winding up the GCRO. In April, the BOA moved to Langham House West, Mill Street, Luton.

Other Developments in the Profession

In 1991 the Society of Osteopaths ceased as a professional organisation and graduates of the ESO were encouraged to join the OAGB.

In 1991, following the London Local Authorities Act (1991), there was concern that certain Boroughs might require osteopaths to licence their premises as 'special treatment premises'. A working party was set up in 1992 to consider exemption. The GCRO wrote to all Boroughs.[31]

The first of a series of intercollegiate research meetings was held in September 1991, hosted by the BSO, to attempt to achieve unity in research effort among the Schools and Colleges and initiate collaborative research. It was considered that this might avoid unnecessary replication, as resources were limited, and might achieve greater success in acquiring external funding. A common research project and joint student project work were discussed.

In May 1994 the GCRO and OAGB issued a joint statement on research. A meeting of the Enabling Group for Osteopathic Research (EGOR) took place on 17 July. 35 osteopaths attended this first working meeting. A further meeting took place in November.[32,33]

The same year, the OAGB produced a booklet on, '*Advice for New Graduates.*'

The King's Fund Report (1991) recommended that the Osteopaths Bill should empower the new GOsC to impose a ruling that, 'Continued registration should be conditional on continued osteopathic education'. Consultation with, registered osteopaths and 'such persons as the Council considers appropriate' was necessary.[34] To facilitate the process, the GCRO set up a Continuing Professional Development (CPD) working party chaired by John Sketchley, its Educational Adviser, which had its first meeting in January 1992. All existing osteopathic educational institutions and other osteopathic organisations were invited. A voluntary CPD scheme was planned. In 1995 the CPD Council issued a paper to all members of the profession, describing its mission, how it intended to operate and the need for funds.[35]

From 1992 there was developing interest in working in the National Health Service. The BMA Report, '*Complementary Medicine— New Approaches to Good Practice*' was published in 1993, in which Osteopathy was held as exemplary. By 1994 osteopaths were gaining employment within the NHS. Three were working in the Physiotherapy Outpatients Department at the Central Middlesex Hospital, as Senior II Physiotherapists.[36,37]

In October 1995, '*Osteopathy and the NHS*' was sent by Lowe Lindsey, Marketing Consultants, with a personalised letter, to almost 3,000 senior partners of GP fund-holding practices in the UK. 2,500 copies were sent to NHS trusts, Health Commissions, Health Authorities, parliamentarians with a special interest in the health service, Department of Health officials and the national media. In 1996 GP fund holders were empowered to purchase osteopathic and chiropractic services.

In 1997 Alan Milburn, Minister of State for Health, announced that they were inviting applications for 20 primary care-led pilots to begin on 1 April 1998, to explore new approaches to securing high quality health care services for all, by bringing together GPs and other primary care professionals.

From 1992 there was a growing interest in Visceral Osteopathy and Animal Osteopathy. In October a course was held on the osteopathic treatment of dogs at a Veterinary Centre in Guernsey.[38] In 1993 the

GCRO announced an intent to produce a list of MROs who treat or have an interest in treating animals. Greg Currie recollected treating a cat that was grossly overweight and constipated when he was clinic superintendent at the BSO in 1951. 'The cat responded well to Osteopathy plus Homeopathy.'[39] A postgraduate seminar on 'Osteopathy for Dogs' took place in June, and an equine Osteopathy course in November, led by Anthony Pusey. A veterinary research project was set up into the diagnosis and treatment of 'back pain' in horses, over a three year period, by Dr Christopher Colles, a vet, and Anthony Pusey, using infra-red thermographic scanning and radiographic and clinical examination. Assessment of the long-term benefits of osteopathic treatment were to be made.[40] In 1994 the GCRO offered advice for osteopaths practising on animals.[41]

The Visceral and Obstetric Society was formed in 1997, to provide a forum for osteopaths to share their views and ideas regarding the treatment of visceral and obstetric clinical conditions.

In 1994 Dr John Sketchley retired as the GCRO Education Adviser, a post which he had held since 1989.

Since September 1974, cranio-sacral courses had been held only at the BSO. A rift occurred in the British cranio-sacral movement in 1992. One division, the British Sutherland Cranial Faculty, held a five day basic course at the BCNO. It became the Sutherland Cranial College in 1994 and registered as a charity.[42] In 1998 it offered a postgraduate qualification in Osteopathy in the Cranial Field.

The Osteopathic Centre for Children (OCC) arose from modest beginnings in Forest Row, due to, 'A chance meeting between Stuart Korth, Patricia Ferrall and a French horn'. By January 1993 it had moved from the Royal Homeopathic Hospital, where it had been 'camping out' for 18 months, to Cavendish Square. In addition to seeing many infants and children, some seriously ill, women were checked during and just after pregnancy and babies routinely examined. The clinic also had an educational role, providing postgraduate supervision in Paediatric Osteopathy.[45]

In 1988, one year after the 'Sweet Pea' Appeal started, the television news reader, John Snow, opened the OCC in Harley Street. It later received one million pounds from the Diana Princess of Wales Memorial Fund.

In 1994 there were concerns about Osteopathy and the law. 'What to do in the witness box' was written by Dr Maree Bellamy.[46]

In December 1994, the Confidential Osteopathic Support Service for Emotional Traumas (COSSET) was initiated, to provide support for those osteopaths troubled, distressed, or in despair, as a result of overwhelming professional or personal problems.[47] The proposal was first made by John Barkworth, Chairman of the GCRO's Ethics Committee at the 50th AGM of the GCRO in November 1993. The suggestion was acted on jointly by the GCRO and OAGB. Counsellors received preparation from the Samaritans. Dorothy Griffiths was the national co-ordinator.

Advice for new graduates was produced in November as the 'New Graduates Manual. Your Osteopathy: Getting your professional message across'. A videotape, 'Osteopaths—Part of the Health Care Team' was shown at the AGM of the GCRO in November 1994. It included interviews with practitioners, showing them treating patients with a wide range of conditions and discussed the benefits of Osteopathy. The education of osteopaths was also covered.[48]

In December 1994 the Clinical Standards Advisory Group report was published on the treatment of low back pain.

The Royal College of General Practitioners' (RCGP) 'Clinical Guidelines for the Management of Acute Low Back Pain' were issued in September 1996 arguing that, 'Manipulation within the first 6 weeks can provide short-term improvement in pain and activity levels and higher patient satisfaction.'[49]

The Sentinel Audit project was initiated in March 1998 by the NHS Executive to audit the RCGP Acute Back Pain Guidelines, with a view to completion in 2000.[50] The NHS Executive sought to encourage the use of multidisciplinary, evidence-based, clinical practice guidelines, with the hope of boosting treatment effectiveness, especially in primary care, by developing audit packages or 'toolkits' for practitioners to use to monitor care against agreed criteria. It provided a grant for such a toolkit to be developed for osteopaths, general practitioners, chiropractors and manipulative physiotherapists.

Diana, Princess of Wales, died in August 1997. She had been the President of the GCRO since 1991 and a great supporter of the OCC. Colin Dove represented the profession and the GCRO at her funeral on 5 September.[51]

Statutory registration in the UK had some impact on the continent. A resolution to launch a process of recognising non-conventional medicine was passed in May 1997 by the European Parliament. Belgium, where it was previously illegal for non-medically qualified practitioners to practise, introduced legislation to regulate Osteopathy.

The VAT (Osteopaths) Order came into force on 12 June 1998, with a concession back to 9 May. Osteopaths were no longer required to pay

7/47 of their fees to HM Customs and Excise, however, they would no longer be able to recover VAT on expenses.[52,53,54]

The Association of Medical Osteopaths was formed in 1998 from members of the old BOA: graduates of the LCOM and USA Colleges of Osteopathic Medicine.

In 1998 there was some debate in the profession regarding whether osteopaths should use the title 'Dr'.[55]

By 1999 a number of specialist groups established themselves, including The Osteopathic Sports Care Association (OSCAR) and Osteopaths in Animal Practice.

The BSO

In 1990 Clive Standen succeeded Sir Norman Lindop as Principal. On 4 April HRH The Princess Royal visited the School, particularly to see the Human Observation and Evaluation Room and to speak to research workers. The BSO started an Advanced Diploma in Osteopathy course. The first Diplomas were awarded in 1992, but shortly after it ceased due to insufficient interest.

In 1991 the BSO was in danger of closing as it had accumulated substantial debts due to rent increases on the Suffolk Street building. Government policy precluding students of independent institutions from receiving mandatory grants made it difficult to recruit new students and also contributed to the financial crisis. There was a concern that if the BSO collapsed it would severely damage the profession, and particularly the prospects of Statutory Regulation. An appeal was launched, but the response was poor. At one point it was feared that the bank would close the building overnight. The School survived and recovered, but for several years the stigma remained that it was in a serious financial state.

In the latter part of 1991 the occupation of a 1.5 acre site close to City University was explored, involving a merger between the BSO and BCNO. Both institutions were interested, but the plan aborted.

The autumn of 1992 saw the demise of the CNAA and the BSO was required to seek degree validation elsewhere. After consideration of a number of universities, it approached the newly formed Open University Validation Services (OUVS), as the latter would not have an interest in the School's assets, thus safeguarding the autonomy of the School. The good reputation of the Open University for developing learning resource materials and an anticipated rigorous validation were also attractions. The BSc (Hons) Degree was validated by the OUVS in 1993.

In 1996 an MSc in Osteopathic Care was validated by the Open

University Validation Services and revalidated in 1999 as an MSc in Health Practice, open to other health care professionals.

A reception was held in St James's Palace in 1992 to mark the 75th anniversary of the School, attended by HRH The Princess Royal.

In 1993 the first Associate Professors were appointed by the BSO: David Seedhouse, Peter Abrahams, Stephen Pheasant, Laurie Hartman and Kim Burton, representing the diverse aspects of osteopathic education. In June of that year, a project was initiated by Martin Collins providing free Osteopathy for the homeless at St Martin-in-the-Fields Social Care Unit, London.

In the summer of 1995 the University of Notre Dame expressed an interest in purchasing the Suffolk Street building from the BSO. A formal offer was made in September and after negotiation it was accepted in principle by the Board in October. During 1996 the School dedicated itself to finding new premises. It had agreed to vacate the Suffolk Street building by December 1996, but this deadline could not be met due to the difficulty of finding alternative accommodation. The University of Notre Dame agreed to postpone relocation until July 1997.

In January 1997, although the BSO had been informed by the vendors of a property in Market Road, London N1 that it was their 'preferred purchaser', a contract was issued to a third party. The BSO then made offers on other properties, but by February the School had been 'gazumped' again, in a space of less than two weeks. Eventually it secured 275 Borough High Street, London SE1, a leasehold property, previously occupied by the Department of Health and Social Security (DHSS), and it relocated in July. On 14 January 1998 HRH The Princess Royal officially opened the building.

In October 1997 Clive Standen indicated his intent to step down as Principal of the School, as from 1 February 1998. The process began of seeking a new Principal. The Executive Management Team suggested that it jointly run the School. The Board of Directors, after some deliberation, eventually agreed to this, with Dr Martin Collins leading the team as 'Principal'. This arrangement was approved formally by the Board of Directors in January 1998 and the appointment made permanent in June.

Other Schools and Colleges

In 1991 Margery Bloomfield became Principal of the ESO, with Simon Fielding and Dr Nic Rowley as Vice-Principals. She had been co-founder and administrative director for 26 years. The ESO initiated a Postgraduate Studies Department, following earlier closure of the equivalent Department at the BSO where it was not financially self-sufficient and had to be maintained by contributions from undergraduate student fees. There was also a proposal that the BSO, ESO and BCNO should contribute towards an autonomous educational board to operate postgraduate studies. The GCRO agreed to provide free accommodation and to hire an education adviser, but the scheme did not develop.

In 1992 the ESO formed the European Society of Osteopaths as an alumnus.

In 1993 the University of Wales validated the BSc Degree course of the ESO. In 1994 a MSc, the profession's first, was developed at the ESO in partnership with the University of Greenwich.[56] Renzo Molinari became Vice-Principal at the ESO, which developed its international links.

In 1995 CIDO gained a partial franchise from the University of Wales to deliver a degree course in conjunction with the ESO. Students could be credited with two years' work at CIDO before entering the ESO.

In October 1996 the ESO purchased Boxley House and moved in January 1997. It became the teaching and administration centre. The official opening took place in July. In September 1997 it announced that Renzo Molinari was to be the new Principal of the School.

In 1990 Dr Ian Drysdale, the Dean, became Principal of the BCNO and the Board of the College set an objective of achieving degree status for the course. They had established a relationship with Paddington College that provided some lecturers. Paddington College merged with the PCL. For this reason and because of geographical proximity in 1989 they were sought as the validating institution for the proposed degree programme, though discussions had taken place with several other universities.[57]

Following negotiations, in 1992 the BCNO's BSc (Honours) Degree was validated by the University of Westminster (previously the Polytechnic of Central London).[7] A postgraduate modular course on Naturopathic Medicine was also approved. It later offered osteopaths with a Diploma from a School/College of Osteopathy recognised by the GCRO an opportunity to undertake a six month conversion course to a BSc (Honours) Degree, validated by the University of Westminster.[58,59] In 1998 it offered an MSc in Health Sciences: Osteopathic Medicine, validated by and jointly taught with the University of Westminster.

In 1996 Glenda Jackson opened Lief House, a four storey building adjacent to the BCNO's Frazer House. In September 1998, Alan

Milburn MP, Minister of State in the Department of Heath opened the BCNO's satellite clinic in the Soho Centre for Health Care, at Parkside Health NHS Community Hospital, where a number of complementary therapies were represented.

At the London School of Osteopathy (LSO), Paul Masters became Principal in 1990 and Dr Peter Spencer in 1994. In 1992 it moved to Lanark Square, London E14 in Docklands. The following year Anglia Polytechnic University validated the degree course.

In 1993 Margaret Bowyer became Principal of COET, Clive Power in 1995, Melanie Coutinho in 1996 and Gareth Holsworth in 1999. In 1997 its BSc (Honours) Degree was validated by Middlesex University.

In 1991 the Oxford School of Osteopathy (OSO) was formed by Ian Swash, who was Chairman of the Guild of Osteopaths to which it became affiliated. Its foundation followed a Complementary Medicine Group Conference held in Oxford in 1990. In 1996 a BSc (Hons) Degree was validated by Oxford Brookes University with the first graduates emerging in 1998. The course was taken over by Oxford Brookes University to become the Oxford School of Osteopathy at Oxford Brookes. In 1996 the Guild of Osteopaths celebrated its 24th anniversary. On 31 March, it was announced that it would merge with the Council of the British and European Osteopathic Association. The Andrew Still College, under the leadership of Malcolm Mayer, joined the Guild.

In 1990 Malcolm Mayer became Principal of the Andrew Still College of Osteopathy and negotiations began with Kingston Polytechnic to offer a Diploma in Osteopathy as from October 1991. In 1992 the CNAA retrospectively validated the course in association with Kingston Polytechnic, but with the demise of the CNAA, Kingston became a University and took over the validation.[60] This was the first part-time course in Osteopathy to gain degree status. Tensions arose with Kingston University regarding what was actually taught. The last group of students to graduate from Kingston University was in 1997. Brunel University took over the validation, but it was not renewed.

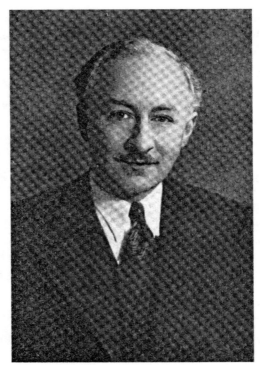

S. ('Sammy') Ball, Chairman GCRO; President BOA

Virginia Wade OBE officially opened the clinic of the John Wernham College of Classical Osteopathy, established at North-East Surrey College of Technology in September 1996.

Deaths

Joyce Canning died in her 90th year in June 1992 treating patients until a few weeks before her death. As Joyce Bishop she was a student at the BSO. She married lecturer and Governor of the School, James Canning, in 1937. Edward Hall was the principal witness at their wedding. Both practised at 50 Cumberland Mansions with J. Martin Littlejohn Jr, and Dr Dorothy Wood (the wife of T Edward Hall). They moved to Farnham, Surrey during the war. With her husband she was an exponent of the Still and Littlejohn long-lever techniques.

Vaughan McDermott of Solihull graduated from the BSO in 1966, and died in 1992.[61] The Birmingham and District Osteopathic Clinic which opened in 1969 was renamed Vaughan McDermott House in 1994. In 1993 R. K. Hardy, Richard Miller, Margot Gore and Jocelyn Proby died.

Stanley Holdich died in 1994. He was born in 1906, graduated in 1928 and was a founder member of the Western Counties group, contributing much to the profession.[62]

In 1996 Barrie Darewski, who had been Secretary to the GCRO from 1974 to 1987 and Stephen Pheasant died. The latter was an eminent ergonomist and supporter of Osteopathy and become one of the Associate Professors of the BSO.

Alec R. Webster died in 1997 aged 84. He practised in Wimbledon, and then at No 1 Harley Street in 1941 before retiring to Eastbourne in 1988. He joined the Society of Osteopaths and then the GCRO in 1946 and was a long standing committee member of the OEF.[63] S. Grierson ('Greg') Currie (See Chapter 9) died aged 82,[64] and Dr C. L. "Johnnie" Johnson, aged 89.[65] The latter was a Kirksville graduate, who worked with Elmer Pheils in Birmingham, before setting up practices in Liverpool, Chester, then in London in Devonshire Street, then Portland Place and Park Lane. He was one of the co-founders of the LCOM.

Profile: Samuel ('Sammy') Ball

Dr Samuel ('Sammy') Ball died in November 1991. He was born in Montreal in 1909. He initially undertook a business course, but after osteopathic treatment for back problems, he decided on a career in Osteopathy. He studied at Kirksville from 1929 to 1933, but not having registered to practise in Quebec, he came to Britain in 1936 and took up a locum position. He was one of the last American-trained Doctors of Osteopathy in Britain. In 1946 he joined the London Faculty of Osteopathy, which developed into the London College of Osteopathy, later the LCOM, and was involved with the teaching, administration and developments of the School and was a member of Osteopathic Trusts. He described himself as a 'ten-fingered osteopath' and his approach was structural, though he had an interest in Cranial Osteopathy. He joined the GCRO in 1947 and was a member of the Council for 34 years and for several years in the 1950s Chairman and served on its Education Committee of which he was Chairman in the 1960s. He strove for high standards of education in the profession and also for its unity.[66,67,68]

Profile: Margot Gore

Margot Gore was born in Ireland in January 1913. The family moved to England for financial reasons, which also precluded a career in medicine. Her second choice of profession was flying and she paid for lessons at Mayland Aerodrome, Essex and later worked as a flying instructor in a private flying club. She was a member of the Civil Air Guard and when war broke out she volunteered for the Air Transport

Auxiliary and became a Commanding Officer, flying planes from the factories to RAF bases. She flew Lancaster bombers, Hurricanes and Spitfires and was awarded an MBE in 1945. After the war she returned to flying, but then chose a career in Osteopathy and graduated with the Gold Medal in 1954, following which she practised in Kensington and later in Oxfordshire. She taught in the BSO clinic and lectured on Nutrition and Dietetics. She was on the OAGB Council and the OEF and the Board of Governing Directors of the School, becoming its Chair in the later 1970s, when the School moved to Suffolk Street. She was a strong believer in 'pure' Osteopathy and opposed 'fringe' Osteopathy and other therapies.[69]

Profile: Tom Dummer

Tom Dummer, who died in May 1998, must rank among the great osteopaths of this century.[70] Born in 1915, he was an osteopathic practitioner who had an interest in homeopathy, naturopathy and radiaesthesia, as well as being a teacher, jazz musician, Buddhist, cook and writer. He graduated as a member of the Institute of Medical Herbalists in the mid 1940s, but then qualified from the British College of Naturopathy in 1952. He founded the clinic at the BCNO, of which he was director for many years.

In 1957 he became associated with a French school under Paul Geny, which affiliated to the BCNO in 1965, before moving to Maidstone in 1971. When the European School of Osteopathy was formed in Maidstone in 1974, he became Principal, a post that he held until 1985. He was co-founder of the Society of Osteopaths with John Wernham, Edward Hall and Peter Blagrave. In 1996 he was awarded an Honorary Diploma of the College D'Etudes Osteopathiques de Montreal. Among his publications are: *Out on the Fringe* (1963) (with Andre Mahe), *Tibetan Medicine* (1988), *Specific Adjusting Technique* (1995) and a two volume textbook on Osteopathy, which went to press at the time of his death.

Profile: Helen Emilie Jackson

Emilie Jackson who, like Sammy Ball, was one of the last osteopaths in Britain to be trained in the US, died in November 1999. She was born Helen Emilie Mercedes Mary Kenney in 1913. Her mother had studied under A. T. Still. Not only were both parents osteopaths, but also her aunt, cousin and sister. Her parents practised close to the Texas/Mexico border. It was claimed that her mother, 'Could shoot a rattlesnake between the eyes at a 1,000 yards and subdued Pancho Villa, the notorious Mexican bandit!' After an initial education at Fort Worth, she studied Osteopathy at Kirksville, where she met and married Philip

Jackson, who like Stephen Ward was British, but preferred to study Osteopathy in the USA. The Jacksons returned to the UK in 1939, Emilie taking the last passenger boat before the outbreak of war. She brought Cranial Osteopathy to Britain and was the first person to teach it here. She became involved with the Osteopathic Institute of Applied Technique in the 1950s. Among her publications were: *Introduction to Osteopathy in the Cranial Field* and *Gravity Assisted Technique*. Initially she practised at Oxford and then at Reading. There are two further generations of osteopaths in her family.[71,72]

References

1. Fielding, S. (1993). Background Information on the Osteopaths Bill/Act. Leaflet. June, 1993.
2. *News Bulletin*. (1992). The General Council and Register of Osteopaths. January, No. 20, 2/92:13.
3. *Newsletter*. (1993). The Osteopathic Association of Great Britain. January/February, 5.1:1.
4. *Newsletter*. (1993). The Osteopathic Association of Great Britain. March, 5.2:5.
5. House of Commons Official Report: Parliamentary debates (Hansard). 216(102): 1170-1205.
6. *Reading Matters*. (1993). The General Council and Register of Osteopaths. June, No. 8, GCR 12/93:2.
7. Chambers, M. M. (1995). The British Naturopathic Association. The first 50 years. (British Naturopathic Association).
8. *Newsletter*. (1991). President's message. The Osteopathic Association of Great Britain. December, 3.12:3.
9. The Osteopathic Association of Great Britain. Report and Accounts for the year ended 31 May, 1992. (London: OAGB).
10. *Reading Matters*. (1993). The General Council and Register of Osteopaths. September, No. 11, GCR 19/93:2-3.
11. *Newsletter*. (1994). The Osteopathic Association of Great Britain. March, 6.3:4.
12. *Newsletter*. (1995). The Osteopathic Association of Great Britain. July, 8.7:6.
13. *Osteopathy Today*. (1997). October, 3.10:4.
14. *Osteopathy Today*. (1997). December, 3.12:8-9.
15. *Osteopathy Today*. (1998). March, 4.03:15.
16. *Osteopathy Today*. (1998). July, 4.07:9.
17. General Osteopathic Council. Report and Accounts 1997-1998:4.
18. *Osteopathy Today*. (1996). February, 2.02:4.
19. *Osteopathy Today*. (1996). March, 2.03:5-9.
20. *Osteopathy Today*. (1996). April, 2.04:5-6.
21. *Osteopathy Today*. (1996). June, 2.06:6-8.

22. *Osteopathy Today*. (1997). February, 3.02:5.
23. *Osteopathy Today*. (1997). February, 3.02:4.
24. *Osteopathy Today*. (1997). April, 3.04:4; 6.
25. *Osteopathy Today*. (1997). May, 3.05:5.
26. *The Osteopath*. (1998). June, 1(6):1-8.
27. *The Osteopath*. (1998). February, 1(3):10-11.
28. General Osteopathic Council. Report and Accounts 1997-1998:10-11.
29. *Osteopathy Today*. (1999). February, 5.02:8.
30. *Osteopathy Today*. (1998). January, 4.01:6-7.
31. *Reading Matters*. (1993). The General Council and Register of Osteopaths. May, No. 7, GCR 9/93:4.
32. *Reading Matters*. (1995). The General Council and Register of Osteopaths.June, No. 31, GCR 8/95:10-11.
33. *Reading Matters*. (1994). The General Council and Register of Osteopaths. September, No. 22, GCR 17/94:3.
34. *Reading Matters*. (1993). The General Council and Register of Osteopaths. July, No. 9, GCR/93:3-4.
35. *Reading Matters*. (1995). The General Council and Register of Osteopaths. August, No. 33, GCR 12/95:3.
36. *Reading Matters*. (1995). The General Council and Register of Osteopaths. May, No. 30, GCR 7/95:4-5.
37. *Reading Matters*. (1995). The General Council and Register of Osteopaths. July, No. 32, GCR 9/95:6-7.
38. *Newsletter* (1993). The Osteopathic Association of Great Britain. January/February, 5.1:11.
39. *Reading Matters*. (1993). The General Council and Register of Osteopaths. May, No. 7, GCR 9/93:5-6.
40. *Reading Matters*. (1993). The General Council and Register of Osteopaths. May, No. 7, GCR 9/93:5.
41. *Reading Matters*. (1994). The General Council and Register of Osteopaths. April, No. 17, GCR 7/94:5-6.
42. *Reading Matters*. (1994). The General Council and Register of Osteopaths. April, No. 17, GCR 7/94:14.
43. Fielding, S. (1993). *News Bulletin*. Annual Report. No. 26, GCR 20/93:1-3.
44. *Reading Matters*. (1995). The General Council and Register of Osteopaths. February, No. 27, GCR 4/95:8-9.
45. *Newsletter*. (1993). The Osteopathic Association of Great Britain. January/February, 5.1:11.
46. *Reading Matters*. (1994). The General Council and Register of Osteopaths. January, No. 15, GCR 3/94:4-5.

47. *Reading Matters*. (1994). The General Council and Register of Osteopaths. December, No. 25, GCR 31/94:3.
48. *Reading Matters*. (1995). The General Council and Register of Osteopaths. February, No. 27, GCR 4/95:2.
49. *Osteopathy Today*. (1996). October, 2.10:11.
50. *Osteopathy Today*. (1998). October, 4.10:20-21.
51. *Osteopathy Today*. (1997). October, 3.10:6-7.
52. *Osteopathy Today*. (1998. August, 4.08:7.
53. *The Osteopath*. (1998). January, 1(2):8-9.
54. *The Osteopath*. (1998). July/August, 1(7):6.
55. *Osteopathy Today*. (1998). January, 4.01:4.
56. *Newsletter*. (1994). The Osteopathic Association of Great Britain. August, 6.8:4-5.
57. Dr Ian Drysdale, Principal of the British College of Osteopathic Medicine. Personal communication.
58. *Newsletter*. (1994). The Osteopathic Association of Great Britain. April, 6.4:15.
59. *Reading Matters*. (1994). The General Council and Register of Osteopaths. May, No.18, GCR 8/94:3.
60. Kingston Polytechnic and The Andrew Still College of Osteopathy. Diploma in Osteopathy. Prospectus (1991).
61. *Newsletter*. (1994). The Osteopathic Association of Great Britain. November, 7.11:8.
62. *Newsletter*. (1994). The Osteopathic Association of Great Britain. December, 7.12:7.
63. *Osteopathy Today*. (1997). July, 3.07:9.
64. *Osteopathy Today*. (1997). May, 3.05:10.
65. *Osteopathy Today*. (1997). April, 3.04:10-11.
66. Dutton, C. (1991). Obituary to Dr Sammy Ball. *The Times*, 3 December 1991.
67. Anon (1992). *Journal of Osteopathic Education*, 2(1):7.
68. From the Secretary. (1992). *News Bulletin*. The General Council and Register of Osteopaths. No. 20, GCR 2/92:4.
69. Smith, A. (1993). *Newsletter*. The Osteopathic Association of Great Britain. October, 5.10:7.
70. *Osteopathy Today*. (1998). June, 4.06:8-9.
71. Jackson, D. (1999/2000). Helen Emilie Jackson. *The Osteopath*, December/January, 2(10):23.
72. Chancellor-Weale, A. (1999). Helen Emilie Jackson, 1913-1999. *Osteopathy Today*, December, 5.12:18.

ABBREVIATIONS

AOA	American Osteopathic Association
ASO	American School of Osteopathy
BAMM	British Association of Medical Managers
BCNO	British College of Naturopathy and Osteopathy
BCOM	British College of Osteopathic Medicine
BEOA	British and European Osteopathic Association
BHFS	British Health Freedom Society
BIOR	British Institute of Osteopathic Research
BMA	British Medical Association
BNA	British Naturopathic Association
BCN	British College of Naturopathy
BNOA	British Naturopathic and Osteopathic Association
BOA	British Osteopathic Association
BSO	British School of Osteopathy
CIDO	College Internationale d'Osteopathie
CNAA	Council for National Academic Awards
COET	College of Osteopaths Educational Trust
CPD	Continuing Professional Development
CPU	Columbia Pacific University
DHSS	Department of Health and Social Services
ENT	Ear, Nose and Throat
EPOC	Extension of the Practice of Osteopathy Campaign
ESO	European School of Osteopathy
GCE	General Certificate of Education
GCRO	General Council and Register of Osteopaths
GLC	Greater London Council
GOsC	General Osteopathic Council
GMC	General Medical Council
GNO	Guild of Naturopathy and Osteopathy
GP	General Practitioner
IAO	Incorporated Association of Osteopaths
ILEA	Inner London Educational Authority
KC	King's Counsel

LCO	London College of Osteopathy.
LCOM	London College of Osteopathic Medicine
LSO	London School of Osteopathy
MP	Member of Parliament
MRO	Member of the Register of Osteopaths
NCA	Nature Cure Association
NESCOT	North-East Surrey College of Technology
NHS	National Health Service
NTA	Natural Therapeutic Association
NTOS	Natural Therapeutic and Osteopathic Society (and Register)
OAGB	Osteopathic Association of Great Britain
OCC	Osteopathic Centre for Children
OEF	Osteopathic Educational Foundation
OSO	Oxford School of Osteopathy
PCL	Polytechnic of Central London
PPP	Professional Profile and Portfolio
RCGP	Royal College of General Practitioners
RQ	Recognised Qualification
SCTF	Sutherland Cranial Teaching Foundation
SORI	Scottish Osteopathic Research Institute
VAT	Value Added Tax

INDEX

590387

Made in the USA